EAI/Springer Innovations in Communication and Computing

Series Editor
Imrich Chlamtac, European Alliance for Innovation, Ghent, Belgium

Editor's Note

The impact of information technologies is creating a new world yet not fully understood. The extent and speed of economic, life style and social changes already perceived in everyday life is hard to estimate without understanding the technological driving forces behind it. This series presents contributed volumes featuring the latest research and development in the various information engineering technologies that play a key role in this process.

The range of topics, focusing primarily on communications and computing engineering include, but are not limited to, wireless networks; mobile communication; design and learning; gaming; interaction; e-health and pervasive healthcare; energy management; smart grids; internet of things; cognitive radio networks; computation; cloud computing; ubiquitous connectivity, and in mode general smart living, smart cities, Internet of Things and more. The series publishes a combination of expanded papers selected from hosted and sponsored European Alliance for Innovation (EAI) conferences that present cutting edge, global research as well as provide new perspectives on traditional related engineering fields. This content, complemented with open calls for contribution of book titles and individual chapters, together maintain Springer's and EAI's high standards of academic excellence. The audience for the books consists of researchers, industry professionals, advanced level students as well as practitioners in related fields of activity include information and communication specialists, security experts, economists, urban planners, doctors, and in general representatives in all those walks of life affected ad contributing to the information revolution.

Indexing: This series is indexed in Scopus, Ei Compendex, and zbMATH.

About EAI

EAI is a grassroots member organization initiated through cooperation between businesses, public, private and government organizations to address the global challenges of Europe's future competitiveness and link the European Research community with its counterparts around the globe. EAI reaches out to hundreds of thousands of individual subscribers on all continents and collaborates with an institutional member base including Fortune 500 companies, government organizations, and educational institutions, provide a free research and innovation platform.

Through its open free membership model EAI promotes a new research and innovation culture based on collaboration, connectivity and recognition of excellence by community.

More information about this series at http://www.springer.com/series/15427

Mohammad Shahid Husain
Muhamad Hariz Bin Muhamad Adnan • Mohammad Zunnun Khan
Saurabh Shukla • Fahad U. Khan
Editors

Pervasive Healthcare

A Compendium of Critical Factors for Success

Springer

EAI
RESEARCH MEETS INNOVATION

Editors
Mohammad Shahid Husain
Information Technology Department
College of Applied Sciences, University of Technology and Applied Sciences
Ibri, Oman

Muhamad Hariz Bin Muhamad Adnan
Universiti Pendidikan Sultan Idris
Tanjung Malim, Malaysia

Mohammad Zunnun Khan
Computer Science and Engineering Department
Integral University
Lucknow, India

Saurabh Shukla
Data Science Institute
National University of Ireland
Galway, Ireland

Fahad U. Khan
Global Health IT Product Consultant
Rhapsody
Auckland, New Zealand

ISSN 2522-8595 ISSN 2522-8609 (electronic)
EAI/Springer Innovations in Communication and Computing
ISBN 978-3-030-77745-6 ISBN 978-3-030-77746-3 (eBook)
https://doi.org/10.1007/978-3-030-77746-3

This Springer imprint is published by the registered company Springer Nature Switzerland AG
The registered company address is: Gewerbestrasse 11, 6330 Cham, Switzerland

We dedicate this book to our parents.

Preface

Pervasive computing is a technology paradigm which enables information services available anytime and anywhere while making the presence of the system invisible to the user. Pervasive computing is expanding its applicability in various domains like Education, Medical, Transport and Sport by allowing much more robust local as well as remote monitoring.

Pervasive healthcare provides solutions for a lot of issues in the healthcare system and is currently a hot research area. The purpose of pervasive healthcare is providing quality medical assistance anywhere and anytime by improving medical information access using ad hoc networks. Pervasive healthcare is a scientific discipline which counters the challenges faced by traditional healthcare system like increasing population, increase in the lifestyle-related diseases, and lack of medical professionals. It helps in providing personalized healthcare monitoring (both long term and short term). The task of pervasive healthcare ranges from incidence identification and management, alarming and handling the emergency situations, monitoring the patients and treat them remotely.

Emerging Need

With the advent of Information and Communication technologies many sectors have started to make use of them. Healthcare industry is way behind in applying sophisticated technologies to support patient as well as medical staff. The use of handheld ICT devices as well as sophisticated tools based on IoT and other sensor devices is increasingly encouraged however, due to issues like lack of technical knowledge of these systems/methods, complex processing, robustness and reliability of applications, fear of information being compromised or loss, lack of time for training to adapt such complex tools/applications. Furthermore, many healthcare providers and hospitals prohibit the usage of sensors or wireless devices within their buildings in fear of interference to more critical medical devices.

Although most of the experts in the healthcare industry believe that with the help of sophisticated techniques, wireless devices, and sensor technologies we can better facilitate the medical staff and give personal care to patients, even effectively monitor patients remotely.

There are several challenges that need to be addressed to make pervasive healthcare a reality.

Purpose

This book will provide in-depth knowledge about critical factors involved in the success of Pervasive Healthcare. The book will deal with the important aspects like challenges, needed infrastructure and security concerns for pervasive healthcare. It will give insights into the pervasive healthcare information system and key consideration related to remote patient monitoring and safety. This book will provide an in-depth discussion of the security issues and protocols for pervasive healthcare.

Audience

This book will explore the concepts/techniques behind the successive Pervasive Healthcare Systems by providing in-depth knowledge about patient empowerment, remote patient monitoring, network establishment, and protocols for effective pervasive healthcare. It will assist individuals as well as organizations in understanding and implementing the smart healthcare system. It will be an ideal resource for researchers, students, and healthcare organizations to get insights about the state of the art in Pervasive Healthcare system.

Emphasis

The proposed book will deal with various aspects of the successive implementation of Pervasive Healthcare in the current scenario including network, information system, protocols, safety and privacy issues, etc.

What You Will Learn

By going through the material presented in this book, you will learn:

- The concept of pervasive healthcare, how it can contribute in providing better record management, patient care, chronic and preventive care.
- The applications of pervasive healthcare techniques.
- Challenges in pervasive healthcare.
- How we can improve the health critical infrastructure of public healthcare system.
- The data privacy in pervasive healthcare.
- How you can apply machine learning approaches and data mining techniques for effective pervasive healthcare system.
- What are the latest trends in pervasive healthcare?
- Use of latest machine learning approaches for different applications like diagnosis of patients, prediction of diseases, and providing remote monitoring of patients.

Book Organization

The early chapters of the book are organized in order to provide conceptual background, starting with an introduction to pervasive healthcare, its importance, the objectives of pervasive healthcare, pervasive healthcare as a scientific discipline, and the current challenges (Chaps. 1–4). This is followed by a chapter on how we can improve the healthcare infrastructure using soft computing techniques (Chap. 5). After this, in the following chapters we discuss the state-of-the-art machine learning approaches which can be applied to solve problems like computer-aided diagnosis, disease prediction, security and privacy. It also provides insights into how we can make use of body sensor networks (BSN), Internet of Things (IoT), cloud infrastructure, machine learning and artificial intelligence in enabling effective pervasive healthcare infrastructure (Chaps. 6-21). Three chapters provide a case study of COVID-19, the pandemic the world is suffering from (Chaps. 10, 19 and 21).

Ibri, Oman — Mohammad Shahid Husain
Tanjung Malim, Malaysia — Muhamad Hariz Bin Muhamad Adnan
Lucknow, India — Mohammad Zunnun Khan
Galway, Ireland — Saurabh Shukla
Auckland, New Zealand — Fahad U. Khan

Acknowledgments

This work was a great experience for us in the field of pervasive healthcare. To make this book project a reality, a lot of people extended their support and helped us. We would like to acknowledge the support and assistance of each individual who helped us in the conception and completion of this book. We want to take this opportunity to offer our profound gratitude to them.

A very special thanks to EAI/Springer Innovations in Communication and Computing (EAISICC) publication team, particularly Eliška Vlčková, Managing Editor, European Alliance for Innovation (EAI); without her continuous encouragement and support, this book would not have been possible.

We also thank our editorial advisory board members Dr. T J Siddiqui, Dr. M Akheela, Dr. Rashid Ali, Prof. Ubaidullah Bokhari, Adil Kaleem, Dr. Arif Siddiqui, and EAI book development team for their guidance and valuable suggestions during the entire journey of book publication.

We thank our reviewers from renowned institutions to spare time from their busy schedule and put a lot of efforts to provide time-constrained impartial and critical review which is very crucial in maintaining the quality and standard of the book and helps us to finish the book in time.

Thanks to our friends and colleagues for providing help wherever and whenever necessary.

This acknowledgment will not be complete until we pay our gratitude and regards to our parents and family members for their unflinching support and encouragement to us in all our pursuits. It is the confidence of our family members in us that has made us the person that we are today. We dedicate this book to them.

Finally, we wish to thank the organizations and individuals who granted us permission to use the research material and information necessary for the completion of this book.

Last but not least we are heartily thankful to almighty God for showering His blessings forever during our entire life.

Contents

Contributors

Ash Mohammad Abbas Department of Computer Engineering, Aligarh Muslim University, Aligarh, India

Syed Haider Abbas Department of Computer Science and Engineering, Integral University, Lucknow, Uttar Pradesh, India

Abdullah Department of Information Technology, College of Engineering and Technology, Adigrat University, Tigray, Ethiopia

Rasha Shakir AbdulWahhab Information Technology Department, University of Technology and Applied Sciences, Suhar, Sultanate of Oman

Afsaruddin Department of CSE, Abdul Kalam Technical University, Lucknow, Uttar Pradesh, India

Tamim Ahmad Department of CSE, AMU, Aligarh, India

Tasneem Ahmed Advanced Computing and Research Laboratory, Department of Computer Application, Integral University, Lucknow, Uttar Pradesh, India

Ravinder Ahuja School of Computing Science and Engineering, Galgotias University, Noida, India

N. Ambika Department of Computer Applications, SSMRV College, Bangalore, India

Solomon Aregawi Department of Information Technology, College of Engineering and Technology, Adigrat University, Tigray, Ethiopia

Sateesh Reddy Avutu Department of Biomedical Engineering, North-Eastern Hill University, Shillong, India, Meghalaya

Alisha Banga Indian Institute of Technology Roorkee, Saharanpur, India

Brijesh Kumar Bhardwaj Department of MCA, DR R M L Avadh University, Ayodhya, Faizabad, India

Amit Kumar Bhasker Department of MCA, Dr. RML Avadh University, Ayodhya, Faizabad, India

Arz Muhammad Brohi Department of Computer Science, Benazir Bhutto Shaheed University (BBSU), Lyari, Karachi, Pakistan

Alakananda Chakraborty Department of Computer Science and Engineering, Amity University, Noida, Uttar Pradesh, India

Prashant Dixit Computer Science and Engineering Department, Jaypee Institute of Information Technology, Noida, India

Mohammad Faisal Advanced Computing and Research Laboratory, Department of Computer Application, Integral University, Lucknow, Uttar Pradesh, India

Haftay Gebrezgabiher Department of Information Technology, College of Engineering and Technology, Adigrat University, Tigray, Ethiopia

Gezahagn Haileslassie Gezahagn Department of Information Technology, College of Engineering and Technology, Adigrat University, Tigray, Ethiopia

Shruti Gupta Department of Computer Science and Engineering, Amity University, Noida, Uttar Pradesh, India

Mohammad Haroon Department of CSE, Integral University, Lucknow, Uttar Pradesh, India

Mahfuzul Huda Saudi Electronic University, Riyadh, Saudi Arabia

Department of Computer Science, College of Computing and Informatics, Saudi Electronic University, Medina, Saudi Arabia

Mohammad Shahid Husain Ibri College of Applied Sciences, University of Technology and Applied Sciences, Muscat, Oman

Geshwaree Huzooree Charles Telfair Campus Curtin University, Moka, Mauritius

Nashra Javed Advanced Computing and Research Laboratory, Department of Computer Application, Integral University, Lucknow, Uttar Pradesh, India

Karan Jetly Information Technology Department, University of Technology and Applied Sciences, Suhar, Sultanate of Oman

Muskan Jindal Department of Computer Science and Engineering, Amity University, Noida, Uttar Pradesh, India

Noorjehan Joonas Ministry of Health and Quality of Life Victoria Hospital Candos, Quatre Bornes, Mauritius

M. H. Khan Department of Computer Science and Engineering, Institute of Engineering and Technology, AKTU, Lucknow, Uttar Pradesh, India

Mohammad Zubair Khan Department of Computer Science, CCSE, Taibah University, Medina, Saudi Arabia

Mohammad Zunnun Khan Department of Computer Science and Engineering, Integral University, Lucknow, Uttar Pradesh, India

Waris Khan Department of Computer Application, Integral University, Lucknow, Uttar Pradesh, India

Zunnun Khan Integral University, Lucknow, Uttar Pradesh, India

Kavi Khedo University of Mauritius, Moka, Mauritius

Mohd. Suhaib Kidwai Department of Electronics and Communication Engineering, Integral University, Lucknow, Uttar Pradesh, India

Akhilesh Kumar MCA Department, I.E.T, Dr. R. M. L. Avadh University, Ayodhya, Faizabad, India

Ilias Maglogiannis Department of Digital Systems, University of Piraeus, Piraeus, Greece

Anshul Mishra Department of IT, BBAU, Lucknow, Uttar Pradesh, India

Department of IT, Baba Saheb Bhim Rao Ambedkar University, Lucknow, Uttar Pradesh, India

Nawazish Naweed University of Technology and Applied Sciences, Ibri, Oman

Sudip Paul Department of Biomedical Engineering, North-Eastern Hill University, Shillong, India, Meghalaya

Andrianos Pavlopoulos Department of Digital Systems, University of Piraeus, Piraeus, Greece

Halima Sadia Department of Computer Science and Engineering, Integral University, Lucknow, Uttar Pradesh, India

Anwar Ali Sathio Department of Computer Science, Benazir Bhutto Shaheed University (BBSU), Lyari, Karachi, Pakistan

Surabhi Saxena Department of BCA, Koneru Lakshmaiah Education Foundation, Guntur, Andhra Pradesh, India

Shqran Shakir Information Technology Department, University of Technology and Applied Sciences, Shinas, Sultanate of Oman

S. C. Sharma Indian Institute of Technology Roorkee, Saharanpur, India

Mohd. Maroof Siddiqui College of Engineering, Dhofar University, Salalah, Oman

Nazish Siddiqui Department of Computer Science and Engineering, Integral University, Lucknow, Uttar Pradesh, India

Nupur Soni School of Computer Applications, Babu Banarasi Das University, Lucknow, Uttar Pradesh, India

Kavita Srivastava Department of Computer Science, SRMU, Lucknow, Uttar Pradesh, India

Nikhil Kumar Srivastava City Collage of Management and Technology, Lucknow, Uttar Pradesh, India

Panagiotis Stavrianos Department of Digital Systems, University of Piraeus, Piraeus, Greece

Teklay Teklu Department of Information Technology, College of Engineering and Technology, Adigrat University, Tigray, Ethiopia

Manish Madhav Tripathi Department of CSE, Integral University, Lucknow, Uttar Pradesh, India

Rama Nandan Tripathi Department of MCA, Dr. RML Avadh University, Ayodhya, Faizabad, India

Hagos Yirgaw Department of Information Technology, College of Engineering and Technology, Adigrat University, Tigray, Ethiopia

Chapter 1
Pervasive Healthcare Computing and its Contribution to Hospitals, Chronic and Preventive Care

Abdullah, Hagos Yirgaw, Solomon Aregawi, Haftay Gebrezgabiher, and Mahfuzul Huda

1.1 Introduction

Pervasive healthcare computing has the prospect to make a key influence in cumulative overall access as well as superiority of healthcare facilities though containing expenses [1–3]. Pervasive computing offers solutions for hospitals, doctors, clinicians, patients, as well as a range of additional caregivers to facilitate them using these problems together with uses and apparatuses to make the recording easy. The following is an observation of fitness data/information:

- Permit message, association also management among the various participants.
- Inspire clinical devotion as well as disease anticipation.
- Facilitate the roaming effort of clinicians and the whole integration of the real as well as digital worlds.
- Allow the expansion of innovative medicinal plans.

In addition, pervasive computing furthermore decreases the paper work by way of removing the requirements of paper-based records and increases the managerial productivity [4–6]. It increases the healthcare services by means of reducing medicinal mistakes by a guarantee that all the healthcare workers have perfect as well as appropriate information [7, 8]. Pervasive healthcare computing in common is progressively more regarded as the greatest encouraging instrument for increasing the total superiority, security, and effectiveness of the health distribution method [9].

Abdullah (✉) · H. Yirgaw · S. Aregawi · H. Gebrezgabiher
Department of Information Technology, College of Engineering and Technology, Adigrat University, Tigray, Ethiopia

M. Huda
Saudi Electronic University, Riyadh, Saudi Arabia

M. S. Husain et al. (eds.), *Pervasive Healthcare*, EAI/Springer Innovations in Communication and Computing, https://doi.org/10.1007/978-3-030-77746-3_1

In excess of the previous few decades, the implementation of pervasive healthcare computing and health information technology has develop progressively shared in healthcare backgrounds [2, 10]. The healthcare sector has a continuous trust on machineries and technologies [2, 4]. The emphasis is to avoid relatively than cure an illness through surveillance of circumstances as well as the advancement of strong performances. This may possibly only be attained once the data associated with the health of the society touches the associated doctor's healthcare authorities, hospitals, policy creators, as well as managers at an exact time wherever and at what time they requisite [3].

1.2 Pervasive Computing for Hospital Care

The wish an increase in patient care initiates the proposal and implementation of novel wireless network and information technologies in the healthcare environment [11–14]. In the previous two decades, there has been a huge investment worldwide in pervasive computing and pervasive healthcare systems [15]. Even although pervasive healthcare systems are frequently leisurelier than other sector industries in accepting novel information and communication technologies, healthcare system has relocated rapidly in the direction of the use of technologies to increase overall patient care and decrease budgets as well as medical errors [11, 16, 17]. Pervasive computing plays a key role in relation to achieving quality healthcare goal to deliver appropriate services that reply directly to their users and backgrounds and in setting up of healthcare main services [3, 5, 18]. The furthermost common are:

1.2.1 Context-Aware Services and Awareness

Medical doctors make decisions that are extremely prejudiced by background information, such as timing, locality, as well as obtainable resourcefulness. Intended, for instance, access to a patients' medicinal information is additionally significant once the physician or doctor is in the obverse of a patient's cot. Consequently, a physician's or doctor's locality is valuable in the decisive kind of record she/he may call for at a given moment [19, 20]. Field trainings of doctor work have been publicized that doctors keep a peripheral device consciousness of persons at work in direction to preserve the temporal outlines or "rhythms" [21–24] of job which is frequently used to organize activities as well as donate to the steady temporal association of the hospital.

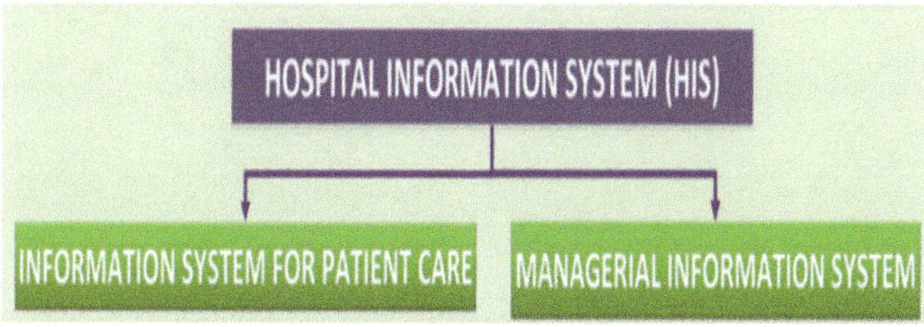

Fig. 1.1 Hospital information system (https://drdollah.files.wordpress.com/2014/07/his2.png)

1.2.2 Hospital Information System

The "hospital information system" is visualized as it comprises dual wide-ranging systems, i.e.:

1. Information system for patient care.
2. Managerial information management system (Fig. 1.1).

Information System for Patient Care

The hospital information management system can be wide-ranging distributed into dual folds:

1. The system intended for the patient care purpose.
2. The information management system intended for managerial purpose.

Conceptual division of systems for patient care (Fig. 1.2).

1.3 Major Goals and Purposes of Patient Care Information Systems

Being a system for supporting processes, these groups of subsystems as well as applications are probable to make use of automation and information technology optimally to appreciate anticipated goals in the subsequent extents:

- Output
- Usefulness
- Suitability
- Competence
- Excellence
- Protection
- Confidentiality and secrecy of information

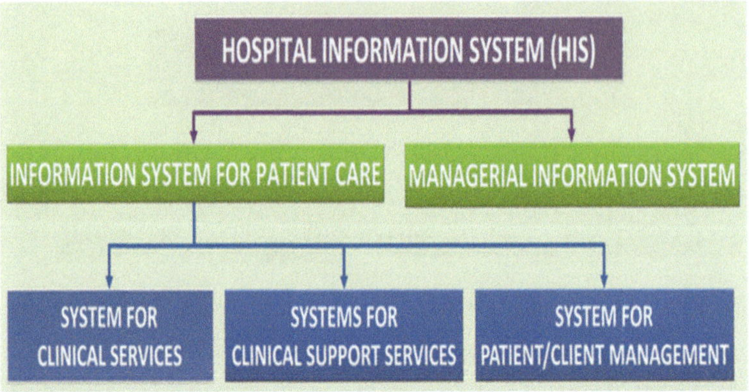

Fig. 1.2 Patient care information system (https://drdollah.files.wordpress.com/2014/07/pcis1.png)

1.3.1 The Associations of the System Are Shown in the Graphic Representation Underneath: Healthcare Information Management System

All the above developed systems are used by healthcare/hospital persons to take care for related patients. Care is here precise as all work doings to provide facilities to patients in reply to their requirements (Fig. 1.3).

Clinical Information System

The clinical information system comprises application units that allow the following:

- Preparation of carefulness (procedure of care plans)
- Setting up of clinical decision support system
- Medical data records (data entry system)
- Quality control mechanism
- Record storing for further use
- Record retrieval and display

Major modules of the clinical information management system (Fig. 1.4).

Clinical Support Systems

Clinical support system mentions facilities that:

- Perform related tests
- Provide supplies timely

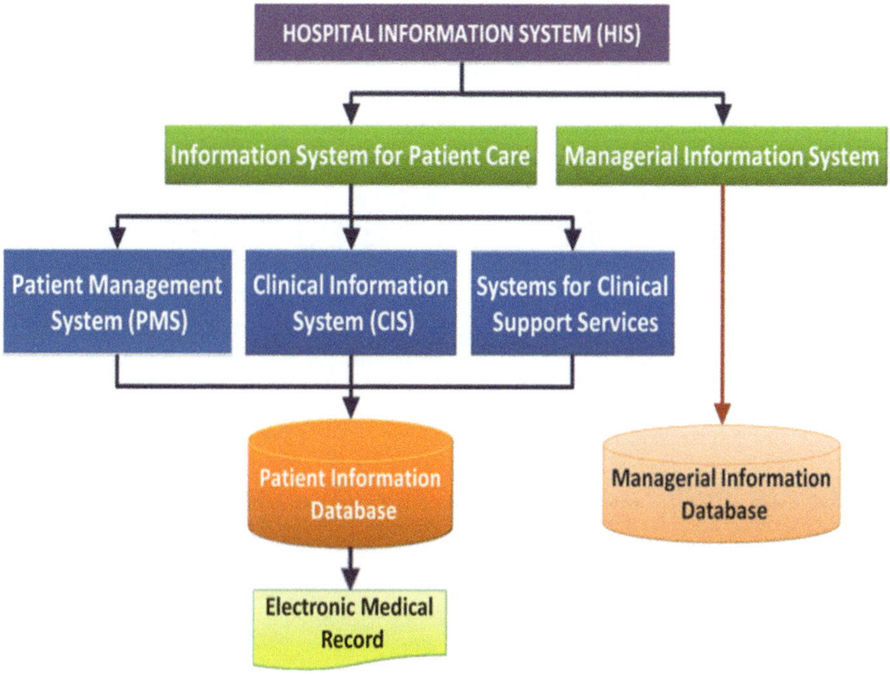

Fig. 1.3 Hospital information system (https://drdollah.files.wordpress.com/2014/07/pcis.png)

Direct healthcare providers demand in lieu of these service areas over the instruction entry functionality. Examination outcomes are submitted to the database management system on or after where they are ready to be available. Prescriptions, sterile supplies, blood products, as well as foodstuff are supplied to persons demanding them. The supplies they received are documented in the database management system (Fig. 1.5).

1.3.2 Electronic Medical Record (EMR)

The electronic medical record provides medical doctors with simultaneous access and retrieval to patient records [2, 4, 25], for example, patient health condition, official visit to health providers, images as well as reports of investigative processes, timetable of facilities, reactions as well as communication information to caregivers, and a whole longitudinal data of care indication founded on judgment support apparatuses that can be applied to support healthcare persons in decision-making.

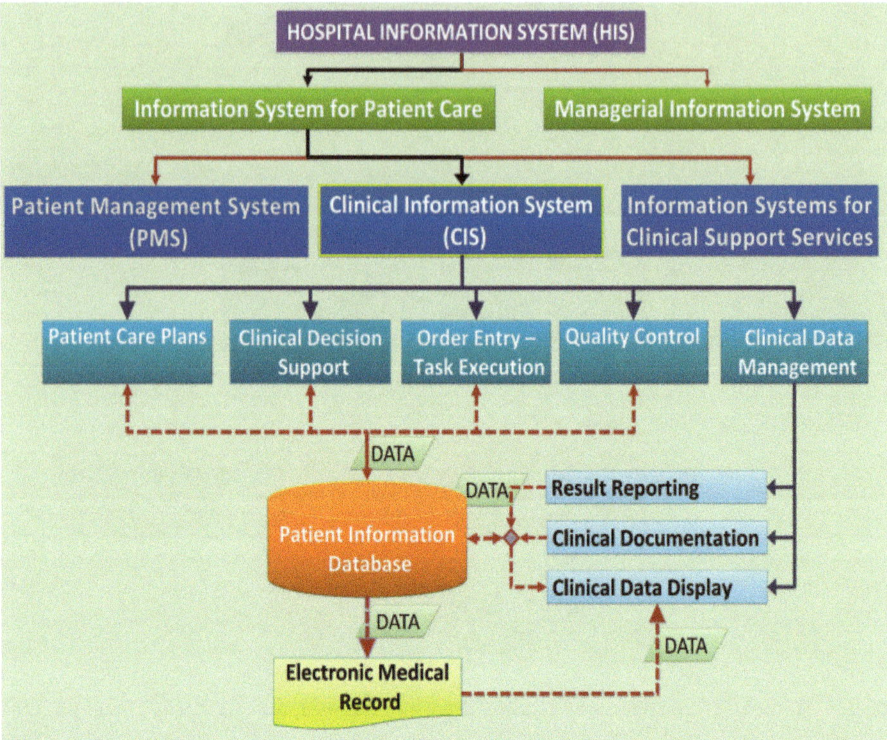

Fig. 1.4 Clinical information system. (https://drdollah.files.wordpress.com/2014/12/cis-latest.png)

1.3.3 Computerized Physician Order Entry

Electronic physician order entry system is a technique of computerized entry system of medicinal physician recommendations for the treatment of related patients underneath his or else her proper care [5, 16, 26, 27]. These instructions are transferred in excess of a computer network to the medical professional or to the related department (like drugstore) accountable aimed at accomplishing the instruction [2, 23]. Computerized physician order entry reductions delay in order completion, decreases an error associated to handwriting, permit order entry at point of proper care or off- site also, offer fault inspection for identical or inappropriate dosages or examinations, and shortens inventory management as well as posting of responsibilities.

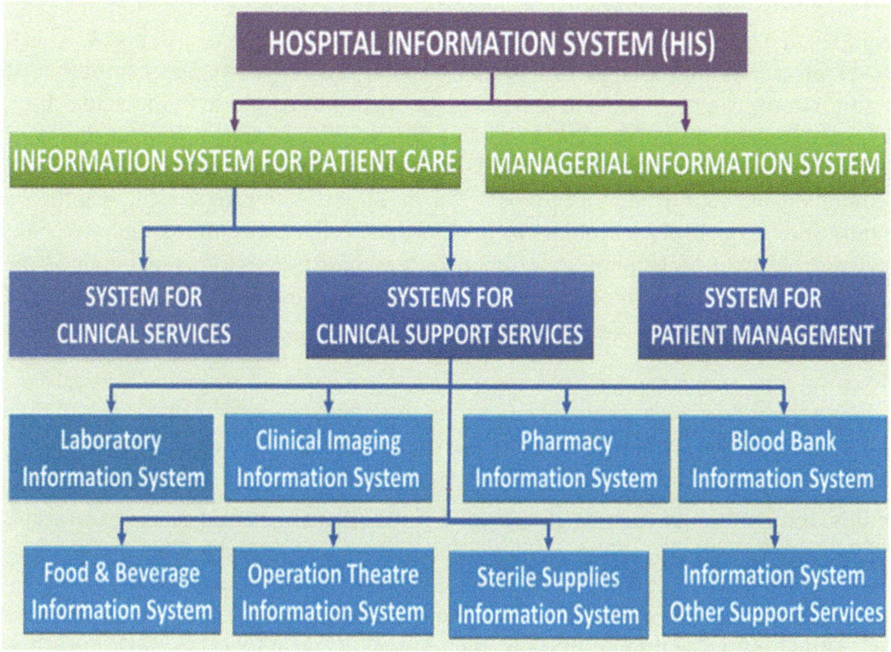

Fig. 1.5 System for clinical support services (https://drdollah.files.wordpress.com/2014/07/support-services.png)

1.3.4 Remote Monitoring

Remote monitoring system is the automated broadcast of healthcare-related information either one entered straight through a patient, otherwise by the use of a medicinal device to a physician's electronic record system, or a related patient's individual health record system [9, 28–30]. The capability for a medical doctor to monitor patient record around analytical, prescription tracing and activities of day-to-day living assessments, apprehended distantly is a significant able for the supervision of chronic health related issues as well as supervision of new circumstances [31, 32].

1.4 Overall Impact of Pervasive Computing on Hospital

Pervasive computing technologies have a superior influence on healthcare-related services as well as study and research [2, 5, 26, 33]. The underneath stated fact deliberate the effect of pervasive computing technologies in the hospitals, patients, service providers, management, investigators, and academician.

Patient-oriented technology is a supporting module to the distribution of health facilities in excess of spaces, offering important apparatuses and systems [4, 9, 34]. Development and acceptance of automatic health records as well as computerized health record system have also enhanced the distribution and also the actual time access of patient record at an assumed fact of time. [22, 35–37]. Clinician-oriented technologies offers trustworthy, important, latest, acceptable, as well as rationally comprehensive data for healthcare providers at all levels to progress the healthcare supply and attainability of countrywide objective [2, 5, 32]. Administrator-oriented pervasive computing technology offers health administrators a means intended for data gathering, processing, and investigation also appropriate for the reportage of the record to their direct level and others.

1.5 Chronic Care Supervision and Supported Cognition

In this unit, we firstly discuss clarifications in facilitating actual time observation, supported steering, as well as community connectedness intended for maintaining bodily as well as psychological happiness of people with chronic disease. Formerly we deliberate current solutions that deliver phase-by-phase assistance to increase the completion of activities of daily living supporting individuals with cognitive disabilities. We lastly précis the pervasive chronic care supervision as well as solutions.

1.5.1 Pervasive Monitoring for Self-Management

One considerable test in lieu of a singular by means of a chronic disease who is living individually alone is the capability to observe physical also social signs at a distance. Developments in pervasive healthcare expertise must allow improvement in observing methods that can constantly identify a person's rudimentary metabolic as well as social factors such as vigorous ciphers, happenings, group collaborations, slumber patterns, as well as other health pointers [38, 39]. Some of these researches [24, 32, 38, 39] have recommended the use of wearable sensors, smart clothing, as well as progressive integrated sensor systems to shape personalized health profiles and quickly inform families and specialized caregivers about the health complications.

1.5.2 Computerized Algorithm-Driven Care

An effective care model should facilitate all the essential components of a chronic care model, namely, a competent delivery system, self-management support, clinical information system (CIS), decision support system, trust on community resources, and health system to improve patients' awareness and increase their engagement and experience [2, 4, 40]. Nowadays, for patients to flawlessly transition between dissimilar facets of chronic care management, effective care delivery systems or an instinctive healthcare platform is necessary to increase coordination among providers and patients [2, 33, 41].

1.5.3 Remote Patient Monitoring

To ease the problem for patients with chronic diseases, remote patient monitoring system makes it stress-free for care teams to track, manage, as well as involve with patients who want extensive and constant care [2, 28, 42]. This evidence-based method can transform primary care crossways to different practice backgrounds to improve consequences. Such program enables and produces actual interactions between care team and patients for real assessment of the patient's health on the genuine time basis. In addition to this, we have a number of health related apps, wearables and in-home devices which are dedicated on general health, workout, wellness and diet [24]. These instruments authorize patients and providers to record the vitals on a systematic basis to produce insights for appropriate advice. The incorporation of such technology with an effective chronic care model makes the wheel rolling for remote care [13, 35]. Inventive technology affords a low price, flexible means to enhance healthcare and reshape chronic care. This kind of mediations can be a powerful way to increase provider practice and support patients with chronic disease like diabetes to live more magnificently [3, 16, 27].

1.5.4 Cost-Effective Treatment

By integrating chronic care through telemonitoring, wearables, and home health clinical devices, patients can decrease the healthcare charge [18, 43]. As there is a shift in the direction of home health, providers have a chance to assimilate digital health tools into treatment plans as well as remote monitoring to support and manage patients with chronic settings and provide proactive care addition to lower the cost. With the help of telemedicine, patients can rapidly consult with their care provider about the new symptom as it seems in real time and in return get recommendation to change the treatment [28, 44]. This confirms that the patient gets the care they want on a timely basis and decreases the chances of a gap in treatment and hospital readmission. This also decreases the cost of care for both patients and care providers [17].

1.5.5 Improved Patient Experience

With an optimum chronic care model, patients do not need to take time off from their job, find conveyance to the doctor clinic, as well as spend money for parking or any of the other loads related with attending a health center appointment. The assimilation of mobile health application in home medical devices can act as a catalyst for effective management of chronic diseases to improve the patient experience and result [42, 44]. The patient appointment tool allows the patient to upload all their medical records/information and episodes. He can view his treatment strategy to comprehend his medication, insulin schedule, or any tests that he wants to take along with his workout regime and food plan.

1.6 Pervasive Computing for Preventive Care

As earlier stated lifespan expectation in developed countries is growing every single year [41, 45–47] as well as along with this bigger long life is a rising "prevalence of chronic conditions and their related pain and disability" [46]. As a result, averting these long-lasting diseases as evolving firstly at home is flattering an added considerable importance. To be sure, numerous nations have shaped defensive plans inspiring well behaviors in an effort to control healthcare budgets on a big gauge. A lot of pervasive computing uses for separate informatics focus on medicine obedience and devotion (e.g., [41, 48, 49]) or convincing technologies aiming at illness deterrence as well as wellness supervision (e.g., [24]). Additional uses highlight on recording therapeutically noteworthy actions designed for long-lasting patients (e.g., [46, 50]) as well as on social health problems. In this section, we discuss several schemes that emphasize on pervasive technologies to assist the automatic and discerning storing of health-related data. We likewise deliberate convincing expertise to facilitate self-monitoring as well as community health to avert cognitive weakening and to uphold bodily as well as mental happiness.

1.6.1 Automated and Selective Capture and Access of Health Information

Handling individual health-related record can be chiefly stimulating for long-lasting patients whose positions length years in addition to are frequently complex [51]. The development of approaches as well as tools used for recording and handling particular health records at hand is still a quantity of exposed queries around in what way persistent technologies can assist the capture, supervision, and handling of health-related information [52]. For that reason, numerous investigation plans have been dedicated on emerging imprisonment and handling tools [40] to assist the administration of health record via numerous stages of physical and programmed capture [53].

1.6.2 Patient Electronic Portals

A patient website is a safe online web-based application that offers patients control as well as access to their personal health record and two method automatic communications by way of providing proper care via a computer system or else a moveable devices [54]. Various research works [21, 55] revealed that patient web-based portals increase the results of defensive care and also disease consciousness and self-management. On the other hand, there is no indication that they increase persistent care consequences.

1.6.3 Persuasive Technologies for Self-Monitoring

Investigators and academicians have initiated toward scrutinizing the usage of convincing technologies [56] intended for inspiring persons to the takings on the accountability of managing, taking, and examining their personal health data and activities. Persuasive tools is normally well defined such as tools that are intended to and developed toward modification of approaches or else overall activities of the handlers via persuading also community inspiration, but not via force [57]. Such type of tools is frequently used in community health, rummage sale, international relations, governments, faith, soldierly exercise, and management as well as may possibly be used in a slightly range of humanoid-to-humanoid or humanoid-to-computer communication [58].

1.6.4 Direct Interaction vs. Mediation

Persuasive technology can also be characterized through whether they amend approaches and activities via straight communication or else over an arbitrating role, on behalf of the instance via human-computer interactions or computer-mediated communications. The illustrations previously stated are the earlier, but there are numerous of the concluding [24, 29, 57, 58]. Communication technology can encourage or else intensify the persuasion of another by renovating the community collaboration, as long as it is a joint feedback on communication, otherwise a rearrangement of communication methods [29, 52, 56, 58].

1.6.5 Persuasion by Social Motivators

Previous researcher works has too used on community instigators alike struggle for persuading[30].By means of relating a handler with other handlers, his/her social group, associates, families as well as other relatives. A convincing solicitation can smear social persuaders on the handler to care personal behavior changes [15]. Social networking sites such as Facebook, LinkedIn, as well as Twitter similarly ease the expansion of such type of systems [59]. It has been revealed that community influence can consequence in better performing vicissitudes than the situation where the handler is out of the way.

1.7 Conclusions

The healthcare area is quickly varying very fast. To begin with, the necessity intended for better efficiency, overall health quality, less cost, as well as safety and security in hospital backgrounds is motivating the requirement for improved connection among record keeping, observation, and patient care systems. Next, there is an increasing movement to enable the patient to control their health in a supplementary active way, welcoming the expansion of a range of individual fitness applications designed for movable devices and home-sensing platforms plus applications. Finally, there is an increasing focus on giving additional active precaution in lieu of patients through long-standing chronic environments and speaking about health as well as wellness matters above long-life parts that are mostly agreeable to the solicitation of unescapable healthcare tools. This chapter has covered pervasive computing methodologies to facilitating several features of health deliveries, in specific concerns. We have defined the usage of universal healthcare tools in favor of hospital care system, to care for supported alive as well as long-lasting illness management and as part of individual health plus wellness management in lieu of preventive care.

References

1. Guest Editorial. (2004). M-Health: Beyond seamless mobility and global wireless healthcare connectivity. *IEEE Transactions on IT in Biomedicine, 8*(4), 405–413.
2. Wan, J., Zou, C., Ullah, S., Lai, C., Zhou, M., & Wang, X. (2013). Cloud-enabled wireless body area networks for pervasive healthcare. *IEEE Network Magazine, 27*(5), 56–61.
3. Bardram, J., & Christensen, H. (2007). Pervasive computing support for hospitals: An overview of the activity-based computing project. *IEEE Pervasive Computing, 6*(1), 44–51. https://doi.org/10.1109/mprv.2007.19
4. de Moraes, J. L. C., de Souza, W. L., Pires, L. F., & do Prado, A. F. (2014). An architecture for health information exchange in pervasive healthcare environment. *International Conference on Enterprise Information Systems, 1*, 385–401.

5. Lin, C., Chiu, M., Hsiao, C., Lee, R., & Tsai, Y. (2006). A wireless healthcare service system for elderly with dementia. *IEEE Transactions on Information Technology in Biomedicine, 10*(2), 696704.
6. Varshney, U., & Sneha, S. (2006). Patient monitoring using ad hoc wireless networks: Reliability and power management. *IEEE Communications Magazine, 44*(4), 49–55.
7. Go, K., Carroll, J., & Imamiya, A. (2000). Family ware: Communicating with someone you love. In *IFIP HOIT conference.*
8. Davis, H., Skov, M. B., Stougaard, M., & Vetere, F. (2007). Virtual box: Supporting mediated family intimacy through virtual and physical play. In *Proceedings of the Australasian conference on computer-human interaction: Entertaining user interfaces* (pp. 151–159).
9. Boric-Lubecke, O., & Lubecke, V. (2002). Wireless house calls: Using communications technology for health care and monitoring. *IEEE Microwave Magazine, 3*(3), 43–48.
10. Freed, N., Burleson, W., Raffle, H., Ballagas, R., & Newman, N. (2010). User interfaces for tangible characters: Can children connect remotely through toy perspectives? In *DC '10: Proceedings of the international conference on interaction design and children.*
11. Fratiglioni, L., Wang, H.-X., Ericsson, K., Maytan, M., & Winblad, B. (2000). Influence of social network on occurrence of dementia: A communitybased longitudinal study. *The Lancet, 355*(9212), 1315–1319.
12. Giles, L. C., Glonek, G. F. V., Luszcz, M. A., & Adrews, G. R. (2005). Effect of social networks on 10 year survival in very old Australians: The Australian longitudinal study of aging. *Journal of Epidemiology and Community Health, 59*, 574–579.
13. House, J. S., Landis, K. R., & Umberson, D. (1988). Social relationships and health. *Science (New York, N.Y.), 241*(4865), 540–545.
14. Cornejo, R., Favela, J., & Tentori, M. (2009). Ambient displays for integrating older adults into social networking sites. In *Collaboration researchers international working group* (pp. 321–336).
15. de Belvis, A., Avolio, M., Sicuro, L., Rosano, A., Latini, E., Damiani, G., & Ricciardi, W. (2008). Social relationships and HRQL: A cross-sectional survey among older Italian adults. *BMC Public Health, 8*(1), 348.
16. Axisa, F., Schmitt, P., Gehin, C., Delhomme, G., McAdams, E., & Dittmar, A. (2005). Flexible technologies and smart clothing for citizen medicine, home healthcare, and disease prevention. *IEEE Transactions on IT in Biomedicine, 9*(3), 325–336.
17. Stanford, V. (2002). Using pervasive computing to deliver elder care. *IEEE Pervasive Computing Magazine, 1*(1), 10–13.
18. Pattichis, C., Kyriacou, E., Voskarides, S., Pattichis, M., Istepanian, R., & Schizas, C. (2002). Wireless telemedicine systems: An overview. *IEEE Antennas and Propagation Magazine, 44*(2), 143–153.
19. Joon, K., Young-Gul, K., Brian, B., & Gee-Woo, B. (2007). Encouraging pa ticipation in virtual communities. *Communications of ACM, 50*(2), 68–73.
20. Pillai, J. A., & Verghese, J. (2009). Social networks and their role in preventing dementia. *Indian Journal of Psychiatry, 51*(5), 22–28.
21. Kruse, C. S., Bolton, K., & Freriks, G. (2015). The effect of patient portals on quality outcomes and its implications to meaningful use: A systematic review. *Journal of Medical Internet Research, 17*, e44.
22. Hayes, G. R., Hirano, S., Marcu, G., Monibi, M., Nguyen, D. H., & Yeganyan, M. (2010). Interactive visual supports for children with autism. *Personal and Ubiquitous Computing, 14*, 663–680.
23. Cornejo R., Favela J., Tentori M. (2010) Ambient Displays for Integrating Older Adults into Social Networking Sites. In: Kolfschoten G., Herrmann T., Lukosch S. (eds) Collaboration and Technology. CRIWG 2010. Lecture Notes in Computer Science, vol 6257. Springer, Berlin, Heidelberg. https://doi.org/10.1007/978-3-642-15714-1_24

24. Garcia-Vazquez, J. P., Rodriguez, M. C., Tentori, M., Saldana, D., Andrade, A. G., & Espinoza, A. N. (2010). An agent-based architecture for developing activity-aware systems for assisting elderly. *Journal of Universal Computer Science, 16*(12), 1500–1520.
25. Middleton, K. R., Anton, S. D., & Perri, M. G. (2013). Long-term adherence to health behavior change. *American Journal of Lifestyle Medicine, 7*(6), 395–404. https://doi.org/10.1177/1559827613488867
26. Frohlich, D., Kuchinsky, A., Pering, C., Don, A., & Ariss, S. (2002). Requirements for Photo ware. In *Proceedings of the 2002 ACM conference on computer supported cooperative work* (pp. 166–175). ACM.
27. Evjemo, B., Svendsen, G. B., Rinde, E., & Johnsen, J. -A. K. (2004). Supporting the distributed family: The need for a conversational context. In *Proceedings of the Nordic conference on human-computer interaction.*
28. He, D., et al. (2012). ReTrust: Attack-resistant and lightweight trust management for medical sensor networks. *IEEE Transactions on Information Technology in Biomedicine, 16*(4), 623–632.
29. Fischer, C. (2008). Feedback on household electricity consumption: A tool for saving energy? *Energy Efficiency, 1*(1), 79–104. https://doi.org/10.1007/s12053-008-9009-7
30. Caraban, A., Ferreira, M. J., Gouveia, R., & Karapanos, E. (2015). Social toothbrush: Fostering family nudging around tooth brushing habits. In *Adjunct Proceedings of the 2015 ACM international joint conference on pervasive and ubiquitous computing and proceedings of the 2015 ACM international symposium on wearable computers, UbiComp/ISWC'15 adjunct* (pp. 649–653). ACM. https://doi.org/10.1145/2800835.2809438
31. Rubenstein, L. Z., Powers, C. M., & MacLean, C. H. (2000). Quality indicators for the management and prevention of falls and mobility problems in vulnerable elders. *Annals of International Medicine, 135*(56), 686–693.
32. Dychtwald, K. (1999). *Age power: How the 21st century will be ruled by the new old.* Putman.
33. Wilmini, N. (2013). Pervasive computing and healthcare. In *Healthcare delivery in the information age*. Springer. https://doi.org/10.1007/978-1-4614-4514-2_2
34. Consolvo, S., Paulos, E., & Smith, I. (2007). *Mobile persuasion for everyday behavior change* (p. 166). E. F. a. E. Eckles (Ed.). Stanford Captology Media.
35. Judge, T. K., Neustaedter, C., Harrison, S., & Blose, A. (2011). Family portals: Connecting families through a multifamily media space. In *CHI '11: Proceedings of the 2011 annual conference on human factors in computing systems.*
36. Hirano, S., Yeganyan, M., Marcu, G., Nguyen, D., & Hayes, G. R. (2010). Sked: Evaluation of a system to support classroom activities for children with autism. In *Proceedings of the international conference on human factors in computing systems (CHI) 2010* (pp. 1633–1642).
37. Belvis, A. G. D., Avolio, M., Sicuro, L., Rosano, A., Latini, E., Damiani, G., & Ricciardi, W. (2008). *Social relationships and HRQL: A cross-sectional survey among older Italian adults.* http://www.ncbi.nlm.nih.gov/pmc/artcles/PMC2569037/?tool=pubmed
38. Bardram, J. E. (2008). Pervasive healthcare as a scientific discipline. *Methods of Information in Medicine, 47*(3), 178–185.
39. Massey, T., Gao, T., Bernstein, D., Husain, A., Crawford, D., White, D., Selavo, L., & Sarrafzadeh, M. (2006). Pervasive triage: Towards ubiquitous, real-time monitoring of vital signs for pre-hospital applications. In *Proceedings of the international workshop on ubiquitous computing for pervasive healthcare.*
40. Locke, E. A., & Latham, G. P. (2002). Building a practically useful theory of goal setting and task motivation: A 35-year odyssey. *American Psychologist, 57*(9), 705–717.
41. Kientz, J. A., Arriaga, R. I., Chetty, M., Hayes, G. R., Richardson, J., Patel, S. N., & Abowd, G. D. (2007). Grow and know: Understanding record-keeping needs for tracking the development of young children. In *Conference on human factors in computing systems.*
42. Suzuki, T., & Doi, M. (2001). Life minder: An evidence-based wearable healthcare assistant. In *Proceedings of the ACM conference on human factors in computing systems* (pp. 127–128).

43. Rodgers, M. M., Pai, V. M., & Conroy, R. S. (2015). Recent advances in wearable sensors for health monitoring. *IEEE Sensors Journal, 15*, 3119–3126.
44. Boukerche, A., & Ren, Y. (2009). A secure mobile healthcare system using trust-based multicast scheme. *IEEE Journal on Selected Areas in Communications, 27*(4), 387–399.
45. Kaushik, P., Intille, S., & Larson, K. (2008). Observations from a case study on user adaptive reminders for medication adherence. In *Proceedings of second international conference on pervasive computing technologies for healthcare.*
46. Lopez-Norris, M., Pazos-Arias, J., Garcia-Duque, J., & Blanco-Fernandez, Y. (2008). Monitoring medicine intake in the networked home: The iCabiNET solution. In *International conference on pervasive computing technologies for healthcare.*
47. Jeong, H., Park, S., & Zimmerman, J. (2008). Opportunities to support parents in managing their children's health. In *Extended abstracts of CHI 2008.*
48. Kaye, J., & Zitzelberger, T. (2006). Overview of healthcare, disease, and disability. In J. Bardram, A. Mihailidis, & D. Wan (Eds.), *Pervasive computing in healthcare* (pp. 3–20). CRC Press.
49. Olshansky, S. J., Carnes, B. A., & Desesquelles, A. (2001). Demography: Prospects for human longevity. *Science, 291*, 1491–1492.
50. Oeppen, J., & Vaupel, J. (2002). Broken limits to life expectancy. *Science, 296*, 1029–1031.
51. Truong, K. N., & Hayes, G. R. (2009). Ubiquitous computing for capture and aceess. *Foundations and Trends! R in Human–Computer Interaction, 2*(2), 95–171.
52. Baranowski, T., Buday, R., Thomson, D. I., & Baranowski, J. (2008). Playing for real: Video games and stories for health-related behavior change. *American Journal of Preventive Medicine, 34*(1), 74–82.
53. Pratt, W., Unruh, K., Civan, A., & Skeels, M. M. (2006). Personal health information management. *Communications of the ACM, 49*(1), 51–55.
54. Office of the National Coordinator for Health Information Technology. *What is a patient portal?* https://www.healthit.gov/providers-professionals/faqs/what-patient-portal
55. Nagykaldi, Z., Aspy, C. B., Chou, A., & Mold, J. W. (2012). Impact of a wellness portal on the delivery of patient-centered preventive care. *Journal of American Board of Family Medicine, 25*, 158–167.
56. Prochanska, J. O., di Clemente, C. C., & Norcross, J. C. (1992). In search of how people change: Applications to addictive behaviors. *American Psychologist, 47*(9), 102–1114.
57. Thieme, A., Comber, R., Miebach, J., Weeden, J., Kraemer, N., Lawson, S., & Olivier, P. (2012). "We've bin watching you": Designing for reflection and social persuasion to promote sustainable lifestyles. In *Proceedings of the SIGCHI conference on human factors in computing systems CHI '12* (pp. 2337–2346). ACM. https://doi.org/10.1145/2207676.2208394
58. Froehlich, J., Dillahunt, T., Klasnja, P., Mankoff, J., Consolvo, S., Harrison, B., & Landay, J. A. (2009). UbiGreen: Investigating a mobile tool for tracking and supporting green transportation habits. In *Proceedings of the SIGCHI conference on human factors in computing systems, CHI '09* (pp. 1043–1052). ACM. https://doi.org/10.1145/1518701.1518861
59. Jadad, A. R., Enkin, M. V., Glouberman, S., Groff, P., & Stern, A. (2006). Are virtual communities good for our health? *British Medical Journal, 332*(7547), 925–926.

Chapter 2
The Imperative Role of Pervasive Data in Healthcare

Anwar Ali Sathio and Arz Muhammad Brohi

2.1 A Brief History of Pervasive Computing

The healthcare Emerging technological change emphasized Researchers, to rethink about the more advanced and low cast technoogical methods and innovative systems like improvement in electronics technology (hardwrae devices) which are responsible to auto sensing capabilities (sensors), to measure all physical entities of real world and manipulate the data for further research studies. Similarly, telecommunication technologies avail high speed of Internet connectivity for traditional desktops, laptops, smart phone as well as embedded devices to ensure scalability, data transferring rates and connectivity of devices while sending data over network. Such enhancements in all afore-mentioned fields have opened door for researchers that innovated new dimension in the field of computer science called pervasive/ubiquitous computing. The words "pervasive" and "ubiquitous" are used interchangeably to describe the same concept.

Pervasive computing is the cutting-edge technology for the contemporary era. The pioneer of pervasive computing/ubiquitous computing was Mark Weiser [1], in PARC (Palo Alto Research Center) in America. Mark Wiser describes the concept of pervasive computing as "Inspired by the social scientists, philosophers and anthropologists at PARC, we have been trying to take a radical look at what computing and networking ought to be like. We believe that people live through their practices and tacit knowledge, so that the most powerful things are those that are effectively invisible in use. This is a challenge that affects all of computer sciences. Our preliminary approach: Activate the world. Provide hundreds of wireless

A. A. Sathio (✉) · A. M. Brohi
Department of Computer Science, Benazir Bhutto Shaheed University (BBSU), Lyari, Karachi, Pakistan
e-mail: anwar.sathio@bbsul.edu.pk; ariz.muhammad@bbsul.edu.pk

M. S. Husain et al. (eds.), *Pervasive Healthcare*, EAI/Springer Innovations in Communication and Computing, https://doi.org/10.1007/978-3-030-77746-3_2

computing devices per person per office of all scales (from 1″ displays to wall-sized). This has required new work in operating systems, user interfaces, networks, wireless, displays and many other areas. We call our work 'ubiquitous computing.' This is different from PDAs [personal digital assistants], Dynabooks or information at your fingertips. It is invisible, everywhere computing that does not live on a personal device of any sort but is in the woodwork everywhere". Pervasive computing has changed the entire world as we perceive. Pervasive computing-enabled Internet of Things (IoT) allow the device to perform action while understanding the context. One of key features of pervasive computing is that it eliminated interaction of the user with application and performed all task on behalf of the user which made it as an invisible servant. These are the main features of pervasive computing according to its nature of working, context awareness, adaptation, scalability, and heterogeneity.

2.2 Main Features of Pervasive Computing

2.2.1 Context Awareness

According to Henricksen et al. [2], an application will be accomplished by reducing input from users and replacing it with a knowledge of context. Context awareness is a software component which exploits information such as activities in which the user is engaged, proximity, to other devices and services, location, time of day and weather conditions. This all information will change application behaviour according to users' condition.

2.2.2 Adaptation

Adaptation is another feature of pervasive computing which is directly related to the user interface for pervasive computing environment that must be highly adaptable in order to respond to changes in the available input and output devices.

2.2.3 Scalability

In the pervasive computing , the factor of scalbility play an important role for healthcare fascilities such factors like time complexity, cost effectiveness, resources managment, hardware and software systems' synchroization, these are very effective parameters for further detailed studies in the context.

2.2.4 *Heterogeneity*

Heterogeneity is related to the combination of different computing devices.

Ubiquitous computing provides two unique parameters anytime and anywhere for anyone which means the user can perform his or her task from anytime and anywhere by using one of the backbone services of pervasive computing called networking, which enable the user to control and perform task according to their need anytime and anywhere. Pervasive/ubiquitous computing covers a wide range of technologies to accomplish its invisible silent servant needs such as distributed and mobile computing, sensor networks, wireless sensor networks, human-computer interaction, artificial intelligence knowledge, etc. [3]. This technology has produced a great impact and brought several changes in every field of domain, because pervasive/ubiquitous computing means everywhere and anytime. This invisible servant work is accomplished by a small, tiny hardware called sensor which senses the physical phenomena and converts that data into the electrical form for further action. These sensors always have limited energy capability to live. The challenges of pervasive computing devices has been literatured by the researchers, they had identified, some are very importants like energey consumption, dat security& trust, data transmission & management and across the board heterogeneous capability. Therefore, there are lots of applications in each domain of life such as environmental monitoring (e.g. weather forecast, forest fire detection), natural disasters (e.g. flood detection and monitoring, earthquake), military (e.g. military equipment monitoring/surveillance, battle field management), business (e.g. product monitoring and tracking), and smart homes (e.g. monitoring and controlling home appliances) [4], and healthcare [5] (measure temperature, heart rate, blood pressure, blood and urine chemical level, breathing rate and volume, sugar level, and patient activities, etc.). Ubiquitous computing has brought great revolution especially in the medical field to change the way of traditional treatment from self-treatment. To automated treatment by using different sensors and actuators, monitoring devices are designed regarding the disease, which enable doctors to monitor each activity of patient such as patient name and location (room number, time, date) as well as to assist the patient from anywhere at anytime if emergency will occur and suggest specific medication for the patient to prevent the impact of disease as well as recover patient health. Many applications are designed in pervasive computing in the healthcare field to make patient treatment easier than traditional treatment. According to literature in traditional treatment, the writing error of doctors would be the cause of patient death [6], and medical error will be imposing substantial cost in national economy.

2.3 Pervasive in Healthcare

The pervasive computing has produced a great impact on every domain of life and has improved the working style of their traditional way atmost level by increasing their performance and as well as cost effcetiveness in the respective field. It is because it will save time and cost of the nation as well as individual person, and in emergency medical situation, medical support will be sent quickly and reduce death ratio of humans because pervasive computing automatically monitors the patient every activity and update doctors if any emergency occurred. Also, it provides real-time data in each second which is used to evaluate the health condition of patients who are suffering from critical health issue specially heart attack, diabetes, and cancer. Therefore, doctors and hospitals needed records of such patient(s) frequently to monitor their condition and also change the treatment if necessary. Accordingly, all fields of life have started integration of pervasive computing functionality.

2.4 Pervasive Applications in Healthcare

The pervasive computing in the context of application, there are many functionality attributes, taking more focussed on patients care, such as information security, automation, web services, monitoring etc. The following are several applications of pervasive computing in healthcare domain from different corporations:

1. *Measure temperature*: Use sensors to continuously measure the patient's temperature to prevent the highest level of temperature that would be the cause of the patient's death.
2. *Heart rate*: Likewise use pervasive computing to measure heart beat fluctuation in the form of an uninterrupted manner and patient heart rate to avoid serious and uncontrolled health condition, because the patient faces sudden and extreme critical health condition.
3. *Blood pressure*: Measuring blood pressure of each patient is a normal route task, but the major concern of this parameter is regarding the more critical condition of the patient with diabetes or those patients who are suffering from blood pressure. It is necessary to continuously measure this parameter of the patient to avoid the flow of blood in high-frequency rate that will burst the veins of the patient.
4. *Blood and urine chemical level*: Similarly, measure the blood as well as urine level of those patients who are suffering from the chemical level in blood as well as urine, if the urine chemical level crossed its highest level that will cause kidney stone. Automatically measure and control the urine and blood level to prevent critical condition of the patient.
5. *Breathing rate and volume and sugar level*: Pervasive computing is also used to monitor breathing rate and volume as well as the sugar level of the patient to recover from a health condition as soon as possible, but these all monitoring and measuring activities will be achieved without human interaction. Also ensure to ring alarm for doctors and nurses if any critical condition occurred.
6. *Lung cancer*: According to WHO reports, and its alarming that mostly cancer deaths observed due to smoking in the world. Smoking fog slowly damage the working capability of lungs and patient therefore, the key attributes shall be con-

sidered such as to monitor the lung cancer, recovery stage data and these data shall be analyzed in real time mode through sensors.

7. *Patient activities*: Patient activities can be classified into two types: one is auditor based and second is gesture based. Auditor activities are used to monitor the movement of patients whether he/she do the same activities which is prevented by the doctor or not indicating the attitude of patient towards instructions given by doctor, that must be followed by patient, other case all activities such as unconscious or partially hit patients.

Measuring heart rates of the patient in critical condition is important for doctors to analyse real-time improvements in patient's health. Similarly nowadays people have acquired more stress which could be the cause of blood pressure. The record of heart patients, such as blood pressure, heart beat rate, temperature, weight, medicine and other related factors monitored for getting the analysis report of the patient recovery. Impure utilization of water would be the cause of kidney disease and block the urine veins. Likewise all these disease treatment will be done when doctor(s) attain real-time data of patient(s) and activities according to the disease that needs proper treatment. These applications of healthcare indicate the importance of pervasive computing in healthcare to provide a quick response to patient to save his/her life. Using pervasive computing to implement recognition of activity of daily life (ADL) using different classifiers and decision-making algorithms provide better healthcare and lifestyle management as well as exploit the machine learning algorithms to predict any disease and provide preliminary stage medication to the patient.

2.4.1 Security Features for Patients' Data

In medical perspective the security feature is one of the key role factors about patient data, because the entire medicine will be prescribed based on the gathered data. Therefore, security of patient data is more critical because the entire decision is based on the gathered data. If the data is accurate and secure, then decision will be correct, and the doctor will prescribe the appropriate medicine for the patient. Otherwise doctors will make such erroneous decision about the patient's treatment due to the gathered forgery-based data, which might be the cause of critical health condition of the patient or death. Therefore, secure confidential-based gathered data will make the doctors and hospitals gain confidence in taking decisions about patient treatment to recover from his/her health condition as soon as possible. Several security approaches have been designed and implemented for ensuring data integrity and confidentiality of patient data [7–10]. Because patient data are always important which are gathered by using body wearable network devices and using wireless sensor networks as an intermediary layer to transmit data over the network, WSNs are an open environment; therefore, it could be easy for attackers to apply any kind of attack (attacker may apply either passive attack which can see and analyse sensitive data but not able to modify it, and it discloses all confidential data, but active attacker can analyse as well as modify sensitive data and resend to the receiver) to modify the data [9]. Therefore, authentication and authorization of data along with integrity and confidential are more reliable and trustworthy data [4], which helps doctor(s) write proper and accurate medicine for the patient to save his/her life.

According to the working nature of pervasive computing technology, avaibility of resources and capability of monitoring through networks over internet invites many threats and attacksers. There are several types of attack, but a few of them are important. The common attacks are as follows:

1. *DOS (Denial-of-Service) Attack*
   The DoS attack was developed first time for testing of the network bandwidth capacity, but later this service attack is used to exploit the entire bandwidth capacity and prevent the access of authenticated user for their desired resources from the network for temporary or infinite time. Due to sending many requests over the network to keep the server busy as well as to consume complete bandwidth, DoS attack cannot be thwart through technical means alone [11]. In September 1996 the first-time attack was applied on *Panix*, the third-oldest ISP service provider in the world. This kind of attack is difficult to prevent through technical means alone because of how to identify which packets would be the cause of DoS attack.
2. *DDOS (Distributed Denial-of-Service) Attack*
   Distributed denial service attack is another type of DoS in this multiple systems that initiate attack to flood bandwidth or resource of target machine and ensure unavailability of resource from an authenticated user for temporary or intended time.
3. *Man-in-the-Middle Attack*
   Man-in-the-middle attack is the type of active attacker which intercepts between two communication parties either observing or modifying sensitive data.
4. *Node Cloning Attack*
   This attack is very difficult to find because all nodes which are cloned mean that they have compromised on security issue. An adversary physically captures a sensor node to extract all the secrete cryptographic from and reprogram it and again deploy that cloned node on the network to apply a variety of inside attacks on the network. This attack is applied on mobile or wireless sensor networks [12, 13].
5. *Sniffing Attack*
   This is another type of network attack which is common. In this attack adversary will capture the network traffic and steal important information such as password. A file also compromises the confidentiality of the security aspect [14].
6. *Packet Drop Attack*
   This is another type of attack which is applied by adversary on the wireless sensor network which is deployed in hostel and unattended environment which easily becomes the victim of an adversary. The malicious node will drop packet

to prevent its further propagation. Therefore, an adversary does not drop each packet, but it drops selective packets [15–17].

There are many pervasive computing systems that have been designed as well as implemented in healthcare system. A few of the systems have been described in this section, such as Intelligent Heart Disease Prediction System (IHDPS) for detecting heart disease proposed by different classifiers like Decision Tree Naïve Bayes and Neural Network to predict and identity the significant impact of attributes of heart disease, and many other propose approaches have been used to achieve the healthcare aim and also many applications regarding to healthcare [18]. Another one is Ubiquitous Healthcare Information System (UHIS) which enables the patient to access healthcare services anywhere and anytime for further reading to see [19].

2.4.2 *Lifecycle of Pervasive Healthcare Data*

The concept of this lifecycle with respect to pervasive healthcare data may be described in the following six major domains. This is a proposed lifecycle model for pervasive healthcare data:

1. Control systems (sensors, databases, management systems)
2. Tool (apps, data mining, monitoring, communication systems, reporting)
3. Extract transform load (ETL) tool (integration, filtrations of data)
4. Dynamic selections (data schemas, labelling of data)
5. Patient's activities-monitoring
6. Patients' behaviour assessment/mood readings

As per the need of healthcare system, we have enlisted the above stages for our proposed model for healthcare which is known as *lifecycle of pervasive healthcare system*. Because without these stages, any proposed system would not be implemented as per the nature of pervasive computing. Therefore, all the above list of stages fall in the healthcare lifecycle of pervasive computing which is represented in pictorial form in Fig. 2.1. Each stage consists of certain components and tasks to perform several actions and send that data as input for the next stages which also perform a necessary task and then send that output as input to another stage, etc.

1. *Control System (Sensors, Databases, Management System)*

   The control system depends on four core objects as given above. The sensor is a tiny device which is responsible for sensing physical phenomenon and sending that gathered data either for processing purpose or storage purpose which is entirely based on purposed system and how it will exploit gathered data. Similarly database is a tool which is capable of storing data for future requirement according to the need. Because database data is also important when the same patient will come back again in the hospital, his/her demography will help the doctors take quick steps to save his/her life. The whole control is being managed by the administrators by helping in supporting the staff further which is classified into:

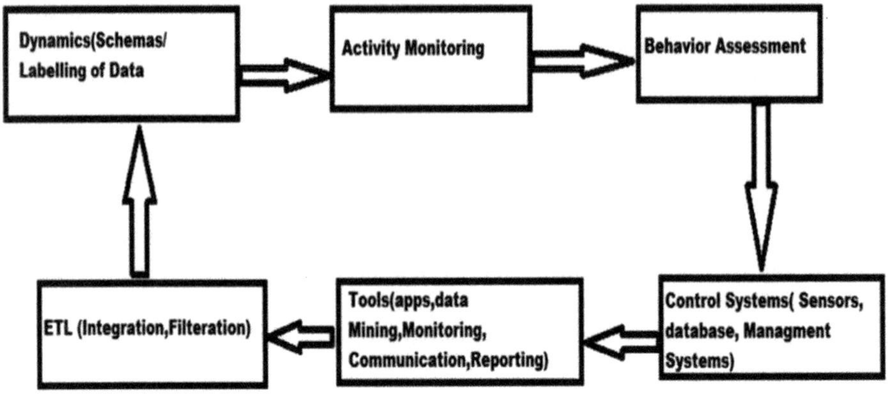

Fig. 2.1 Lifecycle of pervasive healthcare data

(a) Devices (pervasive/sensor-based) manager
(b) Database manager
(c) Host network manager
(d) Communication systems (satellite) manager
(e) Application software manager

2. *Tool (Apps, Data Mining, Monitoring, Communication Systems, Reporting)*

   Tool is the second stage of healthcare lifecycle which consists of six major components that enable the healthcare lifecycle to perform meaningful task. App is indicating any application that is responsible for receiving data from any sensor, and it is front-end for the doctors to analyse fluctuation of receiving the data which gives an entire improvement of clue of the patient's health. This fluctuation data exploits data mining functionality because data mining extracts data on pattern base and produces knowledge discovery report (which is called meaningful data extracted from the gathered data) [20–22]. Monitoring is also front-end for doctors, nurses, and hospital paramedical staff while they continuously monitor the patient's health. The communication system is the soul of the gathering data because it works as the intermediary layer to increase scalability of network and to ensure data transmission over the network. The bandwidth also plays a key role in communication system which affect the data transmission rates if data transmission rates are slow which directly emit an impact on system performance due to high latency. Reporting is the last component of tool it generates the final report that will be used for making decision. It is necessary for reporting that data must be extracted by data mining techniques.

   The concept of tools is generic, but here we have limitation to the following:

(a) Application of front-end tools
(b) Database system and visualization tools
(c) Network tools
(d) Communication tools

(e) Operating system tools
(f) Sensor device controlling and data extraction tools
(g) Data warehousing tools
(h) ETL tools

3. *Extract Transform Load (ETL) Tool (Integration, Filtrations of Data)*
   This is used to integrate the ETL tools with application. As ETL will be integrated with the existing application tool/systems to keep the connection with source data for getting the information or fields/labels, this works like a supporting module with middleware application for extracting the required data, transforming it according to the design of data warehouse, and loading it in the suggested mart if required.
   The ETL tool is available as open source with SQL Server 2012 and the latest versions with special wizard: SQL Server Integration Services (SSIS). Before getting in the process, data sources may be classified in these MySQL, TEXT, XML, Excel, CSV, and SQ-DB types. These sources may be live or offline data sources, according to the nature of the data provider.
4. *Dynamic Selections (Data Schemas, Labelling of Data)*
   In this stage, the system deals with dynamics of all data, including the design of data whether star schemas, snowflake, or galaxy, OLAP framework in synchronous data, data warehousing, and further data mart design. This shall need labelling of data to extract and filter the data attributes of all dynamics like personal profiles, medical staff, and management systems either retaining the same labelling or changing with the suggested labels to better understand the dynamics of data.
5. *Patient Activities (Monitoring (Auditory and Gestured))*
   The fifth stage of healthcare lifecycle deals with patient activities to avoid the prohibited things as well as activities. For example, if the doctor restricted the patient not to smoke, then it is necessary for him to monitor the patient's activities as he/she might be smoking. Auditory data deals with voice communication of patient, whereas gestured data belongs to the patient's movement regarding eye flipping, hand raising, finger movement, etc. All these data are also important in the health perspective.
6. *Patient Behaviour Assessment/Mood Reading*
   Patient assessment is an important factor in the healthcare domain. On the bases of assessment, doctors and nurses predict improvement in the patient's health. This health improvement is entirely based on the patient moods because if the patient gets well, then he/she feels happy and feverish. Mood or behaviour may be classified into two types: one may be positive mood and second may be negative mood. The measurement of these moods is divided into at least two parameters according to the situation and timestamp. Using these parameters, we can calculate whether the patient is in which mood, either in positive or negative mood.

2.4.3 Classification of Pervasive Healthcare Data

The classification of pervasive healthcare data is a very complex subject; however, this can be classified into different types of data: text, images, audios, and videos oriented in online transactional processing (OLTP). These types further can be classified in some domain areas where it has correlation with each type of pervasive healthcare data. The following are the important pervasive healthcare data specifications:

1. Personal profile (patients, doctors, nursing staff, account/management staff, pharma staff, IT staff)
2. Hospital management systems (monitoring, management, control, evaluation systems, updating)
3. Nursing facilities (availability of required nursing facilities, staff, resources, etc.)
4. Medicine (online complete data of stock and valid information)
5. OPD data (recording OPD data and mining the same)
6. Hospitalized data (patient's hospital history data storage)
7. Home arrangement data (home service monitoring and analysis data history)
8. Testing data (keep all records of patients' test data for ready reference)

2.4.4 Dynamics of Pervasive Healthcare Data

The following key components may be involved in the pervasive healthcare data dynamics:

1. Patients
2. Doctors
3. Nursing staff
4. Hospital management
5. Applications/sensor tools
6. Laboratories/testing tools
7. Medicine
8. Sensor systems/machines
9. Diseases classifications
10. Networks/communication technologies
11. Cloud technologies/data mining/data warehousing

2.4.5 Dynamics Labelling Process for Healthcare Data Designing

The data is a real asset for any kind of knowledge, in the pervasive healthcare data, specially depending on how accurate and complete the data is. This data shall be integrated through valid labels for analysing and monitoring the record of all dynamics, as patients, doctors, etc. This large data set is to be generated round the clock, and this activity is monitored by sensor machines automatically. The valid data collection is a very complex job, as well as very expensive, too. Authors Cruz-Sandoval et al. [23] presented two approaches in monitoring the patient's activity through online systems for data extraction:

1. Measuring the burden on the user (gesture-oriented activity), who is performing and annotating the activity
2. Counting the lack of accuracy due to the user (auditory data-oriented) labelling the data (minutes/hours every activity)

The labelling may vary into labels like behaviour, timestamp, etc. It also seems like a segmentation and labelling [24]. The main reason for the labelling of data is to conclude and summarize the facts for knowledge extraction. There are many approaches to get labelled data by using algorithms and techniques. This labelled data can be processed and utilized in many ways for live running sessions as well as future assessment and analysis. The pervasive data by nature is a kind of live data such as online transactional processing (OLTP) data to save the precious lives of the patients. It may either in a synchronous or asynchronous manner depending on the situations. This data may further be utilized and warehoused for future use, and it also can be mined for research and artificial intelligence purposes. In the context of pervasive data, new emerging techniques are used to label the data. Some are mentioned here to understand the labelling concept and its importance in the field of pervasive healthcare data.

2.4.6 Pervasive Healthcare Data Labelling Techniques

The following approaches/techniques can be referred to data labelling with respect to one of the dynamics of pervasive healthcare data [25–33]:

1. Temporal labelling (synchronous/asynchronous)
2. Annotator (observer)
3. Scenario
4. Tool annotation mechanism
5. Survey-based tool annotation mechanism

The data is the backbone of all pervasive systems, so this is a complex dynamic and shall be addressed and mainly cared for to handle the devices as well as persons engaged with the systems. The pervasive healthcare data is a very sensitive and big asset that needs a lot of attention regarding security, integration, consistency, transparency, and being available for all stakeholders. We tried to focus our attention on healthcare data and its behaviours relating to the systems integrated with data and communication systems. The model we suggested in this study shall be effective to compose the theory about pervasive computing in detail. In this model, six components are involved to carry on the complete processing of pervasive healthcare data.

Missing of at least one would damage the structure of pervasive computing theory. The patient and sensor-based device technologies are key factors and play an important role in the pervasive technologies. Patient care is the major activity, with supporting factors like medical staff, IT support team, and sensor devices as well as the main entities in the pervasive health data. The control systems become the starting layer in the process, being physical and logical architecture. It depends on this process and after this next shall be the tool process to handle the situations and make taking care of the patients possible. This suggested model loop will carry on the whole pervasive system smoothly and effectively till it is achieved.

References

1. Weiser, M. (1991). The computer for the 21st century. *Scientific American, 265*(3), 94–104. https://doi.org/10.1038/scientificamerican0991-94
2. Henricksen, K., Indulska, J., & Rakotonirainy, A. (2001). Infrastructure for pervasive computing: Challenges. In GI Jahrestagung (1) (pp. 214–222).
3. Rastegari, E., Rahmani, A., & Setayeshi, S. (2011). Pervasive computing in healthcare systems. *World Academy of Science, Engineering and Technology*, 2011(59).
4. Brohi, A. M., Malkani, Y. A., & Chandio, M. S. (2018). Data provenance in wireless sensor networks (WSNs): A review. In *International conference on computing, mathematics and engineering technologies* (pp. 1–5). https://doi.org/10.1109/ICOMET.2018.8346374
5. Brown, I., & Adams, A. A. (2007). The ethical challenges of ubiquitous healthcare. *International Review of Information Ethics, 8*, 53–60.
6. Miao, Z., & Yuan, B. (2005, November). Discussion on pervasive computing paradigm. In TENCON 2005-2005 IEEE Region 10 Conference (pp. 1-6). IEEE.
7. Ali, S. T., Sivaraman, V., Ostry, D., & Jha, S. (2013). Securing data provenance in body area networks using lightweight wireless link fingerprints. In *Proceedings of the 3rd international workshop on trustworthy embedded devices - trusted '13* (pp. 65–72). https://doi.org/10.1145/2517300.2517303.
8. Hussain, S. R. et al. (2014). Secure data provenance compression using arithmetic coding in wireless sensor networks. In S. R. Hussain, C.Wang, E. Bertino, S. R. Hussain, C. Wang, S. Sultana, & E. Bertino (Eds.), *Secure data provenance compression using arithmetic coding in wireles*.
9. Zhang, G. H., Chung, C., Poon, Y., & Zhang, Y. T. (2011). A review on body area networks security for healthcare. *International Scholarly Research Network, 2011*(1), 692592. https://doi.org/10.5402/2011/692592
10. Sultana, S., Shehab, M., & Bertino, E. (2012). Secure provenance transmission for streaming data. *IEEE Transactions on Knowledge and Data Engineering, 25*(8), 1890–1903.
11. Hasan, R., & Winslett, M. *The case of the fake Picasso: Preventing history forgery with secure provenance* (pp. 1–14).
12. Qabulio, M., Malkani, Y. A., & Keerio, A. A. (2015). On node replication attack in wireless sensor networks. *Mehran University Research Journal of Engineering and Technology, 34*(4), 413–424.
13. Qabulio, M., Malkani, Y. A., & Keerio, A. (2015). *Securing mobile wireless sensor networks (WSNs) against clone node attack* (pp. 20–21).
14. Kulshrestha, A., & Dubey, S. K. (2014). A literature review on sniffing attacks in computer network. *International Journal of Advanced Engineering Research and Science*, (2), 67–73.
15. Sultana, S., Bertino, E., & Shehab, M. (2011). A provenance based mechanism to identify malicious packet dropping adversaries in sensor networks. In *Proceedings - interna-*

tional conference on distributed computing systems (pp. 332–338). https://doi.org/10.1109/ICDCSW.2011.54

16. Wang, C. (2016). Provenance for wireless sensor networks: A survey. *Data Science and Engineering, 1*(3), 189–200. https://doi.org/10.1007/s41019-016-0017-x
17. Wang, C., Hussain, S., & Bertino, E. (2015). Dictionary based secure provenance compression for wireless sensor networks. *IEEE Transactions on Parallel and Distributed Systems, PP*(99), 1. https://doi.org/10.1109/TPDS.2015.2402156
18. Sarkar, P., & Sinha, D. (2017). Application on pervasive computing in healthcare – A review. *Indian Journal of Science and Technology, 10*, 1–10. https://doi.org/10.17485/ijst/2017/v10i3/110619
19. Omary, Z., Mtenzi, F., Wu, B., & Driscoll, C. O. (2011). Ubiquitous healthcare information system: Assessment of its impacts to patient' s information. *International Journal of Information Security Research (IJISR), 1*, 71–77.
20. Jothi, N., Aini, N., Rashid, A., & Husain, W. (2015). Data mining in healthcare – A review. *Procedia - Procedia Computer Science, 72*, 306–313. https://doi.org/10.1016/j.procs.2015.12.145
21. Durairaj, M., & Ranjani, V. (2013). Data mining applications in healthcare sector: a study. *International Journal of Scientific & Technology Research, 2*(10), 29–35.
22. Dey, M., & Rautaray, S. S. (2014). Study and analysis of data mining algorithms for healthcare decision support system. *International Journal of Computer Science and Information Technologies, 5*(1), 470–477.
23. Cruz-sandoval, D., et al. (2019). Semi-automated data labeling for activity recognition in pervasive healthcare. *Sensors, 19*(14), 3035. https://doi.org/10.3390/s19143035
24. Yordanova, K., et al. (2017). Challenges in annotation of user data for ubiquitous systems. *Arduous*, 1–25.
25. Cruciani, F., Cleland, I., Nugent, C., Mccullagh, P., & Synnes, K. (2018). Automatic annotation for human activity recognition in free living using a smartphone. *Sensors, 18*, 2203. https://doi.org/10.3390/s18072203
26. Kipp, M. (2001). Anvil-a generic annotation tool for multimodal dialogue. Proc. 7th European Conference on Speech Communication and Technology (Eurospeech 2001). pp. 1367–1370.
27. Tonkin, E. L., et al. (2018). Talk, text, tag? Understanding self-annotation of smart home data from a user's perspective. *Sensors, 18*(7), 2365. https://doi.org/10.3390/s18072365
28. Lasecki, W. S., Song, Y. C., Kautz, H., & Bigham, J. P. (2013, February). Real-time crowd labeling for deployable activity recognition. In Proceedings of the 2013 conference on Computer supported cooperative work (pp. 1203-1212).
29. Verhagen, S. J. W., Hasmi, L., Drukker, M., Van Os, J., & Delespaul, P. A. E. G. (2016). Use of the experience sampling method in the context of clinical trials. *Evidence-Based Mental Health, 19*(3), 86–89.
30. Intille, S. S., Rondoni, J., Kukla, C., Ancona, I., & Bao, L. (2003, April). A context-aware experience sampling tool. In CHI'03 extended abstracts on Human factors in computing systems (pp. 972-973).
31. Husain, M. S. (2020). Critical concepts and techniques for information retrieval system. In *Natural language processing in artificial intelligence* (p. 29). Apple Academic Press.
32. Khan, M. Z., & Husain, M. S. (2020). Introduction to email, web, and message forensics. In *Critical concepts, standards, and techniques in cyber forensics* (pp. 174–186). IGI Global.
33. Suaib, M., Akbar, M., & Husain, M. S. (2020). Digital forensics and data mining. In *Critical concepts, standards, and techniques in cyber forensics* (pp. 240–247). IGI Global.

Chapter 3
Pervasive Healthcare Computing: Applications, Challenges and Solutions

Abdullah, Gezahagn Haileslassie Gezahagn, Teklay Teklu, Hagos Yirgaw, and Mahfuzul Huda

3.1 Introduction

The scope of the use of pervasive computing is very big [1]. Evolving pervasive computing technologies are valid in several parts of life such as healthcare, game as well as education. Pervasive computing provides a convincing apparition of unremarkable, practical aids to our day-to-day life that differ with and are suitable to our locality and doings [2–4]. In several respects, pervasive computing goals at moving outside the desktop computers to pile itself into the identical fabric of our environments are obtainable for use as soon as required. Taking the operational circumstances for doctors in a hospital into account, this idea is mainly engaging. Hospital general practitioner work in a background that is basically different from the workplace they are tremendously mobile besides repeatedly do not even individual counters or personal laptops.

In such backgrounds, pervasive computing notions as well as tools appear to provide smart consequences [2, 4–6]. One can simply generalize Weiser's groundbreaking pervasive computing idea into a hospital background wherever pads (equal to PDAs), tabs (equal to tablet PCs) and live boards (equal to interactive smart boards) would be reachable in large numbers everywhere [7]. These electronic devices would all be smoothly linked in a wired and wireless network to carry locality and context awareness, reachable for all to use in any place, any time. For example, a nurse would pick up a pad in a patient's chamber and use it for slight, rapid jobs like recording medicine handouts, and a general practitioner would pick up a

Abdullah (✉) · G. H. Gezahagn · T. Teklu · H. Yirgaw
Department of Information Technology, College of Engineering and Technology, Adigrat University, Tigray, Ethiopia

M. Huda
Saudi Electronic University, Riyadh, Saudi Arabia

M. S. Husain et al. (eds.), *Pervasive Healthcare*, EAI/Springer Innovations in Communication and Computing, https://doi.org/10.1007/978-3-030-77746-3_3

tab while incoming at the patient ward, be mechanically recognized and at that time use this pad throughout the hospital/ward round. A radiologist would be capable of approaching and also presenting radiology imageries in medical score quality on a random live board in some of the meeting as well as conference halls in a medical hospital, and cooperative application software system for collocated plus scattered cooperation about patients and their treatments should be accessible in altogether three (3) devices [8–10]. Taking pervasive healthcare computing into the hospitals may possibly significantly increase the thoughtful of necessities for non-office backgrounds, and the chapter concludes with a summary of the significant points that were offered as well as expects the upcoming direction of pervasive healthcare computing in all hospitals.

3.2 Pervasive Healthcare Applications

The pervasive healthcare system consists of pervasive healthiness checking, smart disaster management system, pervasive healthcare information retrieval and pervasive moveable telemedicine [1, 2, 11]. Some key use in pervasive healthcare system, called complete healthiness checking, is obtainable in noteworthy particulars via wireless networking answers of wireless LAN arrangements, cellular, 3G structure-oriented mobile networks and ad hoc wireless network system [8, 12–14]. The use of pervasive computing and intelligent tools to our public life is moving in together with excessive depth as well as scope; in addition it will increase the complete healthcare system as fine [3, 15, 16]. In the next one or two decades, tiny term improvements in mobile and wireless expertise such as the capacity to supply a noteworthy quantity of data on a moveable device and a network of body sensors can be applied to support pervasive healthcare system [17–20]. Furthermore to the present applications, novel pervasive healthcare applications might become probable due to the wireless plus mobile communication technologies (presenting in Fig. 3.1).

3.2.1 Modern Computer Technologies in Hospitals

Computer system and Internet technology are constantly growing in all hospitals. Incorporating separate solutions for patients observing and analysis such as ECG monitors and x-rays system. Wireless communication system permits distributed hospital management systems (DHMS), attached picture archiving and also communication systems, automatic patient record management system and networked intensive care observing systems. Such categories of systems are very common in entirely contemporary and big hospitals these days [11, 21–24].

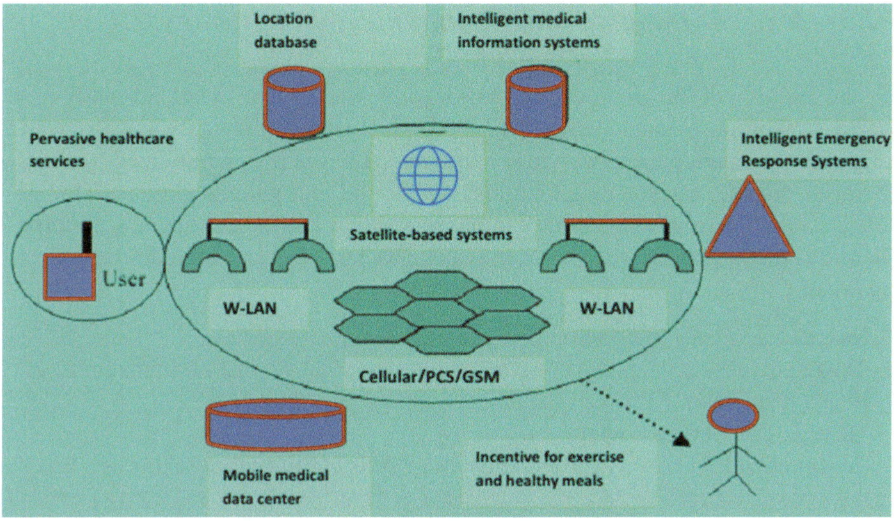

Fig. 3.1 Several existing and evolving pervasive healthcare applications

Hospital communication is moving in the direction of wireless solutions which are progressively significant for together managerial and medical applications [15, 25–27].

3.2.2 Hospital Information System and Electronic Patient Record Management

A complete hospital information/management system commonly includes areas like patient recordkeeping, discharge, medical records, index, billings system, ward information, stores management, drugstore, food, salary, etc. [3, 28, 29]. Today, almost 40% of hospital information system data is administrative data, although medical data have a portion of approximately 60% only [30–32].

A common example of administrative purposes comprise of the following:

- Supply and chain management system
- Resource supervision
- Equipment repairs
- Monetary super
- Human resource system

Hospital clinical systems comprise of the following:

- Electronic patient records
- Drug organization systems
- Medical appointment as well as reservation systems
- Laboratory plus pharmacy supervision systems

3.2.3 *Medical Imaging and Communication Systems (MICS)*

For the duration of the previous one decade, computer systems were normally used for great resolution image creation [14, 33, 34]. Devoted hardware technology and software system are prerequisite to produce such images in computerized tomography scan, magnetic resonance imaging, ultrasound and gamma cameras [19, 35, 36]. Developing from standalone radiology system, MICS are actuality incorporated into the healthcare information system background and include the following areas:

- Image attainment: Interfacing using digital attainment devices
- Image processing: Whichever at the attainment point or post-attainment phase
- Image inspecting: At investigative, consulting, recording
- Storage: For storage devices
- Communication: Mainly through hospital LANs but furthermore through WANs

3.2.4 *Clinical Laboratory Computing*

The major goal of a clinical laboratory system is to offer correct results in small period. Clinical laboratory examination comprises blood chemistry, microbiology, etc. [32, 37, 38]. Results must tie by patients' unique ID particulars and should be valid. Rapid access to clinical laboratory system can donate to proficient patient care system.

3.3 Present-Day Uses and Problems in Pervasive Healthcare Computing

Presently, the use of wireless technologies in healthcare system is partial [1, 15]. Even though healthcare authorities are progressively praised to use handheld electronic devices to retrieve patient data and information, electronic prescription system send gentle reminders to related patients as well as enter analysis and payment codes for pervasive healthcare-related facilities [7, 9, 15, 39]. The actual related problems are:

- Absence of complete coverage of wireless networks as well as mobile networks
- Consistency of wireless network infrastructure
- Common restrictions of handheld electronic devices

3.3.1 In Relation to Information Systems, the Subsequent Problems Need to Be Resolved as Follows

- Coverage of wireless networks and networking devices in all hospitals
- Relational database management system and its availability
- Development and use of online website for all patient healthcare-related history
- Management of overall pervasive healthcare systems comprising privacy and safety

3.3.2 Technological Issues

The wireless network issues in pervasive healthcare system include:

- Wireless network support such as location tracing
- Use of moveable devices for healthcare data storing
- Keep posted as well as broadcast
- Creation of ad hoc wireless networks for improved observing of patients
- Handling healthcare reserve vehicles
- Routing as well as network support for moveable telemedicine

3.3.3 Management-Level Issues

Management issues consist of:

- Safety as well as confidentiality in wireless healthcare system
- Preparation of healthcare expert for smooth pervasive healthcare computing
- Handling the incorporation of wireless results
- Increasing availability of healthcare system via wireless tools
- Lawful and governing matters

3.4 Challenges in Pervasive Healthcare Computing

A lot of motivating challenges of pervasive healthcare system, comprising background consciousness, trustworthiness and independent and flexible process, are also offered alongside with a number of great level clarifications. These challenges include a noteworthy amount of medical faults subsequent in thousands of early deaths as well as hundreds of thousands of damages [40, 41], which may possibly be decreased by having every time everywhere access to patients' informations.

Healthcare workers are subject to significant pressure. World-wise, healthcare facilities in countryside and underserved parts are a main challenge [42–44].

3.4.1 Mobility Amongst Heterogeneous Electronic Devices

Medical clinicians are extremely moveable and use several dissimilar computer systems as well as electronic devices as portion of their day-to-day work. Repeatedly it is hard to save track of where an operator was in an episodic job or to handover a user's session amongst different computers. As an outcome, the computational help for clinical jobs must be manually reproduced constantly during a working day. For instance, a nurse might access a desktop computer to record the medications she has as she returns to her previous task, and she might need to log in on a different computer to resume her interrupted task. The nurse may have to review several steps to get to the point she was at before the disruption took place. The problem with the existing desktop computer technology is that applications run in separation on similar devices. Even though moveable electronic devices like *personal digital assistant (PDA)* and personal computer (PC) are increasingly used in hospitals, there is still a prerequisite to use dissimilar computers during a working day [7, 9, 37, 45]. The use of thin client technology is trying to address this challenge; however, the present solutions still suffer from some of the same limitations.

3.4.2 Rapid Context Switching for Patient Caring

Hospital employees are involved in several simultaneous activities and then constantly alternate between these activities. Disturbances are a normal part of hospital work as physicians' and nurses' requirement to take care of numerous patients as well as join to dissimilar tasks. Continuous disruptions and chore exchanging are not exclusive of hospital work. Nearly all employees incorporate their consideration crossways diverse zones of apprehension [32, 38, 41]. As people shift from one job to a new, they want to incorporate wealth related to the novel job. A day-to-day medical round, for example, includes the estimation of numerous patients. To ensure this, the general practitioner in duty and an assembly of inhabitants travel from single bed to bed, collecting data starting medical archives and direct patient inspections to deliberate as well as choose on the strategy of care for the whole day.

3.4.3 A Precise Summary of Major Challenges and Related Technologies

Furthermost, the major issues included in this summary table are précised in the below-given Table 3.1.

3.5 Scientific Solution of Pervasive Healthcare Challenges

The existing as well as evolving wireless tools [13, 46] may possibly increase the whole superiority of facility for patients together with towns and countryside zones, decrease the pressure and straining on healthcare workers even though improving their output, remembering as well as overall eminence of life as well as decrease the whole budget of healthcare facilities in the extended period perspective. The required medicinal data can be prepared accessible at any time any place via refined electronic devices and generally installed wireless as well as mobile networks [25, 46, 47]. The wireless and mobile system technologies can be used efficiently via equivalent infrastructure abilities to healthcare requirements.

3.5.1 A Heterogeneous Wireless Architecture Intended for Pervasive Healthcare Applications

Figure 3.2 displays my recommendation for an incorporated wireless structural design for advanced pervasive healthcare applications. The structural design is proposed to be autonomous of a solitary wireless technology solution even though permitting the use of a number of miscellaneous moveable and wireless networks to facilitate the necessities of pervasive healthcare applications. This structural design will progress as the deviations in wireless as well as mobile technologies take place using improved bit rate, coverage area and network reliability. The structural design is established by means of numerous distinctive abilities and functionalities of the existing and developing mobile and wireless network devices and wireless networks and middleware. These purposes can facilitate numerous novel healthcare uses, locality tracing of patients as well as devices, intellectual crisis response system and moveable telemedicine. The wireless structural design would decrease extended term budget of healthcare and wished as well as outcome in an improved production of healthcare workers (Table 3.1).

The subsequent sections explain particulars of the recommended structural design via numerous facets such as handling range plus scalability, reliability, appropriateness for pervasive healthcare uses as well as changeability. The structural design is developed to deliver wireless area coverage together with countryside as well as metropolitan zones for mutually internal and outside atmospheres. This

Table 3.1 An outline of major challenges as well as technologies

Challenges	Explanation	Technological support	Concerns
Mobile as well as travelling work	Hospitals' job is extremely mobile, and most of the workers do not have counters to place computers on	Mobile devices	Portable and small Strong hardware Wireless communication system Minor displays
		Shared embedded devices	Immobile and large Influential devices Needs application nomadic
Collaboration and management	Most work in hospitals is highly cooperative and also needs much Management crosswise space and organization	Coordination, booking, scheduling, workflow	Unambiguous coordination Work planning and reservation
		Teleconferencing	Actual time video conferencing crossways distance
		Joint medical archives	By means of data entry for harmonization Promising for revolution events
		Social awareness	Common consciousness of the status of mutual work Interpretation observable concerns in work that may be appropriate to others
		Device composition	Stress-free sharing of resources like screen, files, etc.
Mixed device nomadic	No device fits all jobs in a hospitals and consequently handler's necessity to move between mixed devices often	Web-based uses	Normal technology Partial functionality and responsivity
		Application nomadic	Adaptation to dissimilar devices Necessitates intricate middleware
Patient observing	Observation of dynamic body ciphers is increasingly completed wirelessly even though being incorporated with other systems	Wireless monitors Ad hoc medical sensor network	Moveable patients Patient credentials Wireless communication system Patient location management

(continued)

Table 3.1 (continued)

Challenges	Explanation	Technological support	Concerns
Fast background switching	Background-aware classifications	Background-aware classifications	Sensors to sense the background Information recovery based on background Aide-memoire based on background
Combination of the digital as well as the physical world		Physical networking	Making associations amongst digital material in addition the physical world
		Increased reality	Integration of the digital as well as the physical in one sight
Operator authentication		Smartcards	Stress-free access Needs physical interaction frequently PIN
		Biometrics	Stress-free access

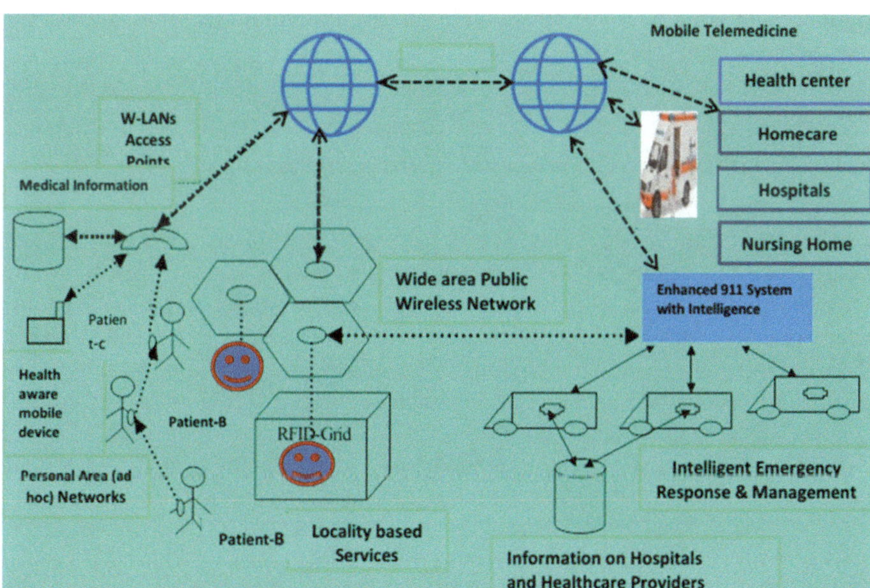

Fig. 3.2 A heterogeneous wireless network structural design intended for pervasive healthcare environment. *RFID* radio-frequency identification

aim is attained by means of unrestricted wide area cellular/mobile network for metropolitan area reportage joined via wireless local area networks in lieu of the crowded inside and outside metropolitan zones. To deliver pervasive healthcare services in countryside ranges that are not enclosed through wide area cellular network, the structural design facilitates one or the other or together with satellite as well as wireless local area networks. This approach to numerous wireless networks improves in cooperation with the coverage area as well as the scalability of the recommended wireless structural design in view of operators, space as well as uses (Table 3.2).

3.5.2 Prioritized Operation Designed for Healthcare Services

Even though it wished be desirable to make available a comprehensive distinct wireless network infrastructure intended for pervasive healthcare applications, the budget needed and unequal designs of use create additional prospectives that the present and developing wireless network technology will be utilized for pervasive healthcare applications. The suggested structural design efficiently facilitates healthcare amenities by assigning advanced urgencies for emergency and catastrophe supervision joint with preventive ability to dismiss non-urgent user traffic flow above mobile wireless networks.

3.5.3 Providing Location-Level Management Support

Pervasive healthcare applications would help as of the place tracing of related patients as well as healthcare service professionals, devices and supplies. It will be very supportive for recognizing persons by means of corresponding blood groups, finding organ donors, providing that post-op care for persons as well as assisting old and psychologically challenged persons in hospitals plus nursing homes. Locality supervision in healthcare background is publicized in Fig. 3.3 by means of numerous apparatuses containing GPS, wireless LANs, cellular/mobile networks and RFID for locality tracing of persons, expedients and also facilities at miscellaneous locality accurateness.

Global Positioning System and A-GPS Support

Satellite-based methods such as Global Positioning Satellite-system can be applied aimed at locality tracing. In this method, satellites transmission oblique locality information, which is at that time received as well as handled by Global Positioning Satellite-system receivers to decide their localities. The locality correctness attained is in the scope of a few to numerous hundred meters. To decrease the complication

Table 3.2 Particulars of the wireless structural design for pervasive healthcare system

Concerns	Wireless solutions	Observations
Coverage area plus scalability	Use of unrestricted wide area cellular networks for metropolitan range reportage joined with wireless LANs for the overcrowded indoor as well as outdoor metropolitan ranges	The access to numerous wireless networks enhances together with the coverage area as well as the scalability of the in relations of users, space and uses
Dependable and reliable operation	Arranged process on behalf of pervasive healthcare services Refining access by means of several wireless networks Placement of fault-tolerant wireless structure Duplication of medicinal information	Intended to guarantee that it is obtainable and serviceable when desirable
Suitability for healthcare applications	Planned by bearing in mind several necessities of healthcare background including an improved right to use and superiority of pervasive healthcare services Facilitates short- as well as long-term observing, non-emergency and emergency circumstances	The structural design will also facilitate numerous novel healthcare uses, locality tracing of patients plus devices, intelligent spare response method
Practical and implementable	Practical by means of consuming the capabilities of the existing wireless networks as well as mobile networks	It can moreover make use of permitted wireless local area network facility, current wide-area cellular network and additional wireless facility The intermediate bit rate observing facilities can be applied by distribution of wireless local area network capability amongst approachable neighbours
Expandable and modifiable	Designed to be available, dependable Extendible for upcoming use as the necessity transformation or else novel healthcare uses appear owing to in cooperation with the elevated concept as well as design method	It will easily support use of the fourth-generation (4G) wireless networks allowing multi-network roaming

(continued)

Table 3.2 (continued)

Concerns	Wireless solutions	Observations
Otherconsiderationsand limitations	Recognized faintness in wireless safety and security The execution of the architecture may possibly vary noticeably in different nation states	Numerous wireless facility suppliers, controlling organizations and insurance companies in the states of America, even though a solitary body in several other nation states

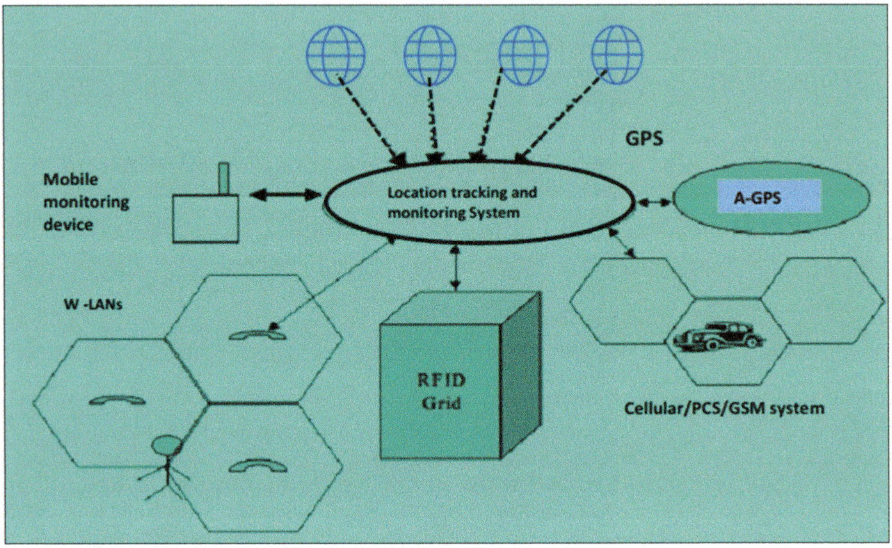

Fig. 3.3 An incorporated tracing and monitoring system

of handler devices, Assisted Global Positioning Satellite-system (A-GPS) may possibly be used (Fig. 3.3). In A- Global Positioning Satellite-system, the dispensation or interpreting of locational info since Global Positioning Satellite-system satellites is mutual amongst hand held devices as well as base stations of cellular networks. This supporting by base stations clues to the term Assisted Global Positioning Satellite-system. Assistance decreases mutually the complication of handler devices in addition the handling delays earlier locational data can be resulting. On the other hand, additional complication is presented in base stations. To increase locality correctness, smooth additional, different Global Positioning Satellite-system can be installed.

Cellular as Well as Wireless Network Support

In cellular network personal communications system as well as Global System for Mobile Communication, locality tracing includes keep posted when the handler travels to a dissimilar locality range (Fig. 3.3). In a broad spectrum, the network system recognizes the locality of handlers by means of precision equivalent to the scope of the locality range. The structural design attains smooth advanced correctness through using a lesser locality area using a condensed cell size and amount of cells. The structural design facilitates smooth advanced locality accurateness via merging minor cells using base station triangulation.

3.6 Conclusions

By means of growing budget of healthcare services combined by using an improved number of patients as well as senior citizens, it is authoritative that technical developments in lieu of current healthcare system be truly measured, specifically once it is clear that additional monetary and humanoid resources are improbable to turn out to be obtainable anytime in a little while. The noteworthy plus on-going improvements in wireless as well as mobile technologies can facilitate the idea of pervasive healthcare by means of refining and increasing the coverage area of present-day services. The growing use of handheld devices by means of healthcare specialists joined through progressively obtainable wireless network will lead to an improved placement of pervasive healthcare system services.

In addition to noticeably enhanced access to pervasive healthcare services, considerable budget savings can be attained to take the entire budget of pervasive healthcare services to an additional adaptable level. In this chapter, we have deliberated pervasive healthcare applications, challenges and solutions and related information system as well as networking concerns.

References

1. Orji, R., & Moffatt, K. (2018). Persuasive technology for health and wellness: State-of-the-art and emerging trends. *Health Informatics Journal, 24*, 66–91.
2. Valarmathi, J., Uthariaraj, D. V. R., Arjun Kumar, G., Subramanian, P., & Karthick, R. (2010). A novel trust management scheme in pervasive computing. In *2010 the 2nd IEEE international conference on information management and engineering (ICIME)* (pp. 141–145).
3. Intille, S. (2016). The precision medicine initiative and pervasive health research. *IEEE Pervasive Computing, 15*, 88–91.
4. Varshney, U. (2003). Pervasive healthcare. *IEEE Computer, 36*(12), 138–140.
5. Starner, T. (2001). The challenges of wearable computing: Part 1. *IEEE Micro, 21*(4), 44–52.
6. Starner, T. (2001). The challenges of wearable computing: Part 2. *IEEE Micro, 21*(4), 54–67.
7. Weiser, M. (1991). The computer for the 21st century. *Scientific American, 265*(3), 94–104.

8. Boric-Lubecke, O., & Lubecke, V. (2002). Wireless house calls: Using communications technology for health care and monitoring. *IEEE Microwave Magazine, 3*(3), 43–48.
9. Varshney, U. (2004). Patient monitoring using ad hoc wireless networks. In *Proceedings of the Americas conference on information systems (AMCIS)*.
10. Pattichis, C., Kyriacou, E., Voskarides, S., Pattichis, M., Istepanian, R., & Schizas, C. (2002). Wireless telemedicine systems: An overview. *IEEE Antennas and Propagation Magazine, 44*(2), 143–153.
11. Fang, R., Pouyanfar, S., Yang, Y., Chen, S.-C., & Iyengar, S. S. (2016). Computational health informatics in the big data age. *ACM Computer Survey, 49*, 1–36.
12. Wan, J., Zou, C., Ullah, S., Lai, C., Zhou, M., & Wang, X. (2013). Cloud-enabled wireless body area networks for pervasive healthcare. *IEEE Network Magazine, 27*(5), 56–61.
13. Lin, C., Chiu, M., Hsiao, C., Lee, R., & Tsai, Y. (2006). A wireless healthcare service system for elderly with dementia. *IEEE Transactions on Information Technology in Biomedicine, 10*(2), 696704.
14. Merico, D., Mileo, A., & Bisani, R. (2009). Pervasive wireless-sensor-networks for home healthcare need automatic resoning. In *Proceedings of the ICST pervasive health*.
15. Mandal, A. K., Sarkar, A., & Chaki, N. (2015). Flexible cloud architecture for healthcare applications. In *Intelligent systems and computing* (Vol. 304). Springer. https://doi.org/10.1007/978-81-322-1985-9_8
16. Sixsmith, A., & Johnson, N. (2004). A smart sensor to detect the falls of the elderly. *IEEE Pervasive Computing Magazine, 3*(2), 42–47.
17. Rodgers, M. M., Pai, V. M., & Conroy, R. S. (2015). Recent advances in wearable sensors for health monitoring. *IEEE Sensors Journal, 15*, 3119–3126.
18. Kern, S., & Jaron, D. (2003). Healthcare technology, economics and policy: An evolving balance. *IEEE Engineering in Medicine and Biology Magazine, 22*(1), 1619.
19. Lupşe, O., Vida, M. M., & Stoicu-Tivadar, L. (2012). Cloud computing and interoperability in healthcare information systems. In *The first international conference on intelligent systems and applications*.
20. Bardram, J., & Christensen, H. (2007). Pervasive computing support for hospitals: An overview of the activity-based computing project. *IEEE Pervasive Computing, 6*(1), 44–51. https://doi.org/10.1109/mprv.2007.19
21. He, D., et al. (2012). ReTrust: Attack-resistant and lightweight trust management for medical sensor networks. *IEEE Transactions on Information Technology in Biomedicine, 16*(4), 623–632.
22. Suzuki, T., & Doi, M. (2001). Life Minder: An evidence-based wearable healthcare assistant. In *Proceedings ACM conference on human factors in computing systems* (pp. 127–128).
23. Chalmers, C., Hurst, W., Mackay, M., & Fergus, P. (2015). Smart health monitoring using the advance metering infrastructure. In *Computer and information technology; ubiquitous computing and communications; dependable, autonomic and secure computing; pervasive intelligence and computing (CIT/IUCC/DASC/PICOM), 2015 IEEE international conference on* (pp. 2297–2302). IEEE.
24. Hansen, T. R., Bardram, J. E., & Soegaard, M. (2006). Moving out of the lab: Deploying pervasive technologies in a hospital. *IEEE Pervasive Computing, 5*(3), 24–31. https://doi.org/10.1109/mprv.2006.53
25. Bardram, J., Mihailidis, A., & Wan, D. (2007). *Pervasive computing in healthcare*. CRC Press.
26. Muras, J. A., Cahill, V., & Stokes E. K. (2006). A taxonomy of pervasive healthcare systems. In *2006 pervasive health conference and workshops*.
27. Ziefle, M., & Rocker, C. (2010). Acceptance of pervasive healthcare systems: A comparison of different implementation concepts, pervasive computing technologies for healthcare (PervasiveHealth), 2010. In *4th international conference on no permissions*.
28. Boukerche, A., & Ren, Y. (2009). A secure mobile healthcare system using trust-based multicast scheme. *IEEE Journal on Selected Areas in Communications, 27*(4), 387–399.

29. Katehakis, D. G., Sfakianakis, S. G., Kavlentakis, G., Anthoulakis, D. N., & Tsiknakis, M. (2007). Delivering a lifelong integrated electronic health record based on a service oriented architecture. *IEEE Transactions on Information Technology in Biomedicine, 11*(6), 639–650.
30. Abowd, G. D., & Mynatt, E. D. (2000). Charting past, present and future research in ubiquitous computing. *ACM Transactions on Computer-Human Interaction, 7*(1), 29–58.
31. Bardram, J. (2004). The personal medical unit – A ubiquitous computing infrastructure for personal pervasive healthcare. In *UbiHealth.*
32. Carlson, V., Klug, T., Ziegert, T., & Zinnen, A. (2006). Wearable computers in clinical ward rounds. In *Proceedings of the 3rd international forum on applied wearable computing* (pp. 1–9).
33. Dishman, E. (2004). Inventing wellness systems for aging in place. *IEEE Computer, 37*(5), 34–41.
34. Forum. (2005). *Federal interagency forum on aging-related statistics.* http://agingstats.gov
35. Stefanov, D., Bien, Z., & Bang, W. (2004). The smart house for older persons and persons with physical disabilities: Structure, technology, arrangements, and perspectives. *IEEE Transactions on Neural Systems and Rehabilitation Engineering, 12*(2), 228250.
36. Bottazzi, D., Corradi, A., & Montanari, R. (2006). Context-aware middleware solutions for anytime and anywhere emergency assistance to elderly people. *IEEE Communications Magazine, 44*(4), 82–90. https://doi.org/10.1109/mcom.2006.1632653
37. Poorejbari, S., & Vahdat-Nejad, H. (2014). An introduction to cloud-based pervasive healthcare systems. In *Proceedings of the 3rd international conference on context-aware systems and applications (ICCASA)* (pp. 173–178).
38. Lina, C. C., Lee, R. G., & Hsiao, C. C. (2008). A pervasive health monitoring service system based on ubiquitous network technology. *International Journal of Medical Informatics, 77,* 461–469.
39. Stanford, V. (2002). Using pervasive computing to deliver elder care. *IEEE Pervasive Computing Magazine, 1*(1), 10–13.
40. Kameas, A., & Calemis, I. (2010). Pervasive systems in health care. In *Handbook of ambient intelligence and smart environment.* https://doi.org/10.1007/978-0-387-93808-0_12
41. IOM. (2000). *To err is human: Building a safer health system, US institute of medicine report.* http://www.nap.edu/books/0309068371/html/
42. Suzuki, T., & Doi, M. (2001). LifeMinder: An evidence-based wearable healthcare assistant. In *Proceedings of the ACM CHI conference.*
43. Pick, J. B. (2004). Geographic information systems: A tutorial and introduction. *Communications of AIS, 14,* 16.
44. Janz, B. D., Pitts, M. G., & Otondo, R. F. (2005). Information systems and health care-II: Back to the future with RFID: Lessons learned - Some old, some new. *Communications of the AIS, 15,* 7.
45. Wilmini, N. (2013). Pervasive computing and healthcare. In *Healthcare delivery in the information age.* Springer. https://doi.org/10.1007/978-1-4614-4514-2_2
46. Varshney, U., & Sneha, S. (2006). Patient monitoring using ad hoc wireless networks: Reliability and power management. *IEEE Communications Magazine, 44*(4), 49–55.
47. Orwat, C., Rashid, A., Holtmann, C., Wolk, M., Scheermesser, M., Kosow, H., & Graefe, A. (2010). Adopting pervasive computing for routine use in healthcare. *IEEE Pervasive Computing, 9,* 64–71.

Chapter 4
Pervasive Healthcare Computing as a Scientific Care Discipline for Patients

Mahfuzul Huda, Mohammad Zubair Khan, and Abdullah

4.1 Introduction

Pervasive computing healthcare technologies have seen significant improvements in recent years, because of the significantly technical developments in modern electronic wireless devices and communication network architectures, electronic sensors instruments, men wearable technologies, and devices. The objective of modern pervasive healthcare facilities is to enable and provide distributed computing systems facilities that are available anytime and anywhere and also provide real-time management services through the use of high-speed communication and information technology [1–9]. Pervasive healthcare service plays an important significance healthcare service in our day-to-day life. It is a very useful treatment service because of the increasing recipient health risk parameters, various types of diseases, and insufficient available resources for expected early-required prevention and care in the many healthcare systems. Subsequently, the recent new developments in the systems serve the extensive use of anywhere real-time patient monitoring and care of health-related risk parameters with high-speed wireless electronic devices [10–13] (Fig. 4.1).

Modern pervasive healthcare treatment and healthcare are important patient's treatment techniques that promote systematic exchange of ideas in a coordinated

M. Huda (✉)
Department of Computer Science, College of Computing and Informatics, Saudi Electronic University, Medina, Saudi Arabia

M. Z. Khan
Department of Computer Science, CCSE, Taibah University, Medina, Saudi Arabia

Abdullah
Department of Information Technology, College of Engineering and Technology, Adigrat University, Tigray, Ethiopia

M. S. Husain et al. (eds.), *Pervasive Healthcare*, EAI/Springer Innovations in Communication and Computing, https://doi.org/10.1007/978-3-030-77746-3_4

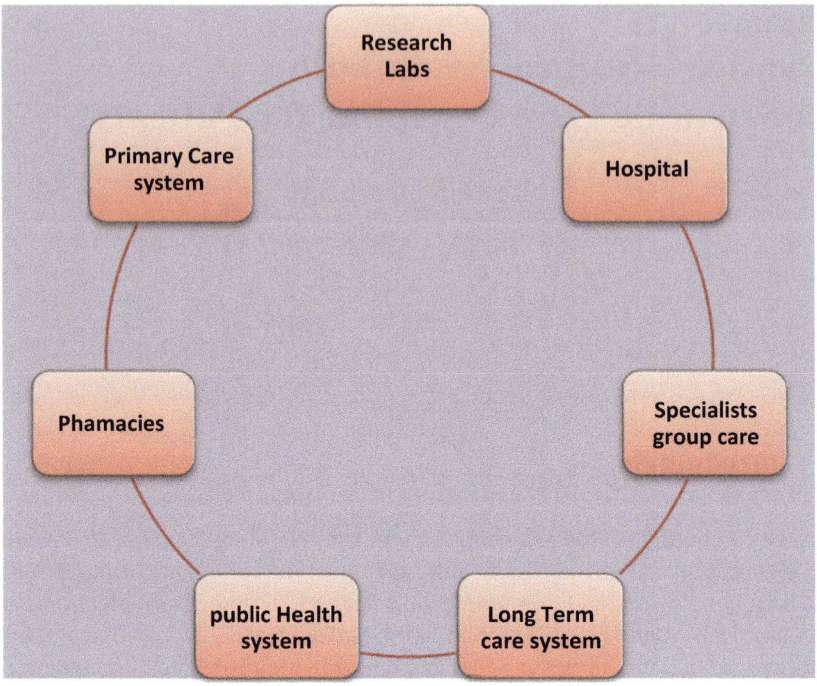

Fig. 4.1 Modern pervasive healthcare computing systems

way during the patients' cares and treatments. An effective care example of this kind of idea coordination has been demonstrated through the creation of pervasive healthcare treatment series as a platform for promoting discussions in this healthcare field. In the past, extended significance work from that platform was identified and available by this journal to provide a good understanding on relevant related work done in the healthcare field. Example of these types of works include a good research related to electronic sensing technologies, modern innovative applications, and visionary treatment roadmaps identifying trends and many opportunities in this healthcare area [14, 15].

4.2 Pervasive Healthcare Computing Systems

Pervasive healthcare computing offers both healthcare professionals and needy ill-patient services, including many new opportunities for better treatments and patient's care services. On one given side, medical healthcare doctors and other many healthcare professionals will get benefit from comprehensive diagnostic and therapeutic treatment opportunities far beyond expectation and what is possible with today's occasional health examinations. They all will have proper access to

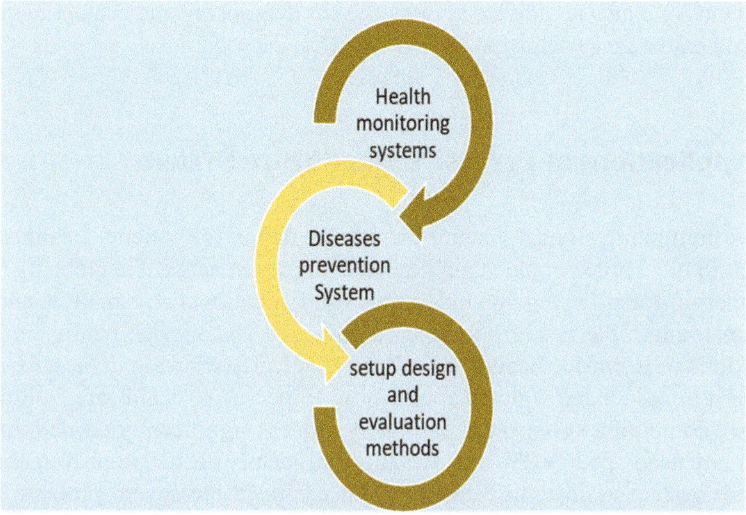

Fig. 4.2 Pervasive healthcare computing setup design and evaluation methods

long-term storage of physiological medical data measured including patient's daily activity and all the situations to which he has been diagnosed to. On the other side, needy patients are properly empowered to take significance and a more active role in their personal healthcare management and better prevention. For example, user feedback data or even personal monitoring and coaching might help a patient adjust his living style parameters to the requirement of his own health [5, 16–22] (Fig. 4.2).

In order to provide healthcare professionals and care seeker patients' services with these new medical opportunities, future research is needed in these healthcare areas:

1. Pervasive treatments and reliable long-term health monitoring systems
2. Disease prevention as the primary element to maintain life-time care
3. A modern healthcare setup structure and comprehensive patients' care methods for pervasive care by the help of patient-centric care

The main element of the first area reflects to the improvement of pervasive electronic sensing. A relevant aspect in healthcare wearable electronic sensing systems is the setup between patients' care and the electronic sensor quality that must be clearly addressed and displayed in order to improve health pervasive electronic sensing treatments to the patients. This system trade-off relationship is further explained in the above healthcare monitoring. Regarding the second-stated issue, details will be provided in the disease prevention systems and evidences that there is a need for care monitoring, including multiple parameters and a need for developing adaptive healthcare systems to enable pervasive healthcare prevention to the patients. Regarding another issue, setup design and evaluation method highlight the requirement for a new healthcare approaches for diagnosing and evaluating modern pervasive healthcare systems [9, 23–28].

4.3 Applications of Pervasive Healthcare System

Pervasive computing clinical systems can be also defined as patients' healthcare and treatment to the whole people at anytime and anywhere across the globe by removing another information, e.g., bounded time limit, locational information, and some other constraints, like needy people care coverage and service quality real care. Applications of pervasive healthcare system are clearly showing in the care system that it must be associated with the applications of pervasive healthcare facilities and healthcare computing systems to completely process significantly needed improvement for any needy people. We can explain significantly needed improvement in the healthcare system as insignificant treatment errors in the severe problem of any clinical healthcare and patients' care systems. For example, medication errors are a severe problem in healthcare systems. In the United States, medication errors are estimated in the treatments which are highly appreciated, due to the reason of 7000 (7 K) people deaths during treatment a year [29, 30]. Such medication errors in severe problem must be considered and tried to be eliminated. This could be possible through introducing pervasive clinical healthcare computing technology and treatment system. Subsequently, many features nowadays will be available, such as electromagnetic radio-frequency identification services that are doing great services in these regards. Eliminating medical type errors is one of the advantages of migrating pervasive computing technology in the healthcare systems and expertise care hospitals [31–35].

4.3.1 Modern Pathological Clinical Methods

Pathological clinical investigation concepts show availability of people's clinical historical data. It is assuring that the implemented methods and concepts of a new medication address the feasibility concept and that further research and disease care date investigation and treatment is reasonably approved by the clinical care authority.

Furthermore, in the pathological clinical methods, the drug approval and commercialization provided required validation data with respect to new indices. The methods used during this clinical proof of concept should be targeted at collecting medical evidence, which clearly demonstrate about adopted treatment technology. It may be relevant to collect initial clinical data evidence for the medical benefit of the adopted technology [36–40].

Pervasive healthcare modern pathological clinical methods for any types of clinical investigation concept are trying to measure some best clinical effects that are essential during the pathological clinical proof of concept. For example, in order to start establishing any pathological clinical effect in the monitoring of hypertension symptoms, blood pressure dataset may be compared over the time span of the clinical proof of concept, and set of questionnaires regarding the target patients' awareness and handling of their blood pressure record may be issued and properly analyzed. The clinical set of evidence may be influenced by different factors and hence not as powerful as would be required in evidence-based medicine treatment [9, 41–44].

4.3.2 Smart Blood Pressure Monitoring System

Hypertension symptom is the most general preventable cause of cardiovascular problem. Home blood pressure monitoring electronic device is a self-monitoring and blood pressure checking tool that can be incorporated into the healthcare service for patients with hypertension disease and is greatly recommended by major guidelines. Hypertension symptom increases the risk of severe heart attack, increasing kidney problems, stroke, and some vital organs failure [45]. Smart blood pressure monitoring system is the leading preventable risk prevention device for global cardiovascular disease problem worldwide. However, the impact of blood pressure on cardiovascular risk has been devoted to the issue of blood pressure measurement and its accuracy [22, 46–49] (Fig. 4.3).

A plane surfaced smart blood pressure patients' details that would automatically measure a patients' blood pressure chart. Pervasive healthcare system aims to discuss the many below-given advantages of home blood pressure monitoring and also examines medical data, aimed at improving its accuracy:

- Can take multiple reading records over a given period of time.
- Predicts cardiovascular disease better than office blood pressure systems.

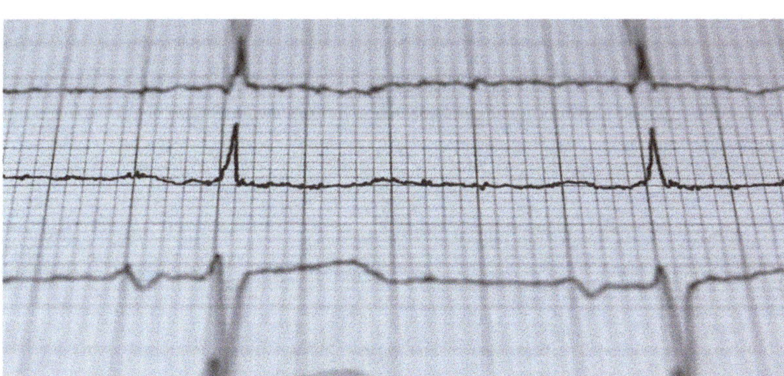

Fig. 4.3 Smart blood pressure monitoring system chart

- Home blood pressure monitoring electronic device allows patients to better understand hypertension and do better management for it.
- It can detect increased blood pressure variability.

According to National Institute for Clinical Excellence's guidelines [50–52] for Home blood pressure monitoring electronic device, recommend that when using Home blood pressure to confirm a diagnosis of hypertension symptom and it is necessary and it is recommended for the use of home blood pressure monitoring to ensure that:

- Blood pressure is recorded two times, morning and evening, on a daily pattern.
- For each blood pressure recording, there is two consecutive measurements that must be taken, at least 60 s apart with the person in a seated position.
- Keep blood pressure recording records continuous for at least 7 days [53–55].

4.3.3 The Future of Pervasive Healthcare

During the last one decade, computers were normally used for high-resolution image cutting-age technologies and field maturing to use as the reasonable parameters of being easily able to implement modern care facilities with the number of patients for estimated and required significant treatment time. The modern pervasive computing health investigators and research experts are doing great efforts on technologies that are often very hard for very large real-time implementation. According to the health experts regarding the extension of deployment in this field, the clinical researchers can identify four important improvement areas for research to allow fast and real-time prototype development, including novel pervasive healthcare technologies and error-free disease diagnosis. The modern pervasive care facilities are doing significant support on patient's personalization and great disease diagnosis to ensuring that they can meet the needs of different kinds of patients: treatment. According to the definition of international treatment and patients' care analogy and healthcare guidelines. It will be facilitated by incorporating these needed aspects into patients' care systems, as pervasive healthcare system research supports, significantly doing positive impact on current and existed patients' care practices. In the clinical care scenarios, the healthcare experts need to do the proper consideration on the real-time diagnosis and treatment transition demands. Subsequently, it is also important and needed because it carries standard dataset to assess and diagnose the values of a healthcare technology in real-world and everywhere settings and it must provide such valuable care information and support to all the people [3, 56, 57].

4.3.4 Adoption and Acceptance

As pervasive healthcare computing technologies fulfil the way for real-time diagnosis and estimating traditional healthcare facilities into a rigorous on time patient's oriented preventive treatment model. The treatment record of patient's illness needs to be further extended and evaluated to make proper consideration an acceptable and significance use of the healthcare systems. The selected or limited use of electronical sensor machines or body fitness devices could lead to the ambiguous results and incorrect inferences, and it finally shows unpredictable effects of the latest technology in the healthcare industry. Considering this, the biased and inappropriate use of healthcare facilities can result in inappropriate input illness information. This information can affect the patents' health and quality of the healthcare service. Finally, it could degrade the perceived clinical care system significances, adoption, and utilization of the pervasive technology. However, it is unethical to always expect real-time perfect data collections and device's dedication from all types of the users. Considering this, the future pervasive clinical care applications must overcome all types of challenges. Nowadays treatment strategies and methods include the care treatment using context-based sensor devices to tag and detect abnormal results during self-monitoring process, considering users' behavior and operational algorithms that get information from incomplete estimated data from diagnosis and always trying to encourage professionalism of users through various operational algorithms and treatment strategies [58–60].

The adoption and acceptance ability to get important task as creating and measuring more reliable digital sensors, modern medical devices, or healthcare systems for patient-care settings. Moreover, to exploit healthcare advancements and facilities for providing real-time required healthcare treatments, a parallel healthcare must be allocated on improving mechanisms on finding the dataset that facilitate the patient's compliance with the suggested and recommended healthcare treatment. Subsequently, tracking and tagging user activities and behaviors in real time can be helpful in the diagnosis and understanding the significance of the collected patients' data sample. Furthermore, eliminating the impairments and issues in the dataset and informing the service through prescribed models [61–63] could validate the input datasets.

All previous research studies and experiments have shown that many factors and inputs such as demographic characteristics and available resources for human populations, lifestyle, and personality along with culture represent strong predictors and patterns, which can be automatically dragged and captured to develop individual care models and diagnosis framework. In addition, future research in healthcare is needed for better and clear understanding of the reasons for special models in specific use of patients' cases. This will certainly help many patients, also it can clearly explain patients' needs and symptoms, and it will further eliminate many obstacles and issues to greater compliance.

It will further explain with example, by defining the latest healthcare strategies for treatment models, such as designing and incorporating fewer complex devices, including automation, comparison with the past, and analysis. Subsequently, most of the existing and available patients' healthcare systems have been developed and designed on targeting and assuming specific patients and diseases without considering valuable features for personalization, and this could be one of the key reasons for the limited acceptability of the care systems. Although many healthcare communities and healthcare centers have been proposing and introducing different concepts of personalization in terms of specific patients and diseases, in practice, there is still a need of individualized technologies and models that would be personalized on specific interaction. To the user's routines, check-up must be appreciated [64].

4.4 Open Data Research in Pervasive Healthcare System

Clinically diagnosed large datasets and inputs and combining all datasets with required information with the needed pattern from other heterogeneous data sources could help research developments in general healthcare by creating new applications and strategies in modern pervasive health systems and making new strategic and treatment policies. Subsequently, progression of computational applications and many techniques in pervasive clinical care computing is the sign of medical data sharing, diagnosing, and the broad availability of healthcare datasets. The need for making healthcare broad availability of healthcare datasets has been strongly recommended by the group of health organizational bodies.

Healthcare models and frameworks that are being invented and used to characterize many types of their data correlation and pattern mapping with symptoms and their pattern symbol within pervasive healthcare frames have a basic requirement, and it must be developed, evaluated, tested, and validated based on test datasets. Validation test datasets can be collected from heterogenous types of patients' covering ranges based on gender, cultural, and social behaviors. Many clinical patients' care research takes the characteristics and features of the digital sensor node index values in the operation and treatments. Furthermore, geographical locations within the organizational bodies, social atmosphere, and the context limitations should be imposed in different environments and experiments [5, 20–22].

Making medical research dataset groups, that are available to the original research team and research groups where they have been diagnosed and generated and experiments, in a responsible within prescribed time frame. Furthermore, considering approved and international trial standards including safeguard criteria will show several significant advantages. From medical research dataset's perspective, collecting and storing such dataset results are critical, expensive, and time-consuming process, leading to the following questions:

- How can dataset be collected ethically with the best practice context?
- How can medical research group ensure that selected standards for dataset management are entrenched and developed and reused effectively?

- Is there any prescribed format or parameter that ensure issues and challenges around dataset are the high-quality empirically validated data in the research?
- What type of research frameworks and models should be designed so that it can support online dataset sharing in real-time repository?

We must address these selected issues in making research dataset repositories for pervasive healthcare systems.

4.5 Conclusions and Future

Pervasive clinical care systems have been proved and defined as modern healthcare to the whole people at anytime and anywhere across the globe by removing constraints such as time limit, locational information, and other constraints including significantly increase in both its service quality and large-scale coverage. Our rigorous work clearly shows that significant and high-level potential mapping in the applications of pervasive healthcare computing systems increases the care process with significant consideration. Pervasive healthcare computing technologies fulfil the way and requirement for transforming currently applicable healthcare systems into a never-ending on-time, large-scale patient's or users' oriented preventive healthcare treatment system. The record of patients' illness needs to be diagnosed and extended and evaluated to consider the significant use of the healthcare systems. The significant and on-going advancement in healthcare treatment systems leads to support and facilitate the acceptability of pervasive healthcare systems. Improving the quality of healthcare services and eliminating medical-type errors are some of the advantages of migrating pervasive computing technology in the healthcare systems and expertise care hospitals. This chapter also shows significantly and approved access to pervasive clinical and healthcare system, including lower cost and real-time health monitoring services to a more generalized level and heterogenous environments. In this chapter, we also highlighted pervasive clinical computing and associated valuable data information systems and their future perspective and uses.

References

1. Stefanov, D., Bien, Z., & Bang, W. (2004). The smart house for older persons and persons with physical disabilities: Structure, technology, arrangements, and perspectives. *IEEE Transactions on Neural Systems and Rehabilitation Engineering, 12*(2), 228250.
2. Lin, C., Chiu, M., Hsiao, C., Lee, R., & Tsai, Y. (2006). A wireless healthcare service system for elderly with dementia. *IEEE Transactions on Information Technology in Biomedicine, 10*(2), 696704.
3. Sixsmith, A., & Johnson, N. (2004). A smart sensor to detect the falls of the elderly. *IEEE Pervasive Computing Magazine, 3*(2), 42–47.
4. Varshney, U., & Sneha, S. (2006) Patient monitoring using ad hoc wireless networks: Reliability and power management. *IEEE Communications Magazine.*

5. Weiser, M. (1991). The computer for the 21st century. *Scientific American, 265*(3), 94–104.
6. Starner, T. (2001). The challenges of wearable computing: Part 1. *IEEE Micro, 21*(4), 44–52.
7. Starner, T. (2001). The challenges of wearable computing: Part 2. *IEEE Micro, 21*(4), 54–67.
8. Fang, R., Pouyanfar, S., Yang, Y., Chen, S.-C., & Iyengar, S. S. (2016). Computational health informatics in the big data age. *ACM Computer Survey, 49*, 1–36.
9. Boric-Lubecke, O., & Lubecke, V. (2002). Wireless house calls: Using communications technology for health care and monitoring. *IEEE Microwave Magazine, 3*(3), 43–48.
10. Varshney, U. (2004). Patient monitoring using Ad Hoc wireless networks. In *Proceedings of the Americas conference on information systems (AMCIS)* (Vol. 44, No. 4, pp. 49–55).
11. Orji, R., & Moffatt, K. (2018). Persuasive technology for health and wellness: State-of-the-art and emerging trends. *Health Inform J, 24*, 66–91.
12. Valarmathi, J., Uthariaraj, D. V. R., Arjun Kumar, G., Subramanian, P., & Karthick, R. (2010). A novel trust management scheme. In *Pervasive computing. 2010 the 2nd IEEE international conference on information management and engineering (ICIME)* (pp. 141–145).
13. Intille, S. (2016). The precision medicine initiative and pervasive health research. *IEEE Pervasive Computing, 15*, 88–91.
14. Varshney, U. (2003). Pervasive healthcare. *IEEE Computer, 36*(12), 138–140.
15. Suzuki, T., & Doi, M. (2001). Life Minder: An evidence-based wearable healthcare assistant. In *Proceedings of the ACM conference on human factors in computing systems* (pp. 127–128).
16. Boukerche, A., & Ren, Y. (2009). A secure mobile healthcare system using trust-based multicast scheme. *IEEE Journal on Selected Areas in Communications, 27*(4), 387–399.
17. Stanford, V. (2002). Using pervasive computing to deliver elder care. *IEEE Pervasive Computing Magazine, 1*(1), 10–13.
18. Kameas, A., & Calemis, I. (2010). Pervasive systems in health care. In *Handbook of ambient intelligence and smart environment.* https://doi.org/10.1007/978-0-387-93808-0_12
19. Wilmini, N. (2013). Pervasive computing and healthcare. In *Healthcare delivery in the information age*. Springer. https://doi.org/10.1007/978-1-4614-4514-2_2
20. Guest Editorial. (2004). M-Health: Beyond seamless mobility and global wireless healthcare connectivity. *IEEE Transactions on IT in Biomedicine, 8*(4), 405–413.
21. Stanford, V. (2002). Using pervasive computing to deliver elder care. *IEEE Pervasive Computing, 1*(1), 10–13.
22. Bardram, J. E., Mihailidis, A., & Wan, D. (2007). *Pervasive computing in healthcare.* CRC Press.
23. Bayraktar, C., Karlik, B., & Demirezen Yamur, F. (2010). Automatic diagnosis of otitis media diseases using wavelet based artificial neural networks. In *1st international symposium on computing in science and engineering (ISCSE).*
24. Varshney, U. (2009). *Pervasive healthcare computing, EMR/HER, wireless and health monitoring*. Springer.
25. Blount, M., et al. (2007). Remote health-care monitoring using personal care connect. *IBM Systems Journal, 46*(1), 95–114.
26. Nelson, M. M., & Illingworth, W. T. (1994). *Practical guide to neural nets*. Addison Wesley.
27. Ozyilmaz, L., & Yildirim, T. (2003). Artificial neural networks for diagnosis of hepatitis disease. *Proceedings of the International Joint Conference on Neural Networks, 1*, 586–589.
28. Yagmur, F. D., Karlik, B., & Okatan, A. (2008). Automatic recognition of retinopathy diseases by using wavelet based neural network. In *First IEEE international conference on the applications of digital information and web technologies.*
29. Kang, K., Woo Lee, J., & Choi, H. (2007). Application binder: Providing instant application runtime for developing healthcare application. *The International Conference on Next-Generation Computing, 1*, 190–194.
30. Wang, K., Sui, Y., Zou, X., Durresi, A., & Fang, S. (2008). Pervasive and trustworthy healthcare. In *AINA workshops 2008* (pp. 750–755).

31. Gumuskaya, H., Gürel, A. V., & Nural, M. V. (2008). Architectures for small mobile communication devices and performance analyses. In *First IEEE international conference on the applications of digital information and web technologies*.
32. Karan, O., Bayraktar, C., Gumuskaya, H., & Karlik, B. Diagnosing illnesses using neural networks and pervasive healthcare computing. In *1st international symposium on computing in science and engineering (ISCSE)*.
33. Poorejbari, S., & Vahdat-Nejad, H. (2014). An introduction to cloud-based pervasive healthcare systems. In *Proceedings of 3rd international conference on context-aware systems and applications* (pp. 173–178).
34. Dishman, E. (2004). Inventing wellness systems for aging in place. *IEEE Computer, 37*(5), 34–41.
35. Wan, J., Zou, C., Ullah, S., Lai, C., Zhou, M., & Wang, X. (2013). Cloud-enabled wireless body area networks for pervasive healthcare. *IEEE Network Magazine, 27*(5), 56–61.
36. Axisa, F., Schmitt, P., Gehin, C., Delhomme, G., McAdams, E., & Dittmar, A. (2005). Flexible technologies and smart clothing for citizen medicine, home healthcare, and disease prevention. *IEEE Transactions on IT in Biomedicine, 9*(3), 325–336.
37. Ghorbani, S., & Du, W. (2013). Personal health service framework. In *The 3rd international conference on current and future trends of information and communication technologies in healthcare (ICTH)*. https://doi.org/10.1016/j.procs.2013.09.045
38. Kern, S., & Jaron, D. (2003). Healthcare technology, economics and policy: An evolving balance. *IEEE Engineering in Medicine and Biology Magazine, 22*(1), 1619.
39. de Moraes, J. L. C., de Souza, W. L., Pires, L. F., & do Prado, A. F. (2014). An architecture for health information exchange in pervasive healthcare environment, *1*, 385–401.
40. *The website for aging and disability statistics*. http://www.census.gov/Press-Release
41. Rafe, V., & Hajvali, M. (2013). Designing an architectural style for pervasive healthcare systems. *Journal of Medical Systems, 37*(2).
42. Lupşe, O., Vida, M. M., & Stoicu-Tivadar, L. (2012). Cloud computing and interoperability in healthcare information systems. In *The first international conference on intelligent systems and applications*.
43. Costlow, T. (2004). RFID monitors help trim health costs. *IEEE Pervasive Computing, 3*(1), 9.
44. Bardram, J., & Christensen, H. (2007). Pervasive computing support for hospitals: An overview of the activity-based computing project. *IEEE Pervasive Computing, 6*(1), 44–51. https://doi.org/10.1109/mprv.2007.19
45. Bottazzi, D., Corradi, A., & Montanari, R. (2006). Context-aware middleware solutions for anytime and anywhere emergency assistance to elderly people. *IEEE Communications Magazine, 44*(4), 82–90. https://doi.org/10.1109/mcom.2006.1632653
46. Chalmers, C., Hurst, W., Mackay, M., & Fergus, P. (2015). Smart health monitoring using the advance metering infrastructure. In *Computer and information technology; ubiquitous computing and communications; dependable, autonomic and secure computing; pervasive intelligence and computing (CIT/IUCC/DASC/PICOM), 2015 IEEE international conference on* (pp. 2297–2302). IEEE.
47. *Cisco context-aware healthcare solution*. (n.d.). http://www.21.com/web/strategy/healthcare/Context-Aware_for_Healthcare.html
48. Hansen, T. R., Bardram, J. E., & Soegaard, M. (2006). Moving out of the lab: Deploying pervasive technologies in a hospital. *IEEE Pervasive Computing, 5*(3), 24–31. https://doi.org/10.1109/mprv.2006.53
49. Muras, J. A., Cahill, V., & Stokes, E. K. (2006). A taxonomy of pervasive healthcare systems. In *2006 pervasive health conference and workshops*.
50. Ziefle, M., & Rocker, C. (2010). Acceptance of pervasive healthcare systems: A comparison of different implementation concepts, pervasive computing technologies for healthcare (PervasiveHealth), 2010. In *4th international conference on no permissions*.
51. Abowd, G. D., & Mynatt, E. D. (2000). Charting past, present and future research in ubiquitous computing. *ACM Transactions on Computer-Human Interaction, 7*(1), 29–58.

52. Abowd, G. D., et al. (2006). Challenges and opportunities for collaboration technologies for chronic care management. In *The human-computer interaction consortium (HCIC)*.
53. Bardram, J. (2004). The personal medical unit – A ubiquitous computing infrastructure for personal pervasive healthcare. In *UbiHealth*.
54. Pal, A., Mbarika, V. W. A., Cobb-Payton, F., Datta, P., & McCoy, S. (2005). Telemedicine diffusion in a developing country: The case of India. *IEEE Transactions on Information Technology in Biomedicine, 9*(1), 59–65.
55. Carlson, V., Klug, T., Ziegert, T., & Zinnen, A. (2006): Wearable computers in clinical ward rounds. In *Proceedings of the 3rd international forum on applied wearable computing* (pp. 1–9).
56. Lina, C. C., Lee, R. G., & Hsiao, C. C. (2008). A pervasive health monitoring service system based on ubiquitous network technology. *International Journal of Medical Informatics, 77*, 461–469.
57. Katehakis, D. G., Sfakianakis, S. G., Kavlentakis, G., Anthoulakis, D. N., & Tsiknakis, M. (2007). Delivering a lifelong integrated electronic health record based on a service oriented architecture. *IEEE Transactions on Information Technology in Biomedicine, 11*(6), 639–650.
58. Merico, D., Mileo, A., & Bisani, R. (2009). Pervasive wireless-sensor-networks for home healthcare need automatic resoning. In *Proceedings of the ICST pervasive health*.
59. Orwat, C., Rashid, A., Holtmann, C., Wolk, M., Scheermesser, M., Kosow, H., & Graefe, A. (2010). Adopting pervasive computing for routine use in healthcare. *IEEE Pervasive Computing, 9*, 64–71.
60. IOM. (2000). *To err is human: Building a safer health system, us institute of medicine report*. http://www.nap.edu/books/0309068371/html/
61. Suzuki, T., & Doi, M. (2001). LifeMinder : An evidence-based wearable healthcare assistant. In *Proceedings of the ACM CHI conference*.
62. Forum. (2005). *Federal interagency forum on aging-related statistics*. http://agingstats.gov
63. Pick, J. B. (2004). Geographic information systems: A tutorial and introduction. *Communications of AIS, 14*, 16.
64. Janz, B. D., Pitts, M. G., & Otondo, R. F. (2005). Information systems and health care-II: Back to the future with RFID: Lessons learned - Some old, some new. *Communications of the AIS, 15*, 7.

Chapter 5
Improving the Healthcare and Public Health Critical Infrastructure by Soft Computing: An Overview

Mohammad Haroon, Manish Madhav Tripathi, Tamim Ahmad, and Afsaruddin

5.1 Introduction

Telemedicine is one of the tools (a combination of software and hardware) that are useful in the healthcare system. The meaning of telemedicine is the use of electronic information to communicate by technology to provide support to healthcare, when the participant or patient is located at a distance. Telemedicine is also referred to as the practice of caring for patients if the patient is not in direct contact with the doctor. Patients are remotely monitored and cared for by the doctor using modern technology. The majority of telemedicine software is used for this kind of operation.

Telemedicine is used by patients who live in rural areas and who cannot easily access of the doctor; they can converse virtually with a physician via the telemedicine software. Physicians and patients can both share their information in real time from one computer screen to another and they can even feel and capture readings from medical devices at a faraway location. The patient can show their diagnostic report and their previous treatment history to the doctor without having to wait for an appointment. The patient can connect with the doctor in the comfort of their own home or at a nearby accessible location. Although the ideas of telemedicine and telehealth are still relatively new, providers and clinicians have emphasized the need for technology adoption in the healthcare system. The backbone of telemedicine consists of information communication technology and the internet of things [1].

M. Haroon (✉) · M. M. Tripathi
Department of CSE, Integral University, Lucknow, India
e-mail: mharoon@iul.ac.in; mmt@iul.ac.in

T. Ahmad
Department of CSE, AMU, Aligarh, India

Afsaruddin
Department of CSE, Abdul Kalam Technical University, Lucknow, India

M. S. Husain et al. (eds.), *Pervasive Healthcare*, EAI/Springer Innovations in Communication and Computing, https://doi.org/10.1007/978-3-030-77746-3_5

What Is Telemedicine Healthcare Telemedicine is simply defined as the remote delivery of healthcare services and systems. Most of the time three main types of telemedicine are used.

Interactive Medicine In this environment patients and physicians communicate in real time. Patients can share their information with the doctor in real-time mode [2].

Store-and-Forward Patient information is captured and stored and shared with the practitioner at a convenient time.

Remote Patient Monitoring In this domain patients can be monitored by tools and technology; the remote patient resides at their home, and their information or data can be collected and shared with the doctor using mobile medical devices. Doctors can diagnose and monitor the patient remotely and prescribes medication [2].

5.2 Information and Telecommunication Technology in Healthcare

Since the introduction of information and telecommunication technology, the healthcare environment has drastically changed. Patient care and the cost of treatment accessibility of healthcare providers and higher quality healthcare services are easily accessible. This improvement is possible just because of the technological innovation by the network system or by the wireless network system or by the wide-area public wireless network system, patients directly reach the practitioner and ask for treatment. Rural patients can easily access the practitioner at their home location. Healthcare providers are subject to considerable stress worldwide, and healthcare services in rural and underserved India are major challenges. Combined with the increased costs of healthcare services so many systems such as policymakers, healthcare providers, hospital insurance companies, patients face many problems accessing resources in the recent scenario. The majority of companies are claiming that the provision of better medical care combined with reduced economic stress is increasing the number of people living significantly longer than ever before [3].

The population rate is drastically increasing; thus, the major challenge is how to provide better and good healthcare services and how to connect or generate a better human network, to increase the number of people using limited financial and human resources. Pervasive healthcare is considered a solution to this problem.

Pervasive healthcare can be defined as healthcare to anyone at any time anywhere by moving location, time and other constraints while increasing both the coverage and quality of healthcare. Broadly, we can define preventive healthcare as including prevention healthcare maintenance and check-ups, short-term monitoring and long-term personalised monitoring. Healthcare monitoring means detection and management of patient health as well as emergency intervention, transportation and treatment. This can be supported by reliable healthcare services and systems. The biomedical information system also plays a significant role in the healthcare system as medical information can be accessed any time anywhere that data can be accessed from mobile devices.

Medical Artificial Intelligence Artificial intelligence devices can assist a physician to make better diagnoses and also to make better clinical decisions in order to get better results. Data in the healthcare system are rapidly increasing and converted into big data; thus, artificial intelligence techniques are used in big data analytics.

In this chapter, we discuss the motivation of the artificial intelligence system and the data analytic technique used in the healthcare system. The various machines used in the generation of the various report in the healthcare system,

To make an effective artificial intelligence system, we have to train using healthcare data, records, and reports (such as the diagnostic record, medical prescriptions, symptoms of disease) so that system responds well, works on a similar group of data, and also maps the association rule on the data (Table 5.1).

5.3 Application of Artificial Intelligence in Healthcare Systems

This section addresses the various ways in which artificial intelligence is affecting healthcare, such as how it is used on and off a computer system, or doing activities that would typically need human intellect, such as object identification, solving complicated issues, and so on. The main benefits of artificial intelligence are that it gives us predictions with an increased level of accuracy, it helps us in decision-making processes, it has to solve complex problems and performs high-level computations. Artificial intelligence (AI) is a technology that makes life simpler by doing high-level computations and solving complicated issues. The introduction of artificial intelligence in 1950 had an impact on various domains, including marketing finance, the gaming industry and even the music. By 2030, the greatest impact will be in the field of healthcare. The reason behind the growth of artificial intelligence in the healthcare industry is that we have huge amounts of medical data in the form of medical history. Whenever we go to any hospitals our history is taken down. Thus, basically, with the availability of data, implementing it becomes much easier. It is based on technologies such as deep learning and machine learning, which require vast amounts of data.

Table 5.1 Computer-based systems used in healthcare systems

S.N	Name of system/device	Application of system/device
1	IBM Watson for oncology	Assisting a diagnosis of skin cancer
2	Bouton et al. developed an artificial intelligence system for neurology	Work as an interface for the neurology system
3	Dilsizian and Siegel proposed an artificial intelligence system for heart diagnosis	MRI or cardiac imaging are used to predict heart disease
4	MYCIN	Diagnosis and treatment of blood bacterial infection
5	INTERNIST-1 and DXplain	For general internal medicine
6	Dendral	Chemical analysis to expect molecular reaction
7	CaDet	Expert system that classifies a tumour at the initial stage
8	PROSPECTOR	Designed for resolving the problem of decision-making in mineral exploration
9	PXDES	System used to determine lung cancer
10	DXplain	Variability of disease based on recommendations of doctors
11	Quotient Health	Reduces the cost of supporting electronic medical records
12	KenSci	Predicts the extent of illness and helps physicians to make a diagnosis
13	Ciox health	Health information management system and modernised workflow
14	PathAI	Helps pathologists to make a quicker and more effective diagnosis
15	Quantitative insights	Improves the diagnosis of the extent of breast cancer
16	Microsoft's Project InnerEye	A system that is used to differentiate between various tumours
17	Pfizer	System used to show how the body's immune system is fighting against cancer
18	Insitro	System used to cure more quickly with lower costs
19	BioSymetrics	Improving accuracy and minimising time in various kinds of tasks, including biopharmaceutical and precision medicine
20	MD Insider	A system used for better mapping of patients with doctors

5.4 Application of Machine Learning Systems in Healthcare

Machine learning is not capable of handling high-dimensional data and particularly the medical data that we have mentioned. It is hard to do this with machine learning, deep learning, and neural networks. With the introduction of speaking it is much easier to keep learning and neural networks specifically focused on solving complex problems that involve high-dimensional data, to develop deep learning and neural networks, a production service provider uses artificial intelligence in healthcare data and to conduct any diagnostic that uses artificial intelligence and machine learning to present or to protect the intent of a particular user. By implementing neurons in an organisation system or an organisation of the workflow, a personalised user experience can be developed [4] that allows the company to make better decisions and that enhances the customer's overall experience. It was benefitting the organisation by collecting, storing and reformatting data in order to provide faster and more consistent access to all the data so that any analysis of any diagnosis can be performed by using machine learning and natural language processing. Based on the attitude gathered during searches, this might be close to invalidating or cancelling the service. It's a rate of the monotonous stars of calling customers and implementing automated systems that will send notifications, medical imaging and diagnostic powered by a fitness more than 40% growth to surpass 2.5 billion US dollars by 2024, so basically, it's a rate of the monotonous stars of calling customers and implementing automated systems that will send notifications, medical imaging and diagnostic powered by a fitness more than 40% growth to surpass 2.5 billion US dollars by 2024. This was something I found in the global market insights; thus, with the help of neural networks and deep learning models, artificial intelligence is revolutionising the field of diagnostic imaging. One application of AI in medical diagnosis is the MRI scan. Medical imaging and diagnostics powered by a student. Imaging and diagnostics in medicine The market for machine learning medical imaging and diagnostics, which is backed by a student, has increased by more than 40% to more than 2.5 million dollars. Scans are the most difficult to analyse because of the amount of information that normal analysis will take. Large and complex results can be analysed. To perform MRI analysis using neural networks is approximately the same as a conventional MRI program will take; thus, you can see that there is a huge difference when you implement these technologies such as learning and neural networks in artificial intelligence in medical diagnosis. Understanding how artificial intelligence has helped to detect diseases as early as possible is very important in the early predictions of medical conditions.

Apple Watches Apple uses the concept of soft computing to build a watch. That watch is used to monitor individual health 24*7, such as personal heart monitoring, breath monitoring while performing various activities, and so on. This watch is also known as a smartwatch; everything is designed according to the concept of the artificial intelligence system. By wearing this watch, health-related data are automatically collected and sent to the server or doctors. Once that the data have been collected, the next step in machine learning is processing, analysing and making predictions from the data.. Furthermore, it builds a model that predicts the risk of a heart attack. And that system is going to protect other individuals. Nowadays, artificial intelligence systems are used in the medical system to save the money and also provide a medical assistant such as a virtual nurse. In a recent survey virtual nursing assistants corresponded to the maximum term value of 20 million US dollar by 2020. The amount of money saved will be 20 million by the end of 2027. So many soft computing approaches such as machine learning, deep learning, neural networks, pattern recognition, speed recognition are going to help healthcare systems. Recently, View has aided in self-care by acting as a virtual nurse. The virtual nurse also assists the patient with their medicine, instructing them on when to take it and whether or not to consume specific foods.

5.4.1 Surgical Robots

Soft computing in the healthcare system, especially in surgery, is also very helpful. It provides many surgical robots that help in surgery. Surgical robots work with the doctor, continuously helping doctors in the operating theatre, and often the surgical robot performs surgery independently without the help of doctors. Using tools and technology errors can be minimised and costs can be reduced. Surgical robot is a smart device that allows professional surgeons to perform complex surgery with better flexibility and control. The Demon Tree is not a robot that perform the surgery; rather, it provides a set of instruments that will help to inform the surgery. Robots are highly capable of performing surgeries on their own. There are a couple of robots, but they require human intervention. These artificial robots are also involved in the decision-making process; using artificial robots we can predict an accurate decision and improve the overall performance of the system. Which is machine learning and deep learning. Machine learning and deep learning are attempts to understand exactly that learning is a subset of artificial intelligence, which provides the machines with the ability to learn automatically and improve from experience without being explicitly programmed. In simple terms, machine learning is an approach in which any intelligent machine reads and interprets a lot of data and takes a legitimate action. Planning is an advanced field of artificial intelligence and machine learning. Planned machine learning uses concepts of neural networks and solves the complex problem and the problem related to a higher dimension.

5.5 Application of Artificial Intelligence System in a Diagnostic Centre

In the recent era, the majority of standard and high-quality diagnostic centres are using artificial intelligence-based devices to diagnose various kinds of diseases [5]. A US study states that 10% of US deaths are caused by medical diagnostic errors. Artificial intelligence system promised to improve the diagnostic process in the healthcare system. After a while, humans commit many mistakes during investigations owing to tiredness and over work [6]. This leads to various errors, but if the diagnostic report is not correct then the patient may die. Incomplete medical history and the large scale of the secondary load of deadly human error can cause loss of life [5, 6].

Pathak Artificial intelligence at maximum accuracy for cancer diagnosis. Artificial intelligence is developing as a medical learning technology that is used by the pathologist in the diagnostic system to make a more accurate diagnostic report. This appliance is used to minimise errors. The artificial intelligence system is used to diagnose cancer.

Developers such as Myers Squibb and organisations such as the Bill and Melinda Gates Foundation have worked with artificial intelligence to expand into the healthcare industry [7].

5.6 Buoy Health

The intelligent device used for symptom checker health is an artificial intelligence-based device to use for the symptom checker and also used to treat the illness, practitioner listen the patient symptom and health comes and then guide the patient to the correct care based on it Diagnostic report many Institutions and medical colleges for allow how to use BIOS artificial intelligence system to help and diagnose and treat the patient more quickly.

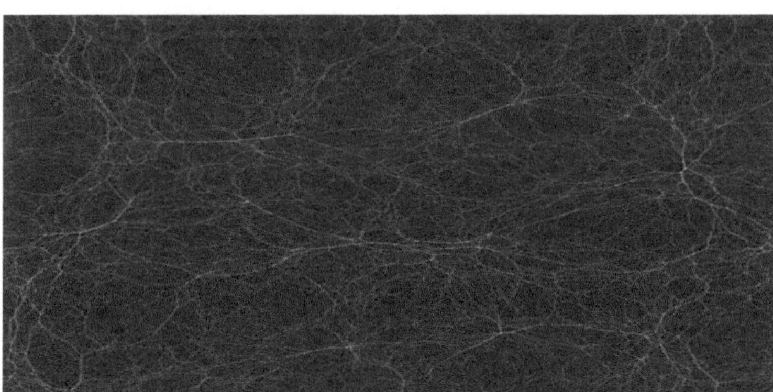

5.7 Enlitic

An artificial intelligence and deep learning-based actionable insight device. Enclitic developed the concept of deep learning medical tools to streamline the radiological diagnosis system. Initially, the deep learning platform is used to analyse the unstructured medical data (radiology images, blood tests, EKG, genomics, patient medical history, etc.) after that. Whatever the particular result that is obtained is directly given to the doctor for a better insight into patient treatment in real time.

Massachusetts Institute of Technology (MIT) named Enlitic the fifth smartest artificial intelligence company producing health devices based on artificial intelligence in the world ranking, over Facebook and Microsoft.

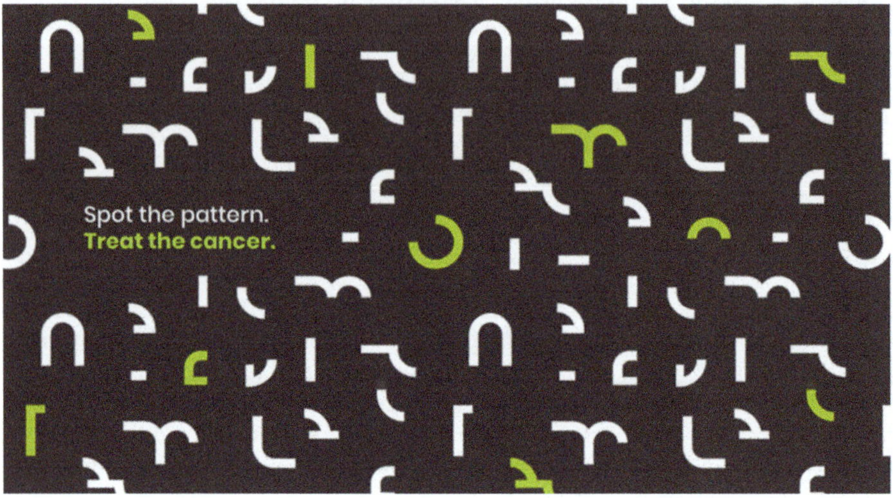

Many more artificial intelligence devices are used in medical diagnostic centres and medical treatment. The majority of artificial intelligence devices, deep learning-based devices, neural network-based devices and machine learning-based devices are helping the medical practitioner as well as the patients. Some devices are used in surgery, some are used for medical diagnostic centres and some are also used as a robot doctors.

5.7.1 Decision Tree

To classify the patient category, i.e. which patients are eligible to receive the telehealth services from the health insurance department or not, we propose a new decision tree algorithm that restricts intelligent decision-based classification and is used to classify the telehealth approach based on data analysis and preprocessing. The decision tree-building model predicts and explains various nodes of the decision tree [9].

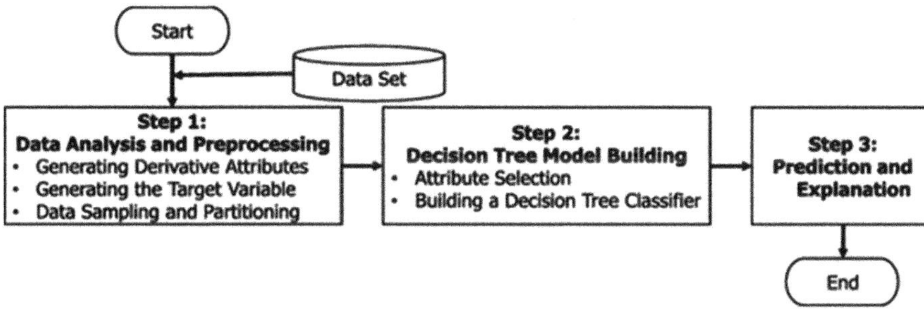

As mentioned in our figure, different challenges are going on. In step 1 all the data analysis and pre-processing work are carried out, generating of the derivation attribute, generating of the target value data sampling, and partitioning.

In step 2 the decision tree model is going to be built. In the decision tree model, attribute selection and the classifier are used.

In step 3 prediction and explanation to the patient take place.

5.7.2 *Making a Decision Tree*

In this part, we describe an interview with three clinical experts in the telehealth and related field. A physician in a medical capacity is expert 1, the social worker in a remote area is expert 2 and the manager at a long-term care centre is expert 3 to identify the target variable of adaptability in the sample data set.

Before the interview we initially introduce all the experts to the data collection and the purpose of data collection. Before the interview we spend at least 10–20 min describing and introducing the purpose of our research. Afterwards, each expert takes 30 min to label the adaptability of each record with a yes or no answer. Finally, the expert explains the correct area they used to make their decision. Then we have used the adaptability criteria for each decision tree, the sample size of the training data set is given, which states the minimum number of records for leaf node to be one, indicating that it contains 0.5% of the data set indicating it a weaker approach to make the decision tree. We make the decision tree as per the data collected from the individual expert and discuss the performance and the rules of each decision tree to all the individual experts. Then, finally, we obtain any corrections and collect all the reports from the expert. Finally, we build the decision tree to test the data set.

Expert one focuses on the clinical record, such as disease, pathology report and frequency of patient admission. The first few branches in the decision tree are related to the clinical attributes. The practitioner also indicates the telehealth services carried out to use the time in the hospital after the equipment has detected abnormal values and that is to minimise the outpatient time [8].

Expert two is fully focused on the welfare-related issues at review such as co-payment exemptions, patient residence, telehealth services can reduce the urban–rural gap and improve the lives of rural residents [8].

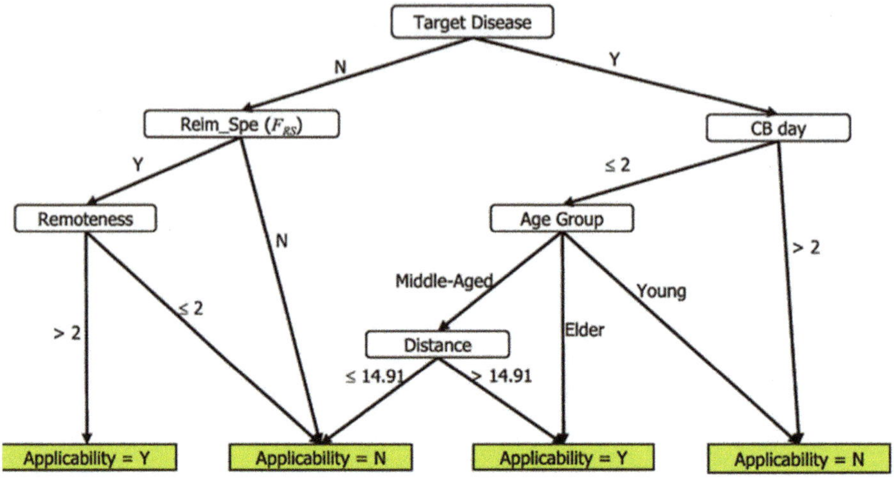

Expert three emphasises the convenience and accessibility of healthcare for the patient and also encourages the early patient to use the telehealth equipment in their long-term care centre frequently; therefore, important attributes for expert three are distance and age [8].

Distance of patient	Drug/day	Economy priority	Target disease	Age group of patients	Applicability
Long distance	More than 4 times	Not defined	Not defined	Any age	Yes
Long distance	Less than 4 times	Not defined	Not defined	Any age	No
Short distance	Less than 4 times	Yes	Not defined	Any age	Yes
Short distance	Less than 4 times	Not defined	Yes	Older age	Yes
Short distance	Less than 4 times	Not defined	Yes	Young or middle-aged	Yes
Short distance	Less than 4 times	Not defined	Not defined	Any age	No
Short distance	Less than 4 times	Not defined	Not defined	Young or middle-aged	Yes

Final decision table

Treatment	Short-distance patient	Distance in km	Age group of patients	Long-distance patient	Insurance status	Applicability
Yes	Not defined	>2	Not defined	>0	Low	Yes
Yes	Not defined	>2	Not defined	>0	Higher or middle	No
Yes	Not defined	>2	Not defined	<0	Not defined	No
Yes	Not defined	<2	Not defined	Not defined	Not defined	No
No	<1	Not defined	Young or middle aged	Not defined	Not defined	No
No	>1	Not defined	Not defined	Not defined	Not defined	No
No	<1	Not defined	Elderly	Not defined	Not defined	Yes

5.8 Decision Support System

In an environment full of uncertainty, it is very tough and difficult to make decisions. When the course goal and how the action will take place are decided, it is easy to move towards the goal. But in uncertain situations the goal is not decided; it is given in terms of probability. It cannot be decided to move forward and action is taken by us to move towards the goal or not. Action can have various possible outcomes. To mention the quality of the actions a utility value is attached to every move. Utility theory and probability theory give rise to the rational decision called decision theory: decision theory = utility theory +probability theory.

The basic idea of decision theory is that a rule is rational if and only if it chooses the action that yields the highest expected value of utility averaged over all the outcomes of the actions. This is called the maximum expected utility.

5.9 Disadvantages of Decision Support Systems

Cost is one of the important factors for a decision support system, setting up the decision support system to monitor costs, analysis of the decision support system, the required advanced data analytics and data statistics. Specialists are required for all purposes; that is why the propositional costs will be increased. Decision support system especially knowledge-driven system are very useful techniques.

For a few years, the decision support system has been incorporated into business to support humans in taking the decision. The decision support system stops the manipulation of the decision, and avoids bias. A lot of uncertainty is associated with decision support systems.

Difficulty in quantifying the data: it is very difficult to analyse data, such as tangible data, intangible data, indefinable data; in reality, some data values may not be very specific. The decision support system quantifies these aspects. The result must be considered by the decision-makers. Decision-makers use their judgement to take the decision.

5.10 Uninformed Assumptions

When the decision support system analyses data for a specific problem, as decision-makers we are unaware of the data and of the assumptions taken by decision support systems. Making decisions without taking uncontrollable situations and factors may be dangerous for the entire system. A decision-maker must comprehend that a computerised decision support system is only an auxiliary instrument. An unstructured or partially structured situation must be considered in-depth and the limitations and assumptions analysed.

5.11 System Design Failure

Systems that assist in making decisions The failure of a decision support system is measured according to the specific demands of a decision maker. It will be difficult to build a decision support system that meets your needs if you don't know what you want it to accomplish or how it should help you. And the outcomes provided by a hazy decision support system aren't what you're searching for. Such circumstances may emerge as a result of a system design flaw.

5.12 Difficulty in Collecting all the Required Data

As decision-makers we can realise a time to capture all related data automatically and mechanically. Although some data are captured and some data cannot be captured, some data automatically are recalled and some data are not automatically recalled, we cannot say that the decision taken by the system is completely correct.

5.13 Lack of Technology Knowledge in Users

A lot of technical knowledge is required to use decision support systems. Although a decision support system is simple, the end user must be technically skilled.

5.14 Conclusion

This is the information age; this information is an important consideration related to the situation that most individual institutions hold their data in electronic form. During the pending and major crisis, we are not obtaining the data easily if the data are not in electronic form. But if the data are in electronic form, we can access them easily in a pandemic situation, like covid-19, flu, etc. We can easily extract the data from the database. It is important to consider what is strategically planned for the use of information and knowledge during the treatment of the patient and the deployment of the medical professionals. The tools and technology are used frequently in health treatment in this era. The majority of pathologists, hospitals, and medical colleges are using intelligent devices for the treatment of the patient, as well as for the taking of samples, and with the telemedicine concept, rural patients are easily connected to the doctor via the technology and they can share their information in real time. Often, doctors can be assisted by the technology in surgery for the treatment of the patient. In the era of information, deep learning, neural networks, artificial intelligence and machine learning play a significant role in taking the decision to treat the patient in various situations.

References

1. Kun, L., Ray, P., Merrell, R., & Kwankam, S. Y. *Joseph Lombardo & David Buckeridge Managing Knowledge through Interoperability*. https://doi.org/10.3395/reciis.v2i1.167en
2. Russell, S. J., & Norvig, P. *Artificial intelligence: A modern approach* (3rd ed.). https://doi.org/10.1016/j.artint.2011.01.005
3. Haroon, M., Srivastava, S., & Bajaj, A. (2013). Web document information extraction using class attribute approach. In *4th International Conference on Computer and Communication Technology (ICCCT)*. IEEE. https://doi.org/10.1109/ICCCT.2013.6749596
4. Ssu-Hsuan, Kuan-Chou, L., & Yang, L. D.-L. Pervasive health service system: Insights on the development of a grid-based personal health service system. In *The 12th IEEE international conference on e-health networking, applications and services*. https://doi.org/10.1109/HEALTH.2010.5556532. Corpus ID: 14207287.
5. Avancha, S., & Baxi, A. Privacy in Mobile Technology for Personal Healthcare. *ACM Computing Surveys (CSUR), 45*(1), 1–54. https://doi.org/10.1109/ISCCSP.2008.4537472
6. Tripathi, M. M., Haroon, M., Jafar, M., & Jain, M. (2010). Maxillofacial surgery using X Ray based face recognition by elastic bunch graph matching. In *International conference of contemporary computing*. Springer. https://doi.org/10.1007/978-3-642-14834-7_18
7. Haroon, M., & Husain, M. (2013). Analysis of dynamic load balancing in multiprocessor system. *International Journal Of Computer Science And Engineering And Information Technology and Research, 3*(1), 398–403.
8. Riyazuddine Khan, Mohd Shahid, Shaid Husain, Afsaruddin, "Adjacent selection method for load balancing in distributed network by artificial intelligence", International Journal Of Advanced Research In Electrical, Electronics and Instrumentation Engineering, 2015 Vol 4, 8, .https://doi.org/10.15662/ijareeie.2015.0408078.7117.
9. Chern, C.-C., Chen, Y.-J., & Hsiao, B. (2019). Decision tree-based classifier in providing telehealth service. *BMC Medical Informatics and Decision Making, 19*(104). https://doi.org/10.1186/s12911-019-0825-9

Chapter 6
An Approach Towards Privacy and Security in Pervasive Healthcare System

Nazish Siddiqui and Syed Haider Abbas

6.1 Introduction

Privacy concerns are regularly addressed in pervasive healthcare system by researchers and end users. Pervasive healthcare systems are tools that can meet the needs of patients anywhere and at any time. Software systems handling user's personal and important data are facing crucial roadblocks while maintaining the high level of data privacy in recent times [1]. A transition in healthcare knowledge is driven by the extensive use of wearable sensor-based technologies. In this regard, medical devices based on sensors may be operated by the multiple associations to feel the patient's record endlessly during the treatment system. However, collected health-related information can only be accessed or used by authorized and approved users, such as medical practitioners, as it often contains confidential and sensitive data. To ensure the safety and protection of users' data, different types of rules and standards were proposed earlier. The Portability and Transparency Act of Health Insurance, proposed in 1996, provides different rules and laws for protecting the confidentiality of personal health records. The EU Safe Harbor Law, the Gramm-Leach-Bliley Act and the Sarbanes-Oxley Act are some examples of these rules [1]. In general, in order to transmit health data, these regulations require strict security measures, and if they do not comply with these laws, they pave the way for strong penalties. More detailed explanations for these EHR-based systems are given in Fernandez-Aleman et al. [2]. In contrast to other schemes, it is essentially on the basis of one unique feature. It is the equivalence between the protection given and the accessibility of medical data. In addition, the entire data of the patient must be available and can also be preserved or circulated so as to distribute it to the healthcare providers based

N. Siddiqui (✉) · S. H. Abbas
Department of Computer Science and Engineering, Integral University, Lucknow, Uttar Pradesh, India

M. S. Husain et al. (eds.), *Pervasive Healthcare*, EAI/Springer Innovations in Communication and Computing, https://doi.org/10.1007/978-3-030-77746-3_6

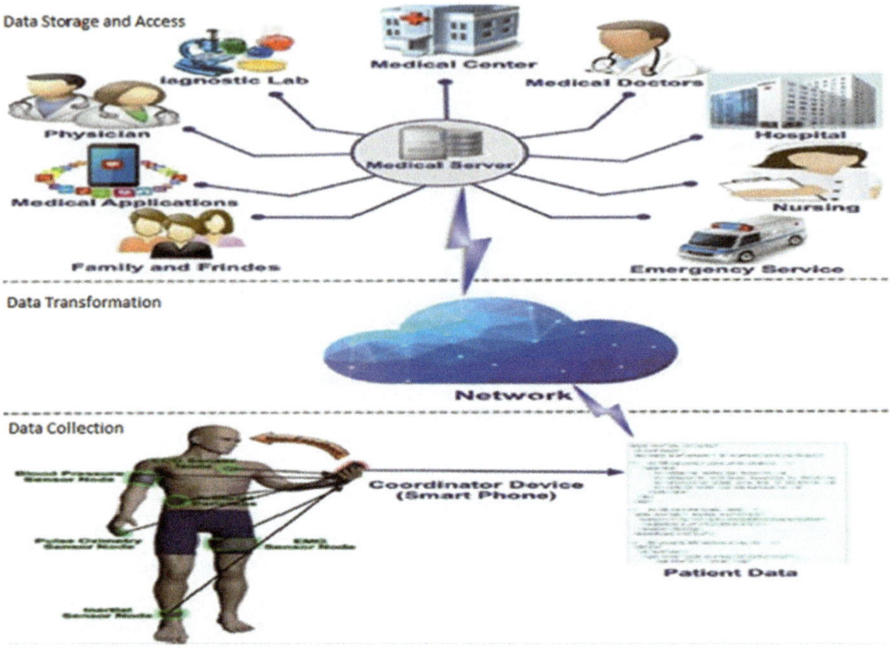

Fig. 6.1 The architecture of healthcare monitoring system

on the expertise. At the same time, for preserving the confidentiality of such data, it must not be readily available and should be considered as private. As a whole, the e-healthcare systems can be defined as the real-time, patient-based digital information which is made available and is maintained by some licensed mainstay. These datasets are generated by collecting different data from various numbers of patients. The healthcare monitoring system consists of three main components: smart server-based sensors for the data collection, i.e., selection of extreme symptoms; a cloud-based network for transformation; and a remote healthcare server for data storage and access (Fig. 6.1).

In these EHR systems, both patients and doctors may be the proprietor of the health datasets. Local or cloud-based servers are used to store and evaluate the health data which is collected and is made accessible to approved users [3]. These network-connected components will serve as an interconnector that links patients with medical personnel so as to improve data transmission and its distribution [4]. Privacy and defense are different. However, in the field of healthcare, data security is the relationship between those two principles (Fig. 6.2).

Although these healthcare systems have more benefits, with regard to the data used in them, there are more therapies for their protection and privacy. These security risks are justified on account of their design [4]. Threats are categorized into different subcategories, such as the level of data collection [5–9], level of transmission [10–13], and level of storage [14–18], which are more explicitly defined in the

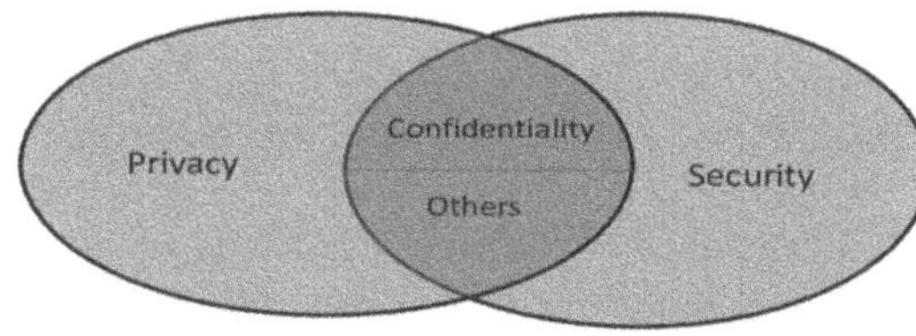

Fig. 6.2 Relationship between privacy and security

next section. Along with the risks listed above, some patients are not ready and do not feel comfortable to use healthcare-based applications. Therefore, without any hesitation, it is important to make sure that the users are comfortable and prepared to use the system. In this article, an exhaustive analysis is carried out to examine the risks that are present while ensuring security and privacy in the healthcare sector. A new smart model for ensuring the enhancement of security and privacy provision in the EHR framework is also proposed.

6.2 Privacy Standards in Healthcare Systems

To ensure high degree of privacy and protection of user data in the EHR system, various criteria must be fulfilled. More than 20 criteria have already been suggested in recent literature by various writers [14–16, 18–23].

1. The process of restricting and monitoring access by licensed users to services is called access control [3]. Three forms of security and privacy specifications listed as identification, authentication, and authorization were used to facilitate privacy and security in access control mechanism [38]. The primary aim of the requirement for identification is to distinguish between the users who can access the datasets. As a result, this approach can be used as a path to classify the users, whether they are authenticated or not [20, 22]. Authentication is the method of offering assurance that the access to information that is requested is genuine and authentic or not. Also, it verifies the assertion of identity prior to accessing the user data [23]. At the same time, it is also ensured that the whole contact process takes place on the communication side and that too with an authorized user [21]. Finally, it decides whether the external requester, breaching the security policies of the system, can be excluded from accessing the data or not. In order to ensure a patient's privacy and to maintain a reasonable balance between the security objectives of confidentiality and availability, it becomes necessary to ensure that a proper and effective access control mechanism exists [16].
2. The phenomenon in which services are open, available, and accessible to authorized users upon request is referred to as availability [23]. This is accessible anywhere at any time through the healthcare server [19]. It must ensure availability and also ensure to prevent the disruption of service due to sudden hardware faults and failures, power outages, and also during the device upgrade process [18].

3. The key role of reliability [43, 45] is to ensure that medical data can be easily retrieved and accessed anywhere and at any time, even if there are possibilities of any threats caused by network failure [15, 24]. In general, due to the risks caused by network problems that can further endanger a patient's life, most of the medical cases face trouble while accessing the data.
4. The method of granting the authority to the unauthorized users whose names are not present in the open list to obtain relevant information in an emergency, so that the life of a patient could be saved, is called flexibility. It is an important feature to make use of the laws of access when it comes to protecting the life of a patient [15].

6.3 Healthcare System Protection

The security of the healthcare systems is always at risk and can be breached by the intruders or from some other users for their personal benefit. The overall performance of healthcare systems is impaired by this unauthorized access [3, 4, 25]. Specifically, in the case of insulin pump sensors, the networks present in hospitals, unauthorized users can easily hack or access health data of individuals [17, 24].

1. *Attacks at the data collection stage:* The various forms of attacks that can be performed at the data collection stage could be jamming, data flooding, de-synchronization, spoofing and collision-based data flooding, selective forwarding, etc. Several other threats like altering the information, dropping, or deleting more relevant data can also be caused at the data collection stage.
2. *Attacks at the data sharing stage:* There are various attacks like patient medical information eavesdropping, man-in-the-middle attack, data tampering attack, juggling attacks, signaling attacks, allocation unfairness, message alteration attack, hello flood attack, data surveillance attack, and wormhole attack. These types of the attacks are causes of many risks, such as altering information, sending extra signals to block the base station, interrupting communication, spying, and networking traffic, during the transmission of data. It is quite simple for an unauthorized programmer to create and design systems that can spy on the patient's information using some wireless technology. Therefore, it becomes a necessity to have an authority or a control mechanism for managing and handling the database of a patient's record. Also, it should serve as a way of protecting and safeguarding the patient's data and hence ensuring security against intruders by reducing unauthorized access [7].
3. *Attacks in the data storage and access process:* There are several attacks that may cause serious threats at the level of data storage and its access process. These include attacks like altering the medical information of patients and changing the configuration settings of the systems, engaged in the monitoring purposes or as servers. Patient information intrusion, malware-based attack, social engineering-based attacks, unapproved access to patient medical informa-

tion, removable delivery media-based attacks, etc. are some other list of attacks that can be conducted for accessing the medical records of the patients at the storage level.

4. *Others issues:* Any breach and interruption in the healthcare system can trigger many hardware and software problems. Hackers are learning and using advanced techniques to find and discover vulnerabilities, even in the newly available software. Besides this, different types of malware attacks like worms, Trojans, viruses, spyware attacks, etc. are most likely to occur in the system [17].

6.4 Security Models in e-Healthcare Systems

It could be spread to more consumers in order to increase the quality of distribution of patient data. As a result, it leads to a disclosure of the privacy of data in the e-healthcare systems. Therefore, the standard approaches used so far in this data exchange are typically encryption techniques. While these encryption methods provide easy access control, they cannot be used for certain complex structures that need different permissions for data access and sharing. Therefore, controlling and protecting the e-health data is a major challenge because of these constraints as large computational load is experienced by using several encryption techniques. Also the vulnerability of attacks on the personal medical information is increased, when it is altered using certain alteration techniques [26]. The elaborated description of various sets of security models at various levels is mentioned below.

1. *The Proposed Security Models at the Data Collection Stage*

   O. G. Morchon and K. Wehrle proposed an enhanced modular-based access control mechanism for the active healthcare applications [27]. Their proposed mechanism is an enhanced version of the popular RBAC method which is already available. There are two key explanations for this system being suggested. Initially, to delegate and share accesses to all the available nodes of a sensor, the policies of different control mechanisms are used. Then, for the purpose of storing current parameters relating to medical data, viz., place, time, health details of patients, etc., and depending on the medical conditions of patients, declaring it as a critical condition, an emergency, or a normal condition, different access control decisions could be taken. The modular-based approach suggested by them helps in improving the device configuration even more efficiently. This approach also minimizes the complexities of regulations and policies which are used for the application of secure and even more efficient medical sensor-based network. But, in case of the arrival of some crucial emergency condition, these restrictions may be overruled. These limitations can be resolved by the sensors for accessing the information which earlier was not permitted, when it was in the normal state. No detection or access control mechanism exists at the time of unfavorable circumstances for the unlicensed entry or sharing of data, which is the key drawback of their proposed mechanism. For the purpose of suggesting a novel method for designing the security model which exhibits the property of being lightweight in nature, there are several security protocols, viz., as LLSP, MiniSec, TinySec, and RC4-based methods, along with several cipher algorithms, viz., as AES, Skipjack, and RC4, that were deeply examined by Amini et al. [28]. Besides this, the authors also researched the different properties of various types of attacks, such as spoofing-based attacks, eavesdropping-based attacks, and data loss-based attacks, in order to reduce the current effects of these attacks and also to further implement them into the cipher algorithms. After performing all these researches, the authors came into the conclusion that for the sake of satisfying and enhancing the confidentiality of the data in the healthcare sector, two cipher algorithms, viz., RC4 and Skipjack, are the most powerful. Maw et al. [29] have suggested an adaptive method of access control model that facilitates several mechanisms of providing access control for accessing medical data linked through networks. Their model provides users with certain benefits of accessing data and over-riding on the occurrence of any unexpected emergency. Therefore, in order to grant permission to access the data, human interference is no longer needed. In order to initialize sessions based on user location, access time, etc., various policies have already been predefined for users. The key drawback of their proposed model, however, is that at the time of a critical situation, there is no mechanism for detecting user access. Another approach for enhancing security in the healthcare systems is the three-tier system, proposed in the research articles [30, 31] which are based on the pair-wise key distribution method. There are two basic keys to their technique. In order to gain network access, one key is for the mobile pool, and the other is a pair-wise key that is basically used to create the connection and link among the sensors present in the device. In context to improving network stability and further reduce the damage and effects on the access nodes by various attacks, an authentication technique between the sensor and the nodes present in it has been developed.

2. *Proposed Security Models at the Point of Sharing*

   A stable framework for data transmission and authentication using encryption techniques was proposed by Boonyarattaphan et al. [26] to enforce two mechanisms: data and channel protection. Using SSL on the HTTP layer, channel protection was provided, while security of data was provided through the SOAP layer lying and installed over HTTP. They stressed on using RBAC along with multi-factor authentication in order to guarantee and ensure proper authentication and authorization. Communication has been split into different layers where, based on stakeholder roles and data sensitivity, several encryption settings and authentication mechanisms can be adapted. The only, but a major drawback here is that it focuses only on the web-based e-health programs to deal with. A new and safe scheme was designed by Kahani et al. [32] that influences both secure authentication of finely grained data access and its scalable control. The zero-knowledge protocol is used for the proposed scheme, in order to verify and preserve the anonymity of the identity of users. The strategy uses a public key system by combining it with a secret session key which is created and obtained by the Derive Unique Key Per Transaction (DUKPT) algorithm for facilitating safe and secure communication among various interacting entities. Here, the access control scheme has been executed in the following two phases: in the first phase, a static authorization method is used to analyze and determine the highest level of accessing rights for the user, while in the second phase, the user is granted access rights, in accordance with the user's intention to access. To keep the confidentiality of user's data against unauthorized access and to minimize collaboration and computational overheads for the owners of the data, it is stored in the cloud in encoded format through encryption. However, by storing the health-related data of patients in the cloud, patients have lost their solo control over their health records. In addition, it has become difficult for obtaining the access control of the patient data in the finely grained, scalable, and properly organized form because of the use of encryption techniques. The security and privacy of the data belonging to the cloud-integrated body sensor networks were advised by Guan et al. [33]. The novel outsourcing scheme for encryption called the Mask-Certificate Attribute-Based Encryption (MC-ABE) was introduced by the combination of seven different encryption algorithms. In this scheme, in order to cover the row data until it is safely processed in the storage service provider (cloud servers), the patient's data encrypts the outsourcing data. In addition, a unique certificate for authentication is implemented for each and every user in order to achieve more efficient access control, which has been checked prior to accessing data. Experimental findings showed that, relative to other common models, the above-proposed scheme incurs very low storage and computing costs. However, achieving finely grained access control is a bit difficult because of the use of encryption methods, and it also requires a high degree of overhead computing. Simplicio et al. [34] suggested a security architecture for Secure Health which is lightweight in nature as it is based on certain frameworks such as TLS/SSL, which in itself is lightweight, in order to ensure safety of data, which could be shared with the server without requiring any extra layer of security. Secure Health offers security services for both stored and distributed data. In addition to this, certain other features enabling security of data, viz., as user authentication and confidentiality of data, are also included. This framework depending on Secure Health was specifically configured and designed to prevent any outsider from illegally accessing or meddling with the system data. Moreover, the managers are also given the authority to identify and determine the misbehavior caused by the insiders.

6.5 Sharing and Access-Level Security Models

The notion of intent for designing a comprehensive usage of an access control model was considered by Lili [35]. In particular, notations have been used to define privacy policies and to grant private data access privileges. This proposed model for access control consists of following eight basic elements, viz., as subject, attributes, objects, attributes of objects, privileges, permissions, obligations, and conditions [35]. Among these core elements, permissions, responsibilities, and conditions are the components of decisions on use control which are used to decide if an object is permitted to be accessed by a subject. The presence of responsibilities and conditions helped address such deficiencies that were prevalent in access control mechanisms. However, the main downside of this model is that it presents just the initial step in the objective data of use control for the authorization model.

In order to encrypt patient's complete health record, another novel attribute-based encryption method was proposed by Shahina et al. [36]. Their methodology allows the patient to provide access control by offering finely grained access control mechanisms based on the semi-trusted servers. For protecting the user's personal health data which are stored on a semi-trusted server, an attribute-based encryption approach is used by them. By this approach, based on the attributes of users, different data access protocols are specified. This essentially allows a patient to communicate with other users by sharing his health record as an encrypted file. Another approach is the novel cloud-based framework which is proposed to facilitate the patients with the authority to safely store their health record information on cloud through some cloud service providers. This method selectively sends and receives health information to various users, such as physicians, family members, or acquaintances. The users here were split into two areas, viz., as the public and the personal domain, to reduce the complexity of key distribution and its management by trusted users. The primary difference that exists between their proposed system and other methods is that using cipher text-based encryption technique, the health information is encrypted. Selvam and Arokia Renjit improved attribute-based encryption [36], which provides protection for healthcare datasets to some extent. In their approach, owners of the data have the right to encrypt them until they are shared on the cloud. The decryption is done according to the requirements of the receiver. This method can certainly be used for securely accessing the data from a healthcare system database. Through this technique, health information is shared more effectively and securely among the users as it allows a patient to share his/her health record in very secure, encrypted file format with other users.

6.6 Intelligence-Based Access Control Security Model

The architecture of intelligence-based access control (IBAC) model for security works on smart agent-based systems to improve and enhance the security features of accessing the data of healthcare sector through finely grained access control techniques. This model proposes a multi-agent framework for the delivery of efficient and safe e-health security services. The architecture of IBAC model is shown in Fig. 6.3. As shown in the proposed method, there are multiple intelligent agents listed as the user interface agent, authentication agent, link establishment agent, and the connection management agent. All these intelligent agents exhibit their distinct and distinguished working characteristics at distinct levels. These types of

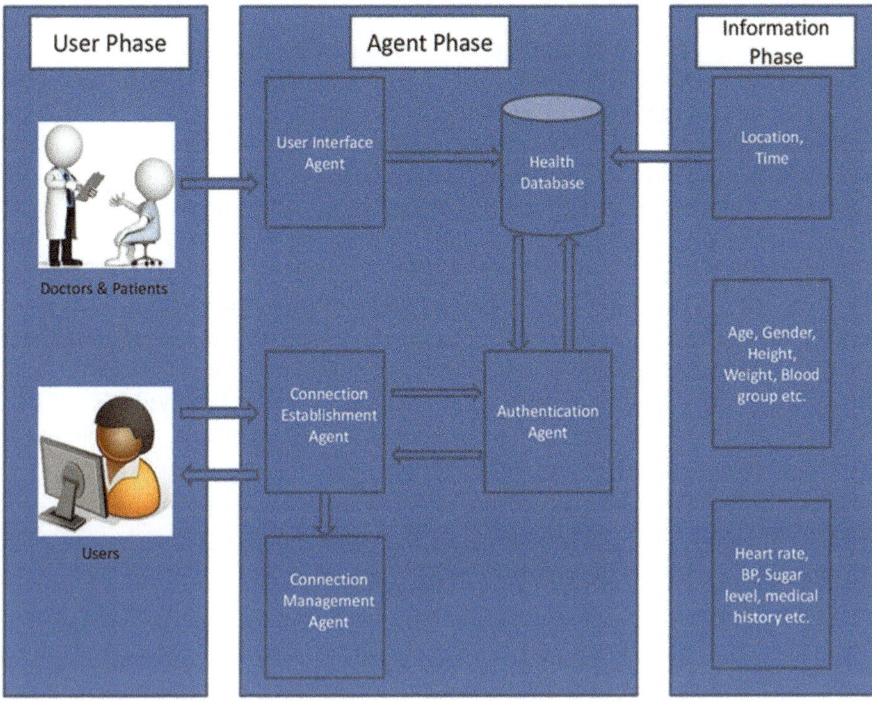

Fig. 6.3 Architecture of the proposed IBAC model

intelligent agents make it simple to use and also enable efficient contact and communication between the users (patients) and e-service providers.

The primary aim of this proposed work is the development of multi-agent system based on intelligence that provides safe and secure access to the information which is stored in the database of healthcare sector. There are several functions, viz., as registration of users, their authentication, establishment of link, and maintenance of the connection, which are carried out effectively by the multi-agent system. Besides all these functions, it also uses a database for storing and retrieving health information, which can be referred to as electronic health record (EHR). The approach envisaged mainly comprises of three different stages, termed as the consumer phase or the user level, the agent phase or the intelligence-based agent level, and the information phase or the database level. All the users who work with this computer make up the user process. Doctors, patients, and specialists allowed to handle and manage the health records for further processing it can be the consumers of the system. The next phase is the agent phase that consists of the multiple intelligent agents who, when obtaining health information, are responsible for maintaining security. The user interface agent has protocols and policies that are defined.

All the usernames and passwords issued and used by the patients, doctors, and approved individual to access and further process data are stored in the health database. In order to verify the user, a user authentication agent is used. It is also used in the health database for the verification of user credentials. Both agents, the first one for connection establishment and the other one for connection management, are used to build and establish a link for providing authentication. The data and information available in the health database present in the information phase consist of the fundamental and all the necessary detailed information about the patient. Besides, having patients' details, it also has environmental details, e.g., the location of the patient and the time details when the data was collected. The patient detail field of the database contains all the detailed information of the patient such as his/her age, blood group, status, weight, height, etc., whereas the current medical details, e.g., heart rate, sugar level, blood pressure, history of service, etc., are present in the current health data field of the database. Along with this, the health database also stores all the usernames and passwords issued and used for accessing and further processing data by the patients, doctors, and approved individuals. A brief description of the functionality and the features of all these agents available in the IBAC model are mentioned in the next section.

6.7 Working Principle of the IBAC Model

The customer request via an interface agent is approved by the suggested intelligence-based access control (IBAC) model. The agent in the IBAC model that provides user interface is directly linked to the people who use or access health records. It accepts usernames and passwords of the users as it is directly linked to a website or mobile device. This agent providing user interface works on certain protocols. These protocols are specified for doctors and patients who are directly associated with the system and frequently upload their health records for storing it on the system's database. In the form of restrictions, all these regulations are then parsed and further stored in a centralized health database. Users, functions, and their permissions compose the database. The agent used for authentication verifies and validates the basic credentials of the customers as their username and password. All the authenticated information will be sent to the position-based multi-agent. The responsibilities for different job operations, including permissions for unique functions, were created by the authentication agent. Specific users are assigned roles and the duties for those roles and allow the specific functions to be performed. In the database, there are three different categories of fields, featuring as the field storing environmental information, the field for storing patient information, and the field for storing current medical information. The information related to the place or time at which the data is collected is stored in the first category of fields in the database; the information related to patients personal details are stored in the second category of fields in the database, whereas the current medical status and the medical history details of the patients are stored in the last category of the database, respectively, as mentioned above. When a user requests data, a link is created by the connection establishment agent between the user requesting for the data and the server providing the services. Requester credentials, entered by the user such as the username and password, are then extracted, referred, and checked from the existing lists of valid and genuine user accounts available in the database. For further reference purposes, descriptions of the relationship established will also be stored in the database so that it can be used. The agent for link management is responsible for establishing and maintaining all the connections that will be used for communication for respective requests and further access to retrieve the data.

After the establishment of the connection, it is the responsibility of the authentication module to validate and authenticate the credentials of the person requesting the data and then finds whether the requested data could be accessed by the user or not. This can be achieved by testing and verifying the credentials of the users with the existing details present in the security database. It also retrieves the applicant's positions as well as the necessary and relevant protocols required for performing the action. Based on the received information, the authentication agent performs the task of further classifying the request of users as usual, emergency, or vital and then determines the access authorization. In certain cases, the patient is able to access the datasets, especially when urgent conditions are required.

6.8 Conclusion and Future Work

Patients' health-related data must be stored safely and securely on medical servers so that it can be accessed and used by the physicians to provide proper care. Intelligent agents are used in this paper to ensure access control. Security models classified at different levels like data collection stage, data sharing stage, and at the level of data storage and access were examined, discussed, and reviewed. Several attacks that could modify the information at these stages change the overall data and render the user unauthorized were discussed. In this article, a novel security model is suggested that aims to avoid these attacks.

This model is new since intelligent agents have been used to provide access control for the whole operation. There are several agents in the proposed model, each of which is in charge of taking on and accomplishing a particular form of mission. The purpose of this agent-driven design is to obtain a simple yet effective access control system which is based on the health situation of the patients and the assigned roles of the applicants. So, in order to protect and ensure the privacy of the e-health data stored in the database of healthcare system, the proposed approach may be more secure since it is entirely based on intelligent systems. Depending on the condition of the patients and the assigned tasks of the claimant, this model aims at a quick, efficient, and effective access control decisions. In order to measure its efficiency and precision, future work may also be applied to the proposed model by using real-time health datasets.

References

1. Barua, M., Alam, S., Liang, X., & Shen, X. (2011). Secure and quality of service assurance scheduling scheme for WBAN with application to e-health. In *Wireless communications and networking conference (WCNC)* (pp. 1–5). IEEE.
2. Fernandez-Aleman, J. L., et al. (2013). Security & privacy in EHR: A systematic literature review. *Journal of Biomedical Informatics, 46*(3), 541–562.
3. Zhang, K., et al. (2015). Security and privacy for mobile healthcare networks: From a quality of protection perspective. *IEEE Wireless Communications, 22*(4), 104–112.
4. Shinde, S. S., & Patil, D. (2015). Review on the security and privacy for mobile healthcare networks: From a quality of protection perspective. *International Journal of Engineering Research, 3*(6), 352–361.
5. Habib, K., et al. (2015). Security analysis of a patient monitoring system for the Internet of Things in eHealth. In *Proceedings of the international conference on ehealth, telemedicine, and social medicine (eTELEMED'15)* (pp.73–78). ARIA.
6. Tang, J., Liu, A., Zhao, M., & Wang, T. (2018). An aggregate signature based trust routing for data gathering in sensor networks. *Security and Communication Networks, Hindawi, 2018*, 1–31.
7. Kumar, P., & Lee, H.-J. (2011). Security issues in healthcare applications using wireless medical sensor networks: A survey. *Sensors, MDPI, 12*(1), 55–91.
8. Saleem, S., Ullah, S., & Kwak, K. S. (2011). A study of IEEE802.15. 4 security framework for wireless body area networks. *Sensors, 11*(2), 1383–1395.
9. Han, S., Zhao, S., Li, Q., Ju, C.-H., & Zhou, W. (2016). PPM-HDA: Privacy-preserving and multifunctional health data aggregation with fault tolerance. *IEEE Transactions on Information Forensics and Security, 11*(9), 1940–1955.
10. Bonab, T. H., & Masdari, M. (2015). Security attacks in wireless body area networks: Challenges and issues. *Academie Royale Des Sciences D Outre-Mer Bulletin Des Seances, 4*(4), 100–107.
11. Partala, J., Keräneny, N., Särestöniemi, M., Hämäläinen, M., Iinatti, J., Jämsä, T., Reponen, J., & Seppänen, T. (2014). Security threats against the transmission chain of a medical health monitoring system. In *2013 IEEE 15th international conference on e-health networking, applications and services (Healthcom)*. IEEE.
12. Chandrasekhar, S., Ibrahim, A., & Singhal, M. (2017). A novel access control protocol using proxy signatures for cloud- based health information exchange. *Computers & Security, 67*, 73–88.
13. Sun, W., Cai, Z., Liu, F., Fang, S., & Wang, G. (2017). A survey of data mining technology on electronic medical records. In *Proceedings of 2017 IEEE 19th international conference on e-health networking, applications and services (Healthcom)* (pp. 1–6). IEEE.
14. Drosatos, G., Efraimidis, P. S., Williams, G. D., & Kaldoudi, E. (2016). Towards privacy by design in personal e-health systems. In *9th international conference on health informatics* (pp. 472–477).
15. Fatema, N., & Brad, R. (2014). Security requirements, counterattacks and projects in healthcare applications using WSNs- a review. *International Journal of Computer Networking and Communication (IJCNAC), 2*(2), 1–9.
16. Santos-Pereira, C., Augusto, A. B., Cruz-Correia, R., & Correia, M. E. (2013). A secure RBAC mobile agent access control model for healthcare institutions. In *Proceedings of the 26th IEEE international symposium on computer-based medical systems* (pp. 349–354). IEEE.
17. Wellington, K. (2013). Cyberattacks on medical devices and hospital networks: Legal gaps and regulatory solutions. *Santa Clara High Technology Law Journal., 30*(2), 139–198.
18. Zhang, R., & Liu, L. (2010). Security models and requirements for healthcare application clouds. In *2010 IEEE 3rd international conference on cloud computing* (pp. 1–9). IEEE.

19. Firouzi, F., Rahmani, M., Mankodiya, K., Badaroglu, M., Merrett, G. V., Wong, P., & Farahani, B. (2018). Internet of-things and big data for smarter healthcare: From device to architecture, applications and analytics. *Future Generation Computer Systems, 78*(pt 2), 583–586.
20. Mare, S., Sorber, J., Shin, M., & Cornelius, C., & Kotz, D. (2011). Adapt-lite: Privacy-aware, secure, and efficient mhealth sensing. In *Proceedings of the 10th annual ACM workshop on privacy in the electronic society* (pp. 137–142). CCS.
21. Saleh, S., Farah, A., Dimassi, H., et al. (2018). Using mobile health to enhance outcomes of non-communicable diseases care in rural settings and refugee camps: Randomized controlled trial. *JMIR mHealth and uHealth, 6*(7), e137.
22. Sharma, S., Chen, K., & Sheth, A. (2018). Towards practical privacy preserving analytics for IoT and cloud based healthcare systems. *IEEE Internet Computing, 22*(2), 42–51.
23. Zubaydi, F., Saleh, A., Aloul, F., & Sagahyroon, A. (2016). Security of mobile health (mHealth) systems. In *2015 IEEE 15th international conference on bioinformatics and bioengineering (BIBE)* (pp. 1–6). IEEE.
24. Wang, J., et al. (2013). A research on security and privacy issues for patient related data in medical organization system. *International Journal of Security and Its Applications, 7*(4), 287–298.
25. Zhang, K., et al. (2014). Sybil attacks and their defenses in the internet of things. *IEEE Internet of Things Journal, 1*(5), 372–383.
26. Boonyarattaphan, A., Bai, Y., & Chung, S. (2009). A security framework for e-health service authentication and e-health data transmission. In *Communications and information technology, 2009. ISCIT 2009. 9th International Symposium on. 2009*. IEEE.
27. Garcia-Morchon, O., & Wehrle, K. (2010). Efficient and context- aware access control for pervasive medical sensor networks. In *8th IEEE international conference on pervasive computing and communications workshops (PERCOM workshops)* (pp. 322–327). IEEE.
28. Amini, S., Verhoeven, R., Lukkien, J. J., & Chen, S. (2011). Toward a security model for a body sensor platform. In *2011 IEEE international conference in consumer electronics (ICCE)* (pp. 143–144). Institute of Electrical and Electronics Engineers.
29. Maw, H. A., & Xiao, H., & Christianson, B. (2013). An adaptive access control model for medical data in wireless sensor networks. In *15th international conference on e-health networking, applications & services (Healthcom)* (pp. 1–8). IEEE.
30. Linciya, T., & Anandkumar, K. (2013). Enhanced three tier security architecture for WSN against mobile sink replication attacks using mutual authentication scheme. *International Journal of Wireless & Mobile Networks, 5*(2), 81–93.
31. Rasheed, A., & Mahapatra, R. N. (2012). The three-tier security scheme in wireless sensor networks with mobile sinks. *IEEE Transactions on Parallel and Distributed Systems, 23*(5), 958–965.
32. Kahani, N., Elgazzar, K., & Cordy, J. R. (2016). Authentication and access control in e-health systems in the cloud. In 2016 *IEEE 2nd international conference on big data security on cloud (BigDataSecurity), IEEE international conference on high performance and smart computing (HPSC), and IEEE international conference on intelligent data and security (IDS)* (pp. 13–23).
33. Guan, Z., Yang, T., & Du, X. (2015). Achieving secure and efficient data access control for cloud-integrated body sensor networks. *International Journal of Distributed Sensor Networks, 2015*, 1–11.
34. Simplicio, M. A., Jr., Iwaya, L. H., Barros, B. M., Carvalho, T. C. M. B., & Näslund, M. (2015). Secure Health: A delay-tolerant security framework for mobile health data collection. *IEEE Journal of Biomedical and Health Informatics, 19*(2), 761–772.
35. Sun, L., & Wang, H. (2011). A purpose based usage access control model for e-healthcare services. In *2011 international conference on data and knowledge engineering (ICDKE)*. IEEE.
36. Shahina, S., Minni, G., & Yasin, S. (2016). Sharing personal health records in cloud with scalable and secure using ABE. *International Journal of Emerging Technology in Computer Science & Electronics, 23*(8).

37. Wang, C.-J., Xu, X.-L., Shi, D.-Y., & Lin, W.-L. (2014). An efficient cloud-based personal health records system using attribute-based encryption and anonymous multi receiver identity-based encryption. In *Ninth international conference on P2P, parallel, grid, cloud and internet computing-IEEE* (pp. 74–81).
38. Siddiqui, N., Husain, M. S., & Akbar, M. (2016). Analysis of security challenges in vehicular adhoc network. In *Proceedings of international conference on advancement in computer engineering & information technology* (pp. s87–s90). IJCSIT.
39. Masood, I., Wang, Y., Daud, A., Aljohani, N. R., & Dawood, H. (2018). Towards smart healthcare: Patient data privacy and security in sensor-cloud infrastructure. *Wireless Communications and Mobile Computing, Hindawi, 2018*, 1–23.
40. Verma, A., Arif, M., & Husain, M. S. (2018). Analysis of DDOS attack detection and prevention in cloud environment: A review. *International Journal of Advanced Research in Computer Science, 9*, 107–113.
41. Mu, K., & Li, L. (2014). An efficient pair wise key predistribution scheme for wireless sensor networks. *Journal of Networks, 9*(2), 277–282.
42. Ramli, S. N., et al. (2013). A biometric-based security for data authentication in wireless body area network (wban). In *15th international conference on advanced communication technology (ICACT)*. IEEE.
43. Siddiqui, N., & Husain, M. S. (2016). CTS: A credit based threshold system to minimize the dissemination of faulty data in vehicular adhoc networks. *International Journal of Control Theory and Applications, 9*, 8499–8508.
44. Husain, M. S. (2020). Nature inspired approach for intrusion detection systems. In *Design and analysis of security protocol for communication* (pp. 171–182).
45. Siddiqui, N., & Husain, M. S. (2016). An approach to minimize faulty data propagation in vehicular adhoc network. *HCTL Open International Journal of Technology Innovations and Research (IJTIR), 21*, 26–38.
46. Sun, W., Cai, Z., Li, Y., Liu, F., Fang, S., & Wang, G. (2018). *Security and privacy in the medical internet of things: A review, security and communication networks*. Hindawi.

Chapter 7
Body Sensor Networks for Healthcare: Advancements and Solutions

Ash Mohammad Abbas

7.1 Introduction

A network of sensor devices that communicate using wireless links and help in monitoring the health of human beings is often called body sensor networks (BSNs) or body area networks (BANs). A BSN or BAN has many applications such as health monitoring of patients, intensive care unit (ICU), monitoring movements, preparing patient histories, etc. A BSN can be used for healthcare of both indoor and outdoor patients. The use of a BSN becomes significantly important in case of pandemics for remote monitoring of patients by physicians and medical staff.

A lot of research is carried out by different researchers pertaining to BSNs from different perspectives. Electromyogram (EMG) is used to sense strain in muscles of a human body. The readings of EMG sensors can be sent over a network using a wireless body area network (WBAN) to physicians for analysis who are at remote locations. A description of such an application is provided in [1]. An energy-efficient algorithm for mobile BSNs with multihop topology is presented in [2]. A contactless system for EEG/ECG using wireless sensors is presented in [3] for BSNs. It consists of electrodes that are capacitative in nature. The system consists of a minimal number of wires on the body.

Traditional method of measuring blood pressure (BP) is based on cuff. Such a method provides better readings; however, it is cumbersome to repeat the measurements frequently. For a continuous measurement of BP, a cuffless method is better suited to measure the BP in a passive manner. Such devices contain sensors and can be worn by patients. With the help of such devices, it is possible to uncover the

A. M. Abbas (✉)
Department of Computer Engineering, Aligarh Muslim University, Aligarh, India
e-mail: am.abbas.ce@amu.ac.in

M. S. Husain et al. (eds.), *Pervasive Healthcare*, EAI/Springer Innovations in Communication and Computing, https://doi.org/10.1007/978-3-030-77746-3_7

variations in BP during various activities of patients. A survey of the research in this direction is presented in [4].

Advancements in sensor technology enabled to produce printable, flexible, and stretchable sensors that are used in ECG, photoplethysmography (PPG) and tonoarteriography (TAG). Note that all these techniques can be combined into a wearable BSN. TAG is a technique that provides a continuous and cuffless measurement of arterial BP. A TAG-based BSN that consists of ECG and PPG sensors is proposed in [5]. The BSN takes into account the effect of change in posture on pulse transit time (PTT) of TAG, ECG and PPG. Further, the correlation among PTTs of these techniques is studied.

A description of cognitive sensing in BSN is presented in [6] containing its features and challenges. The presentation covers bio-inspired sensing and quorum sensing for a self-organized and self-managed network. In a BSN, multiple sensors collect clinical information for enhancement of accuracy. A scheme for separating sources of information using independent component analysis (ICA) is proposed in [7].

The devices might be implanted inside the body, worn or lying in close proximity of the body of a person or a creature. A concept called human body networks (HBN) is presented in [9]. Technology-assisted living is an application of wireless sensor networks that possesses a potential in the market. A description of quality of service (QoS) in BSN from the point of view of aggregator is presented in [8]. A comparison of different schemes for BSNs is provided in Table 7.1.

In this chapter, we present a survey of the research related to BSNs. We point out their applications together with different issues and challenges pertaining to the research in the area of BSNs. We describe the research related to different architectural frameworks of BSNs. We consider both wearable and nonwearable BSNs. We present advancements and schemes related to infrastructure of BSNs. Further, we describe research related to privacy and security in case of BSNs.

Table 7.1 A comparison of different schemes for BSN

Scheme	Basis	Features
EMG [1]	To sense strain in muscles in the body	Sending EMG readings to physicians using WBAN
Energy-efficient algorithm [2]	Mobile BSN	Multihop topology
Contactless system for EEG/ECG [3]	Wireless sensors	Capacitative electrodes
TAG-based BSN [5]	Cuffless measurement of arterial BP	Effect of change in PTT, ECG and PPG
Cognitive sensing in BSN [6]	Bio-inspired and quorum sensing	Self-organized and self-managed network
Source separation [7]	ICA	Enhancement of accuracy
Technology-assisted living [8]	QoS at aggregator	Marketing potential

7.2 Applications, Issues and Challenges

There are many applications of BSNs related to healthcare of people. Some of them are as follows:

- *Intensive care*: A BSN can be helpful in intensive care unit (ICU). It reduces delays in sending notifications related to the conditions of patients. The devices that are part of a BSN may collect different parameters for clinical analysis. It may help doctors diagnose the disease from symptoms and prescribe remedies to patients.
- *Health monitoring*: Using BSNs the doctors and medical staff can monitor the health of patients. The parameters related to health such as temperature, blood pressure, blood sugar, heart rate, etc. can be measured and monitored.
- *Diagnostic tests*: There are tests such as treadmill stress test (TMT) where BSNs can be used for measuring different parameters such as blood pressure, heart rate, ECG, etc.
- *Monitoring of movements*: Using a BSN, the movements of patients with diseases such as Alzheimer's and dementia can be monitored, and remedial measures can be initiated in a timely manner.
- *Monitoring exercises*: In physical fitness centres, one may monitor parameters such as blood pressure, heart rate, etc., so as to monitor the speed of different types of exercises.
- *Patients' history*: The data gathered by different sensor devices can be used to prepare histories of patients in a precise and accurate manner. This may help in diagnosing the cause of illness and the kind of treatment the patient needs.

Additionally, BSNs have other applications. For example, a BSN for applications in sports is presented in [10]. A summary of different applications of a BSN is provided in Fig. 7.1.

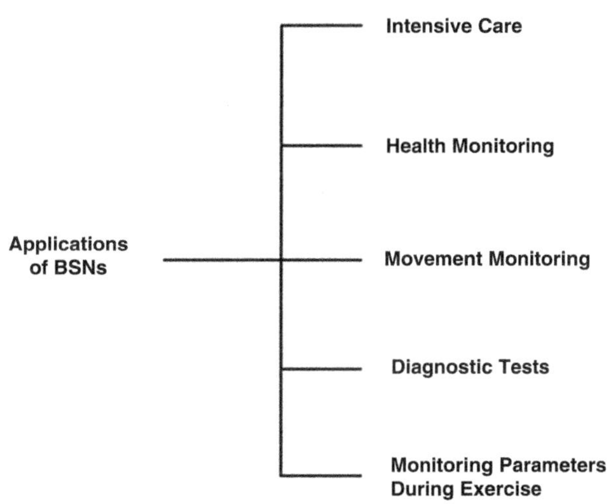

Fig. 7.1 Some applications of a body sensor network

The devices used in forming a BSN are small in size and possess limited resources. There are many issues and challenges pertaining to BSNs. Some of them are as follows:

- *Low power*: The devices used to form a BSN should not consume too much power as the devices are operated through batteries. The depletion of battery power may make the devices useless in a BSN.
- *High bandwidth*: The communication in case of hospital environment is crucial. Therefore, the devices in a BSN should be able to communicate at the data rates as high as possible.
- *Low cost*: The devices needed for healthcare applications should be available at affordable prices. In other words, the devices that are part of a BSN should be available at low cost to ensure their widespread use.
- *Harmless*: The devices used to form a BSN are likely to be in close proximity of the human body; therefore, such devices should be free from all electro-magnetic radiations to avoid harmful effects.

Additionally, sensors that are part of a BSN should be very small in size and inconspicuous. Issues and requirements for BSNs are presented in [11]. Care and monitoring of the patients need to be improved from the point of view of logistic constraints of healthcare professionals and patients. Therein, the components of a BSN such as wireless links, coupling among bodies, and coexistence of BSNs are studied.

7.3 Architecture of BSN

Figure 7.2 shows an architecture of a BSN in a hospital environment. It consists of three major components: (1) patients with sensors spread over their bodies, (2) measurement devices connected to sensors and (3) patient care unit with doctors and related medical staff. The patient care unit is part of the hospital which contains other units as well such as emergency unit, wards, central lab, diagnostic centres, outdoor patient's unit, departments, speciality and super-speciality centres, etc. The data collection in various constituent units of a hospital is computerized. The hospital contains servers and computing facilities to analyse the data.

There can be various types of sensors for measurement of different parameters related to health such as glucose level, blood pressure, temperature, oxygen level, heart rate, pulse rate, EEG, ECG, movement monitoring, etc. The sensors are connected to the respective measurement devices. The measurement devices send the data about different health parameters to a data collection unit that is connected to computing devices or servers. The data is processed using machine learning techniques to extract meaningful information so as to send it to the attending doctors or medical staff in the patient care unit. The human body sensors connected to the respective measurement devices may send the data directly to the attending doctors and medical staff of the patient care unit in case of emergency. Note that we have

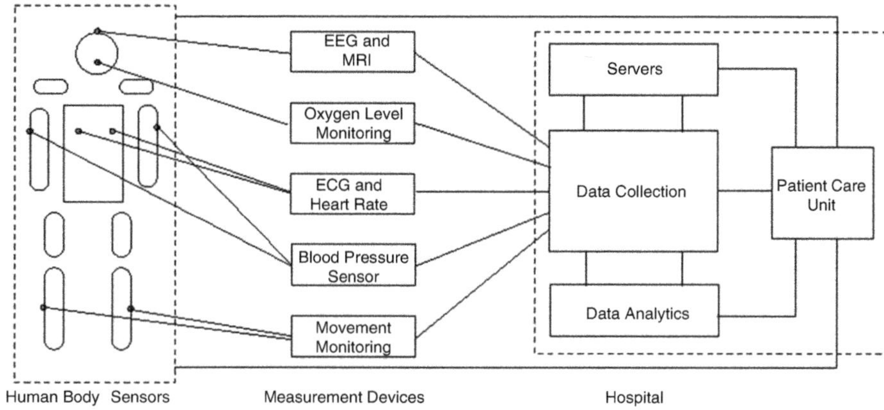

Fig. 7.2 An architecture of a body sensor network in a hospital environment

shown only a single patient in the architecture of a BSN for ease of understandability. The human body sensors and the measurement devices can be replicated for a number of patients in a hospital environment.

A framework called SenseFace is proposed in [12] for sending the data collected by sensors in a BSN to an online social network. It takes into account the mobility of both BSN and the social network. An architecture for monitoring of patients in a BSN called DexterNet is presented in [13, 14] that consists of three layers, namely, body sensor layer (BSL), personal network layer (PNL) and global network library (GNL). A software library called Signal Processing in Node Environment (SPINE) contains an abstraction of BSL and PNL and can be used instantaneously to reconfigure DexterNet.

A three-layered architecture called SENET for wireless body sensor networks (WBSN) is proposed in [15]. Layer 1, the lower most layer, consists of body sensors; layer 2, the middle layer, contains Internet of Things (IoT) devices; and the layer 3, the top-most layer, consists of machine learning techniques running on computers. The performance of machine learning algorithms such as genetic algorithm (GA), particle swarm optimization (PSO), ant colony optimization (ACO) and world competitive contests (WCC) is evaluated. The performance of a system can be enhanced using a multi-core design scheme. An architecture called hybrid wireless network on chip (WNoC) is proposed in [16] for multi-core BSN (MBSN) applications together with an analysis of traffic.

A healthcare IoT may consist of a large number of wearable sensors together with computing elements. Due to a huge amount of data to be processed, an issue is to send data from servers to end users in real time. In other words, the end-to-end delays need to be minimized. A three-tier architecture based on a combination of machine learning and fog computing techniques to reduce delays in healthcare IoTs is proposed in [17]. Further, an analysis of healthcare IoT that consists of reinforcement learning in a fog computing scenario is carried out and is validated through simulations using a simulator called iFogSim. A summary of architectures for a BSN is provided in Table 7.2.

Table 7.2 A comparison of architectures for BSN

Architecture	Basis	Features
SenseFace [12]	Sending data to OSN	Mobility of OSN and BSN
SENET [15]	Three layers	Machine learning algorithms
DexterNet [13, 14]	Three layers called BSL, PNL and GNL	SPINE software library
Hybrid WNoC [16]	Multi-core design scheme	Analysis of traffic
Three-tier architecture [17]	Reduction in delays	Analysis of healthcare IoT using RL

7.4 Body Sensor Networks

In this section, we describe schemes related to wearable and nonwearable body sensor networks.

7.4.1 Wearable BSNs

There is a lot of impact of wireless sensor networks (WSN) on human life, and BSN is a class of WSN where the deployment is the human body instead of a field. Different disorders occurring with aging such as cognitive impairments, dementia, and Alzheimer's can be diagnosed early based on investigations about locomotion. Cloths with wearable sensors can be used for locomotion monitoring. A wearable BSN for locomotion monitoring is presented in [18]. An increasing interest is created in BSN with wearable sensors for enabling healthcare based on technological advancements. The wearable devices can be wireless thermometer, glucometer, pulse and blood pressure meter, hearing and visual aids, etc. A survey of devices that are wearable is provided in [19]. Wearable BSNs based on smart textiles help in monitoring the health of human beings. The challenges faced by wearable BSNs include reduction of the size of sensors and antennas and embedding them into wearable textiles. A survey of research related to wearable BSNs is provided in [20].

A wearable battery-free BSN using near-field-based textiles is presented in [21]. Body sensors are embedded in cloths to be worn by patients for monitoring of different parameters related to their health. Such cloths, often called smart cloths, need to be comfortable. Strategies and solutions related to smart cloths in a European project called MyHeart are described in [22]. A spoof surface plasmon (SSP) clothing for WBAN is described in [23] from the point of view of robustness and energy efficiency. A wearable BSN comprising of metamaterial textiles is presented in [24]. It is capable of transferring the power wirelessly in an energy-efficient manner.

The design of a wearable health monitoring system called LifePebble is described in [25]. It measures the temperature, heart rate, electrocardiogram (ECG) and physical movement in three-dimensional space. It consists of a system on chip (SoC) called Sensium™ customized for the design of wearable BSNs. It is suited for monitoring the lifestyles of patients in early stages of type 2 diabetes. A comparison of schemes for wearable BSNs is provided in Table 7.3.

7.4.2 *Nonwearable BSN*

The effect of placement of body node coordinators (BNCs) in an intra-body sensor network (intra-BSN) is examined in [26]. In a BSN, the data collected by sensors needs to be forwarded to a BNC through an intermediate node called a forwarder. The forwarder is selected based on optimizing a cost function such as the remaining energy and path loss from a sensor to BNC. An intra-wireless body sensor networks (intra-WBSN) is a network with short-range devices and is often used in monitoring health of patients. A protocol called relay-based energy-efficient routing (REER) for intra-WBSN is proposed in [27]. The major issues in such networks are maximizing the lifetime of the network and minimizing the energy consumption. In other words, minimizing the energy consumption leads to maximizing the network lifetime. Sensor devices forward the data to body node coordinator (BNC) through intermediate relay nodes that are embedded in cloths that can be recharged and replaced.

There are chances of inter-user interference (IUI) when two or more BSNs are in close vicinity adversely affecting the speed of transmission of data. The effect of IUI on the performance of BSNs in terms of packet error ratio (PER) is evaluated in [28]. Therein, the effect of transmission power, node density and traffic intensity is studied for deployment of BSNs in a hospital. There are wearable, implantable and ingestible sensors that are often used for diagnostic purposes. Sensors can be connected to cloud to overcome their resource limitations. A description of cloud-enabled BSN together with simulation results is provided in [29].

The use of resources of ambient sensors may help in extending the lifetime of batteries of wearable sensors in a BSN. It may also help enhance the coverage of a BSN and may lead to sensing that is aware of the context. Autonomic sensing allows a BSN to manage its topology depending on the resources of its sensor devices. A self-organizing approach for a network containing a combination of ambient and wearable sensors is proposed in [30] using a clustering scheme. The cluster heads are selected using the Maximum a Posteriori (MAP) scheme taking into account the

Table 7.3 A comparison of schemes for wearable BSNs

Scheme	Basis	Features
Wearable BSN-1 [18]	Locomotion monitoring	To diagnose disorders with aging
Wearable BSN-2 [21]	Near-field-based textiles	Battery-free
Wearable BSN-3 [24]	Consists of metamaterial textiles	Wireless power transfer
Smart cloths [22]	Based on MyHeart project	Strategies and solutions
LifePebble [25]	Sensium SoC	Monitoring diabetic type 2 patients

Table 7.4 A comparison of schemes for nonwearable BSNs

Scheme	Basis	Features
Placement of BNCs [26]	Intra-BSN	Optimization of energy and path loss
REER [27]	Intra-WBSN	Maximizing lifetime of a BSN
Effect of IUI [28]	Packet error ratio	Deployment of BSN in a hospital
Cloud-enabled BSN [29]	Overcomes resource limitations of sensors	Used for diagnostic purposes
Self-organizing approach [30]	Clustering scheme	CH selection using MAP scheme

remaining energy of sensors, connectivity and distance to the sink. A comparison of schemes for nonwearable BSNs is provided in Table 7.4.

7.5 Advancements in Infrastructure of BSNs

In this section, we describe advancements pertaining to the human body sensors and wireless body area networks (WBAN).

7.5.1 Sensors for BSN

Body sensors are devices that operate in the close vicinity of the human body. There are many types of body sensors such as bionic ear, bionic eye, pacemaker, wireless capsule, etc. An overview of sensors used in BSN is provided in [31]. In a BSN, pressure sensors such as force-sensitive resistor (FSR) and piezoelectric sensors (PES) are often used to measure the force exerted by limbs in human bodies. These sensors need to be flexible in order to use them for monitoring movement of human bodies. The design of a FSR-based flexible pressure sensor using composition of electrode and carbon-infused thin film conductive layers is presented in [32].

A BSN should enable remote monitoring for treatment of patients. An Android/OSGi-based mobile gateway for BSNs is proposed in [36] containing data transfer interface, graphical user interface and a server for management of wireless sensors that can be accessed remotely through mobile phones. The design of wireless antennas and wireless sensor node for BSNs using radio frequency of 17 GHz is proposed in [35]. A survey of medium access control (MAC) layer protocols for storing the energy in a BSN is presented in [38].

To address the issue of data availability, a BSN should have a transceiver with multiple radios. Such a system is presented in [33] that enables it to operate using multiple frequency bands. A scheme for communication among sensors of healthcare devices to a central sensor that monitors the health of a patient in a BSN is proposed

Table 7.5 A comparison of advancement in sensors for BSNs

Scheme	Basis	Features
Transceiver with multiple radios [33]	Addresses issue of data availability	Operates in multiple frequency bands
Communication among sensors and sink [34]	Network coding	To mitigate the effect of fading
BSN node [35]	Wireless antenna	Uses a radio frequency of 17 GHz
Pressure sensors [32]	Based on FSR	Use of thin-film conductive layers
Mobile gateway [36]	Android/OSGi	Remote monitoring of patients
CC-IBC [37]	Electro-optical sensor	In vivo communications

in [34]. The scheme is based on cooperation among sensors using network coding and tries to reduce the effect of fading as compared to the direct data transfer schemes.

A promising technology for BSN is intra-body communication (IBC). Its characteristics include low power consumption, higher bandwidth and security for short-distance communication using wireless links. A capacitative coupling IBC-based BSN that uses Mach-Zhender electro-optical (EO) sensor is proposed in [37]. The in vivo experiments are used to verify the frequency response of signals transmitted through different paths. Frequency-division multiple access (FDMA) is used for transmission of signals. The objective is to achieve reliable, economic and high-speed transmission of signals in a BSN. A comparison of advancement in sensors for BSNs is provided in Table 7.5.

7.5.2 *Wireless BAN*

Wireless body area networks (WBAN) are often used for monitoring the health of patients. The body sensors used in a WBAN are operated through batteries with limited power. Persons that are hospitalized are often termed as indoor patients. A WBAN may help in measurement of physiological data and daily care of indoor patients. Also, a WBAN reduces latencies in diagnosing a disease and prescription of remedies by physicians. However, movements of patients during the period of their daily care may affect reliable transmission of signals. A cross-layer reliable transmission scheme (CL-RRS) based on IEEE 802.15.6 is proposed in [42]. It detects a sensor with failed transmission and enhances the probability of successful transmissions.

In [40], creation of a WBAN by spreading tiny sensors on the human body is described. It has been pointed out that with the movement of the body, the distribution of sensors that is assumed to be uniform may change, and there can be holes in the network. A routing scheme using the position information of sensors equipped with GPS devices is presented that takes into account the remaining energy of sensors. Note that such a notion of a WBAN is feasible only when the GPS provides locations up to a precision of centimetres. Generally, the locations provided by GPS are not so precisely specified. Delivering locations up to such a precision can be a direction for future generations of networks.

The objective of a WBAN is to monitor the health of patients and forward the data towards a base station also called a sink. A challenge in routing the data in a WBAN is due to the human body as a medium of transmission. There can be two types of WBANs, namely, on-body and in-body. The latter type of WBAN is more constrained as compared to the former type of WBAN. A survey of routing protocols for in-body WBANs is presented in [44]. An energy-efficient medium access control (MAC) layer protocol for prolonging the lifetime of a WBAN is proposed in [43]. The proposed protocol is a combination of carrier-sense multiple access (CSMA) with collision avoidance (CA) and time division multiple access (TDMA).

A WBAN based on capacitative coupling body channel communication (CC-BCC) incurs less energy consumption as compared to other schemes. In CC-BCC, the human body is used as a medium to forward the signal that results in significantly small path loss. A low-power body communication channel for wearable BAN is demonstrated in [41] that includes micro-inertial measurement unit (μ-IMU), temperature sensor and CC-BCC module. The rise in the temperature may damage the neighbouring tissues in a wireless BSN. A temperature-aware routing protocol for WBSNs is presented in [45] that takes into account movements of patients. A Bluetooth-based WBSN is designed in [46] for recordkeeping applications. It consists of a sensor node and a user interface device to be worn on the wrist of a patient. A group-based reliable data transport (GRDT) protocol is proposed in [47] for WBSN using a combination of time division multiple access (TDMA) and frequency-division multiple access (FDMA) schemes. Designs of WBSN for coal mine applications using genetic algorithms to optimize energy consumption are presented in [48, 49].

The sensors used to form a WBAN are low-power devices that are used to monitor the health of patients. The design of a MAC protocol is a crucial task in case of WBAN because it decides several key functions in a WBAN. A programmable MAC called one command at a time for WBANs using low-power sensors is proposed in [50], which is based on IEEE 802.15.6 standard. The IEEE 802.15.6 standard has a beacon frame structure that is comprised of exclusive access phase (EAP) and random access phase (RAP). A MAC protocol for WBSN based on dynamic EAP is proposed in [51]. A poll-based MAC protocol called PMAC for WBAN is proposed in [52]. It consists of mechanisms for energy efficiency and QoS. An adaptive MAC protocol called AD-MAC is proposed in [53]. It has mechanisms for dynamically assigning priorities, time slots and length.

A scheme for activation of sensors that provides a trade-off between power consumption and the probability of misclassification of health of patients is described in [39]. The flow of information and response of a WBAN are modelled using a Partially Observable Markov Decision Process (POMDP). Further, a learning algorithm is developed to evaluate health state transition probabilities using the data gathered about a group of patients that are monitored using a WBAN. A network

Table 7.6 A comparison of schemes for WBAN

Scheme	Basis	Features
Sensor activation scheme [39]	Health transition probabilities	POMDP model
Creation of WBAN [40]	Routing scheme	Positional information using GPS
Capacitative WBAN [41]	CC-BCC	Includes μ-IMU and temperature sensor
CL-RRS [42]	IEEE 802.15.6	Enhancement of successful transmissions
Energy-efficient MAC [43]	CSMA-CA and TDMA	Prolonging lifetime of BSN

layer protocol called iTALK is proposed in [54] for BSNs with star topology and is based on IEEE 802.15.4 MAC layer. A comparison of schemes for WBANs is provided in Table 7.6.

7.6 Security in BSN

A BSN leads to store information about various parameters related to health status of patients. The data needs to be stored and transferred in a secure manner. A survey of research related to security in BSN is presented in [55]. In case of medical BSNs, a basic requirement pertaining to the security is management of cryptographic keys. The issue is that the management of keys in medical context should conform to the security in healthcare domain together with resource constraints of BSNs. A service for management of keys for hospital BSNs is presented in [56] based on deterministic pairwise key pre-distribution scheme (DPKPS). Therein, it is observed that the security in a BSN is provided economically together with low power consumption.

An architecture for providing security in case of a BSN is proposed in [59]. The major focus is the use of body channel for privacy of data and the use of physiological data in enhancing the security. An enormous amount of research is carried out to use secure and private communication protocols for BSNs. An architectural framework called DependData is proposed in [58] to verify data dependability in BSNs used for monitoring the health of patients. The framework consists of three decision-making (DM) layers to verify dependable data at different levels. The first layer verifies the signal data at the sensors, the second layer verifies the data at each local aggregator and the third layer verifies the data at the remote user level. The verifications at all layers ensure the dependability of data.

Electronic health records (EHRs) enable patients to maintain the record about their health and may share them with others whenever required. However, EHRs are prone to different types of security and privacy attacks during their transmission. An architectural framework called Blockchain-Based Deep Learning as-a-Service (BinDaaS) is proposed in [57] for secure transmission of EHRs. It is a combination of blockchain and deep learning techniques. It contains a blockchain-based authentication and signature technique using lattice-based cryptography and the prediction

Table 7.7 A comparison of schemes for provision of security in BSNs

Scheme	Basis	Features
BinDaaS [57]	Lattice-based cryptography	Electronic health records
DependData [58]	Data dependability	Decision-making layers
DPKPS [56]	Key management for hospital BSN	Low power consumption
Security architecture [59]	Use of body channel	Use of physiological data to enhance security
Security analysis of IEEE 802.15.6 [60]	Elliptic curve cryptography	Vulnerability to attacks

of ensuing diseases using deep learning techniques. IEEE 802.15.6 is an international standard for WBAN that includes elliptic curve-based cryptographic protocols for agreement and generation of keys. Analysis of vulnerabilities of the key generation protocols of IEEE 802.15.6 is carried out in [60]. A comparison of schemes for provision of security in BSNs is provided in Table 7.7.

7.7 Conclusion

Advancements in wireless sensor networks and miniaturization of sensors led to an emergence of a special class of networks called body sensor networks (BSNs). In this chapter, we presented a review of advancements in BSNs pertaining to healthcare applications. We considered wearable as well as nonwearable BSNs together with schemes and solutions. We pointed out issues and challenges pertaining to BSNs. We presented research related to different architectural frameworks for BSNs. We described research related to advancement in sensor technology, protocols and schemes for wireless body area networks. Further, we described research related to privacy and security in case of BSNs.

References

1. Al Rasyid, M. U. H., Prasetyo, D., Nadhori, I. U., & Alasiry, A. H. (2015). Mobile monitoring of muscular strain sensor based on wireless body area network. In *International electronics symposium (IES)* (pp. 284–287). IEEE.
2. Braem, B., De Cleyn, P., & Blondia, C. (2010). Supporting mobility in body sensor networks. In *IEEE international conference on body sensor networks* (pp. 52–55). IEEE.
3. Chi, Y. M., & Cauwenberghs, G. (2010). Wireless non-contact EEG/ECG electrodes for body sensor networks. In *International conference on body sensor networks* (pp. 297–301). IEEE.
4. Pandit, J. A., Lores, E., & Batlle, D. (2020). Cu_ess blood pressure monitoring: Promises and challenges. *Clinical Journal of the American Society of Nephrology, 15*(10), 1531–1538.
5. Ding, X., Dai, W., Luo, N., Liu, J., Zhao, N., & Zhang, Y. (2015). A flexible tonoarteriography-based body sensor network for cuffless measurement of arterial blood pressure. In *2015 IEEE*

12th international conference on wearable and implantable body sensor networks (BSN) (pp. 1–4). IEEE.
6. Yang, G.-Z. (2008). Cognitive sensing for body sensor networks. *Sensors, 2008*, 612.
7. Lo, B., Deligianni, F., & Yang, G. Z. (2006). Source recovery for body sensor network. In *International workshop on wearable and implantable body sensor networks (BSN)* (p. 4). Springer.
8. Zhou, G., Wan, C., Yarvis, M. D., & Stankovic, J. A. (2007). Aggregator-centric qos for body sensor networks. In *IEEE 6th international symposium on information processing in sensor networks* (pp. 539–540). IEEE.
9. Wu, Z., Xiao, D., Peng, X., Xu, H., & Zhuang, X. (2008). Human body network: Network in the future? In *IEEE international symposium on knowledge acquisition and modeling workshop* (pp. 578–581). IEEE.
10. Sabti, H. A., & Thiel, D. V. (2014). Time multiplexing-star shape body sensor network for sports applications. In *IEEE antennas and propagation society international symposium (APSURSI)* (pp. 969–970). IEEE.
11. Davenport, D. M., Deb, B., & Ross, F. J. (2009). Wireless propagation and coexistence of medical body sensor networks for ambulatory patient monitoring. In *IEEE sixth international workshop on wearable and implantable body sensor networks* (pp. 41–45). IEEE.
12. Abdur Rahman, M., El Saddik, A., & Gueaieb, W. (2009). Data visualization: From body sensor network to social networks. In *IEEE international workshop on robotic and sensors environments* (pp. 157–162). IEEE.
13. Bajcsy, R. (2010). A wireless body sensor network for different health related applications. In *IEEE international conference on sensor networks, ubiquitous, and trustworthy computing* (p. 1). IEEE.
14. Kuryloski, P., Giani, A., Giannantonio, R., Gilani, K., Gravina, R., Seppa, V., Seto, E., Shia, V., Wang, C., Yan, P., Yang, A. Y., Hyttinen, J., Sastry, S., Wicker, S., & Bajcsy, R. (2009). Dexternet: An open platform for heterogeneous body sensor networks and its applications. In *IEEE sixth international workshop on wearable and implantable body sensor networks* (pp. 92–97). IEEE.
15. Bulaghi, Z. A., Navin, A. H. Z., Hosseinzadeh, M., & Rezaee, A. (2020). Senet: A novel architecture for IOT-based body sensor networks. *Informatics in Medicine Unlocked, 20*, 100365.
16. Elmiligi, H., Gebali, F., Watheq El-Kharashi, M., & Morgan, A. A. (2015). Traffic analysis of multi-core body sensor networks based on wireless noc infrastructure. In *IEEE pacific rim conference on communications, computers and signal processing (PACRIM)* (pp. 201–204). IEEE.
17. Shukla, S., Hassan, M. F., Jung, L. T., Awang, A., & Khan, M. K. (2019). A 3-tier architecture for network latency reduction in healthcare internet-of-things using fog computing and machine learning. In *Proceedings of the 8th international conference on software and computer applications (ICSCA)* (pp. 522–528). Association for Computing Machinery.
18. Barnes, J., Ramachandra, V., Gilani, K., Guenterberg, E., Ghasemzadeh, H., & Jafari, R. (2008). Locomotion monitoring using body sensor networks. In *International conference on information processing in sensor networks (IPSN)* (pp. 555–556). ACM.
19. Dias, D., & Cunha, J. P. S. (2018). Wearable health devices vital sign monitoring, systems and technologies. *Sensors, 18*(8), 2414.
20. Kim, Y. K., Wang, H., & Mahmud, M. S. (2016). Wearable body sensor network for healthcare applications. In V. Koncar (Ed.), *Smart textiles and their applications* (Woodhead publishing series in textiles) (pp. 161–184). Woodhead Publishing.
21. Lin, R., Kim, H.-J., Achavananthadith, S., Kurt, S. A., Tan, S. C. C., Yao, H., Tee, B. C. K., Lee, J. K. W., & Ho, J. S. (2020). Wireless battery-free body sensor networks using near-field-enabled clothing. *Nature Communications, 11*, 444.
22. Luprano, J., Sola, J., Dasen, S., Koller, J. M., & Chetelat, O. (2006). Combination of body sensor networks and on-body signal processing algorithms: the practical case of myheart project. In *International workshop on wearable and implantable body sensor networks (BSN)* (p. 79). IEEE.

23. Tian, X., Zhang, M., & Ho, J. S. (2019). Robust and high-efficiency wireless body area networks with spoof surface plasmons on clothing. In *IEEE MTT-S International Microwave Symposium (IMS)* (pp. 1507–1510). IEEE.
24. Tian, X., Lee, P. M., Tan, Y. J., Tina, L. Y. W., Yao, H., Zhang, M., Li, Z., Ng, K. A., Tee, C. K., & Ho, J. S. (2019). Wireless body sensor networks based on metamaterial textiles. *Nature Electronics, 2*, 243–251.
25. Silveira, M. H., Nunn, C., Lakhanpal, A., McDonagh, D., McPartland, R., & Burdett, A. (2009). Key considerations and experience using the ultra low power sensium platform in body sensor networks. In *Sixth international workshop on wearable and implantable body sensor networks* (pp. 262–266). IEEE.
26. Rashid, T., Kumar, S., & Kumar, A. (2017). Effect of body node coordinator (BNC) positions on the performance of intra-body sensor network (intra-wbsn). In *4th IEEE international conference on power, control and embedded systems (ICPCES)* (pp. 1–6). IEEE.
27. Rashid, T., Kumar, S., & Kumar, A. (2017). Reer: Relay based energy efficient routing for intra body sensor network (intra-wbsn). In *4th international conference on signal processing and integrated networks (SPIN)* (pp. 222–227). IEEE.
28. Sun, W., Yu, G., & Wong, W.-C. (2012). Inter-user interference in body sensor networks: A case study in moderate-scale deployment in hospital environment. In *IEEE 14th international conference on e-Health networking, applications and services (Healthcom)* (pp. 447–450). IEEE.
29. Yu, R., Mak, T. W. C., Zhang, R., Wong, S. H., Zheng, Y., Lau, J. Y. W., & Poon, C. C. Y. (2017). Smart healthcare: Cloud-enabled body sensor networks. In *IEEE 14th international conference on wearable and implantable body sensor networks (BSN)* (pp. 99–102). IEEE.
30. Yu, R., Yang, G., & Lo, B. P. L. (2014). Autonomic body sensor networks. In *IEEE MTT-S international microwave workshop series on RF and wireless technologies for biomedical and healthcare applications (IMWS-Bio)* (pp. 1–3). IEEE.
31. Yuce, M. R. (2013). Recent wireless body sensors: Design and implementation. In *IEEE MTT-S international microwave workshop series on RF and wireless technologies for biomedical and healthcare applications (IMWS-BIO)* (pp. 1–3). IEEE.
32. Salibindla, S., Ripoche, B., Lai, D. T. H., & Maas, S. (2013). Characterization of a new flexible pressure sensor for body sensor networks. In *IEEE eighth international conference on intelligent sensors, sensor networks and information processing* (pp. 27–31). IEEE.
33. Buckley, J., O'Flynn, B., Loizou, L., Haigh, P., Boyle, D., Angove, P., Barton, J., O'Mathuna, C., Popovici, E., & O'Connell, S. (2012). A novel and miniaturized 433/868mhz multi-band wireless sensor platform for body sensor network applications. In *Ninth international conference on wearable and implantable body sensor networks* (pp. 63–66). ACM.
34. Meng, Y., Qin, T., & Xing, J. (2014). Sensor cooperation based on network coding in wireless body area networks. In *International conference on wireless communication and sensor network* (pp. 358–361). ACM.
35. Rydberg, A., van Engen, P., Cheng, S., van Doremalen, R., Sanduleanu, M., Hjort, K., De Raedt, W., Fritzsch, T., & Hallbjorner, P. (2009). Body surface backed exible antennas and 3d si-level integrated wireless sensor nodes for 17 ghz wireless body area networks. In *2nd IET seminar on antennas and propagation for body-centric wireless communications* (pp. 1–4). IEEE.
36. Wang, Z., Hou, R., & Zhou, Z. (2016). An android/osgi-based mobile gateway for body sensor network. In *15th international symposium on parallel and distributed computing (ISPDC)* (pp. 135–140). IEEE.
37. Zhang, K., Song, Y., & Peng, J. (2018). Research on body sensor network based on the capacitive coupling intra-body communication using a mach-zehnder electro-optical sensor. In *2nd IEEE advanced information management, communicates, electronic and automation control conference (IMCEC)* (pp. 2336–2340). IEEE.
38. Liu, S., Wang, K., Guo, J., Wang, Y., & Qi, X. (2015). Review on mac protocols in energy-harvesting wireless body area networks. In *IEEE international conference on identification, information, and knowledge in the internet of things (IIKI)* (pp. 303–304). IEEE.

39. Geller, T., David, Y. B., Khmelnitsky, E., Ben-Gal, I., Ward, A., Miller, D., & Bambos, N. (2019). Learning health state transition probabilities via wireless body area networks. In *IEEE international conference on communications (ICC)* (pp. 1–6). IEEE.
40. Kim, K., Lee, I., Yoon, M., Kim, J., Lee, H., & Han, K. (2009). An efficient routing protocol based on position information in mobile wireless body area sensor networks. In *First international conference on networks communications* (pp. 396–399). IEEE.
41. Mao, J., Wang, W., Ding, G., & Zhang, Z. (2019). Live demonstration: Wearable body area network system based on low power body channel communication. In *IEEE biomedical circuits and systems conference (BioCAS)* (p. 1). IEEE.
42. Tseng, H., Wu, R., & Wu, Y. (2016). An efficient cross-layer reliable retransmission scheme for the human body shadowing in IEEE 802.15.6-based wireless body area networks. *IEEE Sensors Journal, 16*(9), 3282–3292.
43. Yang, X., Wang, L., & Zhang, Z. (2018). Wireless body area networks mac protocol for energy efficiency and extending lifetime. *IEEE Sensors Letters, 2*(1), 1–4.
44. Romaissa, B., & Eddine, B. D. (2017). In-body routing protocols for wireless body sensor networks. In *IEEE 10th international conference on developments in eSystems engineering (DeSE)* (pp. 160–165). IEEE.
45. Kim, B.-S., Kang, S. Y., Lim, J. H., Kim, K. H., & Kim, K.-I. (2017). A mobility-based temperature-aware routing protocol for wireless body sensor networks. In *IEEE international conference on information networking (ICOIN)* (pp. 63–66). IEEE.
46. Zhong, L., Sinclair, M., & Bittner, R. (2006). A phone-centered body sensor network platform cost, energy efficiency user interface. In *IEEE international workshop on wearable and implantable body sensor networks (BSN)* (p. 182). IEEE.
47. Geng, D., Zhao, Z., Fang, Z., Xuan, Y., Zhao, J., Wu, S., Xu, J., & Du, L. (2010). Grdt: Group-based reliable data transport in wireless body area sensor networks. In *IET international conference on wireless sensor network (IET-WSN)* (pp. 385–392). IEEE.
48. Ma, Y., & Wang, Y. (2009). Optimization design of undermine wireless sensor network based on genetic quantum algorithm. In *2009 Chinese control and decision conference* (pp. 4697–4701). IEEE.
49. Yong, M., Yu, Y., Yan, W., Huludao, L., Gang, L., & Ling, L. (2009). Optimization design of coal mine wireless body sensor network based on genetic algorithm. In *IEEE international conference on networks security, wireless communications and trusted computing* (Vol. 2, pp. 366–369). IEEE.
50. Michaelides, C., & Pavlidou, F. (2019). Programmable mac in body area networks, one command at a time. *IEEE Sensors Letters, 3*(7), 1–4.
51. Enkoji, A., Li, M., Brisky, J. D., & Melvin, R. (2019). Dynamic EAP based mac protocol for wireless body area networks. In *IEEE international conference on computing, networking and communications (ICNC)* (pp. 531–536). IEEE.
52. Bhatia, A., & Patro, R. K. (2016). Pmac: A poll-based mac protocol for wireless body area networks (WBANS). In *IEEE international conference on advanced networks and telecommunications systems (ANTS)* (pp. 1–6). IEEE.
53. Wang, J., Xie, Y., & Yi, Q. (2015). An all dynamic mac protocol for wireless body area network. In *11th IEEE international conference on wireless communications, networking and mobile computing (WiCOM 2015)* (pp. 1–6). IEEE.
54. Schlsser, M., Rzezniczek, L., Akgn, F., Ying, H., Seyrafi, A., & Schiek, M. (2009). Optimized network layer protocol for sensor driven autonomous real-time data fusion in a star bsn. In *IEEE international conference on intelligent sensors, sensor networks and information processing (ISSNIP)* (pp. 279–282). IEEE.
55. Sawaneh, I. A., Sankoh, I., & Koroma, D. K. (2017). A survey on security issues and wearable sensors in wireless body area network for healthcare system. In *IEEE 14th international computer conference on wavelet active media technology and information processing (ICCWAMTIP)* (pp. 304–308). IEEE.

56. Morchon, O. G., Baldus, H., & Sanchez, D. S. (2006). Resource-efficient security for medical body sensor networks. In *International workshop on wearable and implantable body sensor networks (BSN)* (p. 83). IEEE.
57. Bhattacharya, P., Tanwar, S., Bodke, U., Tyagi, S., & Kumar, N. (2019). Bindaas: Blockchain-based deep-learning as-a-service in healthcare 4.0 applications. In *IEEE transactions on network science and engineering* (p. 1). IEEE.
58. Hai, T., Bhuiyan, M. Z. A., Wang, J., Wang, T., Hsu, D. F., Li, Y., Salih, S. Q., Wu, J., & Liu, P. (2020). Dependdata: Data collection dependability through three-layer decision-making in BSNS for healthcare monitoring. *Information Fusion, 62*, 32–46.
59. Bao, S.-D., & Zhang, Y.-T. (2006). A design proposal of security architecture for medical body sensor networks. In *IEEE international workshop on wearable and implantable body sensor networks (BSN)* (p. 90). IEEE.
60. Toorani, M. (2015). On vulnerabilities of the security association in the IEEE 802.15.6 standard. In M. Brenner, N. Christin, B. Johnson, & K. Rohloff (Eds.), *International conference on financial cryptography and data security (FC)* (Vol. 8976, pp. 245–260). Springer.

Chapter 8
Artificial Intelligence Algorithms for Healthcare and Neurorehabilitation Engineering

Sateesh Reddy Avutu and Sudip Paul

8.1 Introduction

Artificial intelligence (AI) is an extensive branch of computer science used to simulate machines' human intelligence processes. The goal of AI is to create systems that can function independently and intelligently. Figure 8.1 shows the brief technical structure of AI. It has to work based on symbolic learning or machine learning. In machine learning, to train the machine, the user has to feed enormous data. Symbolic learning uses images with different symbols to learn the classification and prediction of the data used above techniques. The human brain is a network of neurons. The neural networks replicate the human brain's structure and function, helping to develop the machines' cognitive capabilities. If the neural networks are more complex and more in-depth to learn, use deep learning techniques. The various forms of deep learning machinery have a different way of replicating the individual's anatomy. To scan the input images from top to bottom and left to right for object recognition through computer vision, the convolution neural networks (CNN) are complicated in AI. Recurrent neural networks (RNN) can use to remember the past activities by the machine. The AI uses three kinds of learning techniques named supervised, unsupervised, and reinforcement learning. Goleman et al. sufficiently explained the motivation behind AI development and history [1].

AI finds its place in all the fields such as agriculture, medicine, education, economics, and many more; however, this chapter has devoted to providing comprehensive notes on various rehabilitation devices and testing each device's performance concerning AI. The different algorithms commonly used in several rehabilitation

S. R. Avutu · S. Paul (✉)
Department of Biomedical Engineering, North-Eastern Hill University,
Shillong, India, Meghalaya

M. S. Husain et al. (eds.), *Pervasive Healthcare*, EAI/Springer Innovations in Communication and Computing, https://doi.org/10.1007/978-3-030-77746-3_8

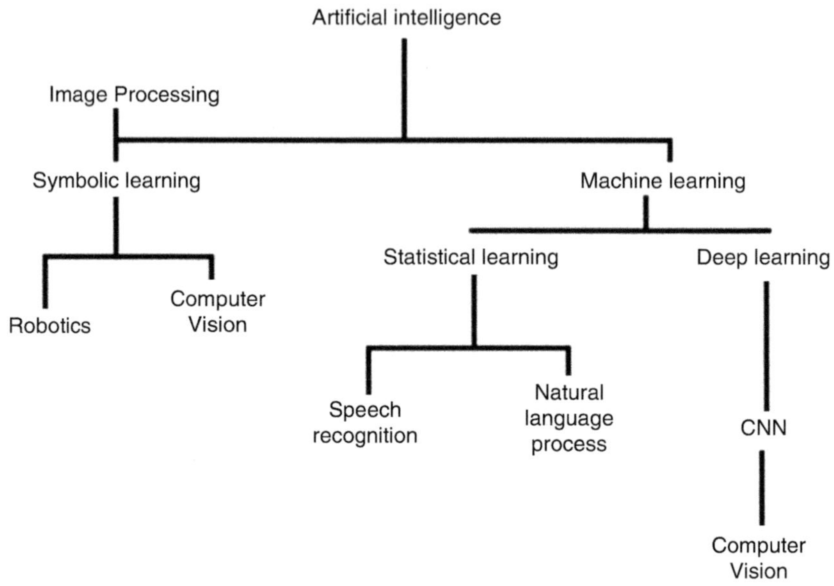

Fig. 8.1 Brief technical structure of AI

devices have been discussed, and the current scenario, future scope, and challenges in front of rehabilitation engineers/scientists have been concluded.

8.2 Artificial Intelligence and Algorithms

An algorithm comprises a step-by-step set of rules to be followed during the calculation or processing to get the expected output. Well-defined inputs and clear, finiteness, workable, language-independent well-defined outputs are an algorithm's characteristics. Figure 8.2 shows the steps involved in implementing the AI algorithm. AI algorithms use three machine learning techniques such as data classification, clustering, and regression to solve the problems. Based on the problem's complexity, a single specific algorithm or combination of algorithms is used to get the desired output. The purpose and subtechniques of each machine learning technique are as shown in Table 8.1.

8.2.1 Data Classification Algorithms

These algorithms have to play with an enormous amount of input data set used to predict a particular class of data by dividing the dependent variable into classes. It can use to predict an output from several fixed predefined outcomes. Support vector

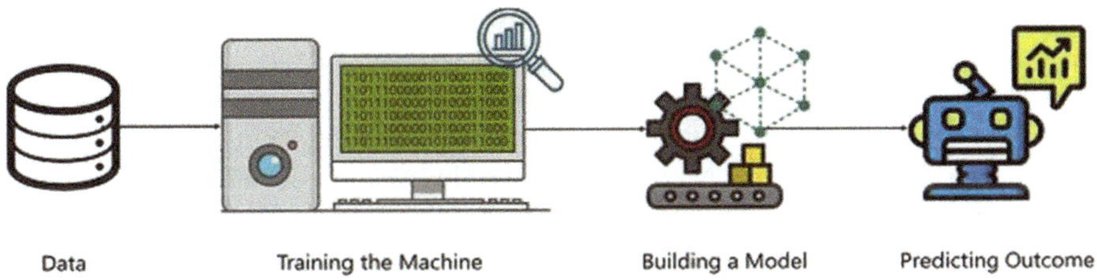

Fig. 8.2 Basic steps for implementation of the AI algorithm

Table 8.1 Purpose of machine learning techniques

Data classification	Regression	Clustering
Supervised learning The output is a categorical quantity The primary aim is to compute the category of the data	Supervised learning The output is a continuous quantity The primary aim is to forecast or predict	Unsupervised learning Assigns data points into clusters The primary aim is to group similar items clusters

machines, random forest, decision tree, Naive Bayes, k-nearest neighbors, and logistic regression are popular algorithms. The problem of data classification has many applications in an extensive selection of mining applications. Because the problem tries to learn the relationship between a pair of attribute variables and a target factor of interest. Since we can express many technical problems as associations among feature and target factors, this gives an extensive assortment of the version's applicability. Classification could be said and presented that a set of training data points and affiliated training labels find out the class tag to get an unlabeled assessment example. I can describe several variations with this problem in various settings. Classification algorithms typically contain two phases:

- Coaching stage: In this period, a version has been assembled in the practice examples.
- Screening period: We use this model to assign a tag to an unlabeled test instance during this period.

The outcome of the classification algorithm might be shown to get a test case in one of two manners:

- Discrete label: During this instance, a tag is coming back to the evaluation case.
- Numerical score: In this case, it returns a numerical score for each category tag and test case mix. Notice that the numerical score can be converted to a different tag for an evaluation example by picking the class with the highest rating for that assessment instance. The advantage of the numerical score is that it now becomes possible to assess the relative propensity of distinct evaluation circumstances to belong to some specific type worth focusing on and rank them whenever desired.

Such approaches can be used frequently in rare class detection problems, in which the initial class distribution is highly imbalanced, and the discovery of several classes is more valuable than the others. Aggarwal [2] gave a comprehensive review of various classification algorithms with applications.

Data mining was used in quite a few applications like promotion, client relationship management, technology, drug investigation, professional outlook, World Wide Web mining, and computing. Naturally, data mining was implemented productively in healthcare fraud, along with discovering abuse instances. Clinical conclusions depend on medical practitioners' experience and instinct instead of the knowledge-rich information concealed inside the database. This clinic contributes to unwelcome biases, glitches, and surplus medical prices that affect sufferers' help. This proposal is assuring because of data modeling and investigation applications, e.g., data mining, and possess the possibility to produce knowledge-rich surroundings, which may significantly enhance the attribute of medical conclusions. Successful data mining software has also given the impetus for its pertinent events to ultimately use these since they have understood that data mining is vital in acquiring invaluable advice for several businesses involved with healthcare-related businesses. Healthcare insurance providers can spot abuse and fraud cases; caregivers can create far better decisions, notably in handling their clients; and also healthcare professionals can supply improved remedies and services. The massive levels of information made by healthcare arrangements are excessively intricate and voluminous to be processed and examined with conventional procedures. Data mining may improve decision-making by detecting tendencies and patterns from considerable quantities of data that is complex. Such an investigation has gotten more and more crucial as monetary stresses have significantly improved healthcare associations' demand to create conclusions dependent on medical and clinical information investigation. Insights acquired from data mining may influence sales, cost, and running efficacy while keeping up a superior maintenance degree.

Healthcare associations that do data mining are far better placed to satisfy their long-term demands. In the last few decades, their peripherals are made more economical and much more easily obtainable, as well as in accord with this evolution of it, many forms of complex data mining processes have now struck on the industry. These new-age data mining methods adopt conventional and latest complex classification calculations. Both equally classification methods are accountable for tackling complex data sets like multidimensionality, person inference, earlier comprehension, site information, data details that induce overfitting of variants and advancement in human skill, noisy cleanup, and mining data sets, along with incremental data sets. Interdisciplinary data mining methods and procedures might be appropriately used for several of the data mentioned above bases, such as forecasting the effect and detecting purposeful connections inside the information together to extract helpful advice for comprehension creation. Laschowski et al. [3] explained how data mining could use on medical data for early detection of various diseases and treatment planning and concluded the comparative analysis of various algorithms in terms of performance, merits, and demerits.

Figure 8.3 shows a stepwise implementation of machine learning algorithms for healthcare. In clinical problem identification, the problem will redefine that are suited to machine learning. The appropriate real-world clinical data will be selected

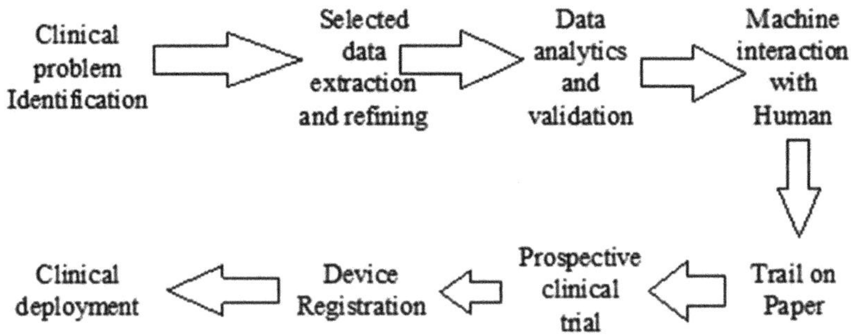

Fig. 8.3 Steps involved in the machine's implementation learning algorithm for healthcare

for data exploration—a suitable machine learning method applicable in data analytics to determine the cross-validation cohorts. Human-machine interaction and machine learning tools on human decisions, including legal and ethical implications on practice, will be verified and tested on the paper to estimate the machine learning tool's proposed model's accuracy. A prospective clinical trial is a real-world model setting with clinician and machine learning. In this stage, review the clinical trial data to make the data model's final adjustment.

A suitable regulatory agency will register the medical device along with the well-defined model. Upon completing registration, the clinicians have trained before, and technical support will provide after launch. Table 8.2 shows the medical data used for various diseases [4].

8.2.2 Regression Algorithms

To predict the output values based on input features from the input data used, these algorithms fall under the category of supervised machine learning algorithms. This algorithm builds a model using features of training data to predict the value of new data. The regression algorithms are classified as:

- Simple and multiple linear regression model
- Lasso regression
- Support vector machines
- Logistic regression
- Multivariate regression algorithm

Simple linear regression model: A statistical study used to study the relationships between two quantitative variables depends on the linear relationship between the input and output variables. The simple or multiple linear regression is depending on the number of input variables.

Table 8.2 Medical data used for various diseases

Name of the disease	Medical data
Eye diseases	Retinal image stores as electronic health record data
Pulmonary diseases	Chest radiographs
Cardiac abnormalities	Magnetic resonance imaging (MRI) of heart ventricles
Fractures	X-ray data
Neurological disorders	Computed tomography (CT) of the brain
Oncology	Computed tomography (CT) of a particular organ

Lasso regression: Least absolute shrinkage and selection operator (Lasso) is used to obtain the subset of predictors with minimal error. It uses the constraint on the model parameters, which leads the value of some variables to word zero.

Support vector machines: It is a robust algorithm based on the Vapnik-Chervonenkis theory used for classification or regression challenges. This algorithm operates natively on numeric attributes used to classify medical images.

Logistic regression: This is one of the commonly used regression techniques used to find fraud detection and clinical trials. It provides the quantified value used to measure the strength associated with the rest of the variables.

Multivariate regression algorithm: This technique is useful for more than one predictor variable in the model. It is one of the simplest supervised machine learning algorithms used to predict the response variable for a given set of explanatory variables. The implementation of this kind of algorithm is easy in Python.

8.2.3 Clustering Algorithms

It is a machine learning technique used to group the data points among the given set of points. It is an unsupervised learning method. The popular clustering algorithms are:

- k-Means clustering
- Density-based spatial clustering
- Mean-shift clustering
- Expectation-maximization clustering
- Agglomerative hierarchical clustering

k-Means clustering: It identifies the k-number of centroids and allocates every data point to the nearest cluster and keeps that the centroid values are as small as possible and used image 2D image segmentation and image compression.

Density-based spatial clustering: This algorithm finds nonlinear structure shapes based on the density. It utilizes the concept of density connectivity and reachability.

Mean-shift clustering: The data points are assigned to the clusters iteratively by shifting points toward the mode, which is the region's highest data points. It has applications in the field of computer vision and image processing.

Expectation-maximization clustering: It is similar to the k-means algorithm. It computes the probabilities of cluster memberships based on probability distributions.

Agglomerative hierarchical clustering: It is a popular hierarchical clustering algorithm used to group objects in clusters based on their similarity.

8.3 Rehabilitation and Devices

Rehabilitation is a process that can help humans get back from illness. It improves cognitive, physical, and mental abilities, which is necessary for day-to-day life. The process of rehabilitation depends on the type of injury, gender, and place. The rehabilitation process may contain a single device or a group of different healthcare professionals—the professionals trace out the needs, treatment plan, and goals of rehabilitation. The assistive devices are the tools which help people overcome movement-related issues. Cognitive skills like memory, learning, planning, thinking, and decision-making can be improved using rehabilitation therapy techniques. Occupational therapy is preferred to improve daily activities; physical therapy strengthens the muscles and nerves.

Recreational therapy uses games, arts, and crafts to improve emotional skills—the problems treated with speech-language therapy associated with speaking, understanding reading, writing, and swallowing. Vocational rehabilitation will help reframe the skills for different environments such as school, office, home, and many more. According to the World Health Organization (WHO) [5], by year 2030, the burden of the world due to neurological disorders raised by 0.5%. Cerebrovascular disease occupies the first place among the other neurological disorders such as Alzheimer's, migraine, epilepsy, tetanus, meningitis, Parkinson's, and multiple sclerosis. Rehabilitation devices are tools or equipment that utilizes the engineering principles to improve the abilities of disabled people. Table 8.3 shows the classification of neurological and physical medicine devices [6] and branch devices.

Table 8.3 Classification of neurological and physical medicine devices

Rehabilitation devices	Neuro-interventional devices	Neuro-diagnostic and neurosurgical devices
Wheelchairs, walkers Electrical stimulators Massagers and vibrators Powered muscle stimulators Brain-computer interfaces Orthoses, exoskeletons	Embolization coils Flow diverters Guidewires and catheters for the neuro-vasculature Neuro-vascular and cerebral interventional devices Cerebrospinal fluid shunts	EEG and non-EEG diagnostic devices Surgical instruments and tools for the neuro-vasculature Neurocognitive diagnostic devices

8.3.1 Walkers and Wheelchairs

Wheelchair and walkers provide the solution for movement disorders. The selection of either wheelchair or walker depends on the nature of the disability, age, gender, and environment. In the olden days, blind people and wheelchair redundant patients depend on a helper to do their regular activities. Tremendous development in technology leads to innovation devices. The walker is a light stick or frame used to enhance stable walking. The people with blindness, age-related physical restrictions, and temporary movement loss due to minor injuries will prefer the walkers, and walking stick, frame walker, front-wheeled walker, hybrid walker stick, and rollator are shown in Figure 8.4. The hybrid walker has a height-adjustable mechanism and foldable frame.

Any smart assistance falls under the sensor-based, vision-based, or smartphone-based category. The sensor-based approach utilizes the sensor fusion techniques and microcontroller to alert the users about surrounding environments. In the vision-based approach, various cameras as a sensor and the processing unit are embedded with precession algorithms to maintain good accuracy. In the smartphone-based approach, all the sensors are embedded in the phone to observe the real world, and after processing the sensor data, it will send the alert signal. Islam et al. [7] gave the summary of smart assistance-based walking devices. They criticized and tabulated the work done by the various authors around the globe. Kaur and Garg [8] wrote a comprehensive review of sensors and camera-based assistive devices for blind people and concluded several algorithms' performance and accuracy. A smart-assembled Nav-Cane is developed [9] with 15 different sensors. The disadvantage of the above is that it failed to recognize the objects in unfamiliar indoor environments. The machine learning algorithms may be the solution to the above problem. The onboard computers provide a free hand to an engineer to use the complex algorithms. It will occupy less space and less power compared with the traditional computing machines. However, these systems are not reliable in terms of accuracy.

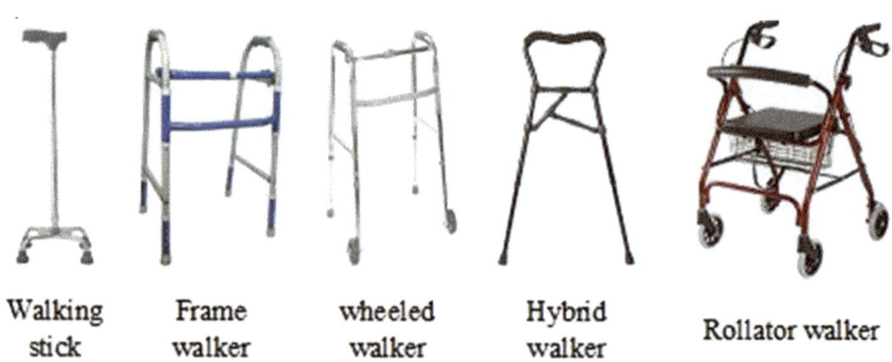

Fig. 8.4 The classification of walkers

For the past two decades, the researchers focused on the wheelchair investigation for further improvement. Scientists worldwide are working to utilize advanced technology to address the wheelchair's problems in the design, autonomous navigation, add-on devices, and user comfort. It is a painful research to bring a tradeoff between patient comfort, quality, and device cost. The AI algorithms will manufacture add-on devices such as autonomous navigation modules and detachable robotic arms. The Global Positioning System (GPS) is the tool that can make the wheelchair user take him to a desirable location.

Nevertheless, most users want to move independently within the indoor atmosphere to keep their self-respect. The GPS cannot give accurate location within the 3-m range. Artificial intelligence algorithms are the right solution for the above problem. The autonomous navigation is achieved with and without bacon. Irrespective of bacon utility, the autonomous navigation task can be simplified into the following task:

- Localization
- Obstacle detection and escape
- Goal identification

Localization is the identification of its current position concerning the environment. The environment may be structured or unstructured. Obstacle detection is a crucial part of navigation. The system has to identify the obstacles in 360°, and it has to decide to avoid that path. Goal identification is similar to localization; the system has to check itself whether it reached its destination or not. Bluetooth low energy (BLE), wireless fidelity (Wi-Fi), pedestrian dead reckoning (PDR), ultra-wideband (UWB), magnetic, sound, radio-frequency identification (RFID), and vision are popular techniques used for localization. Independent of the technology used, the following are the common principles employed with technology in the indoor positioning system (IPS).

Time of arrival (TOA): It calculates the signal's journey time between the transmitter and receiver. It helps calculate the propagation speed of signals such as sound or radiofrequency concerning transmission medium.

The difference in arrival (TDOA) time: It calculated the difference in TOA of signals from various transmitters, which helps estimate the distance between the transmitters.

Received signal strength (RSS): It indicates the intensity of the transmitted signal. The distance between the transmitter and receiver, interference, and attenuation are factors which affect the signal strength.

The angle of arrival (AOA): It is the angle at which the signal reaches the receiver used to fix the moving object's position.

Fingerprinting: Used to compare the Wi-Fi signal intensity received from an arbitrary point. Radio map.

Channel state information (CSI): It is known as the properties of a communication link. It will describe signal propagation from transmitter to receiver.

Table 8.4 The advantages and disadvantages of different localization techniques

Technique name	Advantage	Disadvantage
TOA	Localization accuracy is high; it does not require any fingerprinting	Time synchronization and multiple antennas are required between transmitter and receiver. Line of sight is mandatory for performance
AOA	Localization accuracy is high; it does not require any fingerprinting	It requires complex hardware and directional antennas and complex algorithms
Fingerprinting	Ease to use	It is required when there is a minor variation in the space
TDOA	It does not require clock synchronization and fingerprinting among the device	The performance in short-ranger measurements may be affected due to processing delay
CSI	More reliable on multipath and indoor noise	The implementation is difficult
RSS	It is cost-efficient and compatible with several technologies	More sensitive to multipath fading and environmental noise. Accuracy is low and requires fingerprinting

Table 8.4 shows the advantages and disadvantages of different localization techniques [10] compared to the performance of different wireless technologies for localization in power consumption and maximum throughput and maximum range.

In the absence of beacons, complex artificial algorithms such as Dijkstra's, Dijkstra's* (D*), and A* are used to achieve autonomous navigation. Koubaa et al. [11] explained the various path planning algorithms.

8.3.2 *Electrical Stimulators*

Electrical stimulation (FES) is used to activate the paralyzed muscles through electrical pulses to help grasp, transfer, breathe, stand, walk, and assist bowel and bladder's function. The electrical stimulators are classified based on the application and place where the simulation has to be applied. Some famous electrical stimulators are:

- Transcutaneous electrical nerve stimulation (TENS)
- Electrical muscle stimulation (EMS)
- Neuromuscular electrical stimulation (NMES)
- Functional electrical stimulation (FES)
- Interferential current (IFC) electrical stimulation
- Russian stimulation

Takeda et al. [12] reviewed and concluded the various stimulation devices and their clinical trials' performance. Each method has its advantages and disadvantages. McCaughey et al. [13] did the meta-analysis and systematic review to

Table 8.5 The purpose of various electrical stimulators

Stimulator name	Purpose
TENS	It will give temporary relief from the pain due to sore, aching muscles, and chronic. It has a limited function, which makes it cheap
EMS	Design to strengthen the muscles, muscular endurance, and muscle size. It can accelerate muscle recovery and makes the muscle contract forcefully used for athletes
NMES	In this method, muscle spasms are relaxed to prevent muscle atrophy intended for therapeutic use. It will help improve the blood circulation, range of motion, and re-educating the neuromuscular system
FES	It works the same as NMES and useful for neurological rehabilitation. This stimulation helps turn the muscle contractions into functional movements. It is incorporated with exercise or bracing
IFC	Design to reduce pain due to chronic, acute, post-traumatic, and post-surgical pain. Compared with TENS, it has more functions that lead to costlier and more effective
Russian stimulation	Its purpose is similar to EMS. It works based on the high-frequency, sinusoidal stimulation waveforms

determine the effect of stimulators on spinal cord injury (SCI) patients. Table 8.5 shows the purpose of the above stimulators.

8.3.3 Brain-Computer Interfaces

The brain-computer interface (BCI) establishes a connection between the machine and the brain's neural parts to prevent and detect diagnosis and rehabilitation in the medical field. Abdulkader et al. [14] explained the various components involved to make the BCI and concluded the various applications and challenging tasks. Lotte et al. [15] reviewed the classification of algorithms for EEG-based BCI. Figure 8.5 shows the data classification process in the EEG-based BCI system. To make the exploration easy, they divided the algorithms into four groups: adaptive classifiers, transfer learning methods, matrix classifiers, and deep learning. In general, the BCI algorithms are classified as:

- Linear classifiers
- Nonlinear Bayesian classifiers
- Neural networks
- Nearest neighbor classifiers
- Combination of classifiers

The AI-based BCI is the reinforcement learning (RL) method, which translates the neuronal information into meaningful commands to control the external device. The structure of a BCI system with AI is shown in Fig. 8.6.

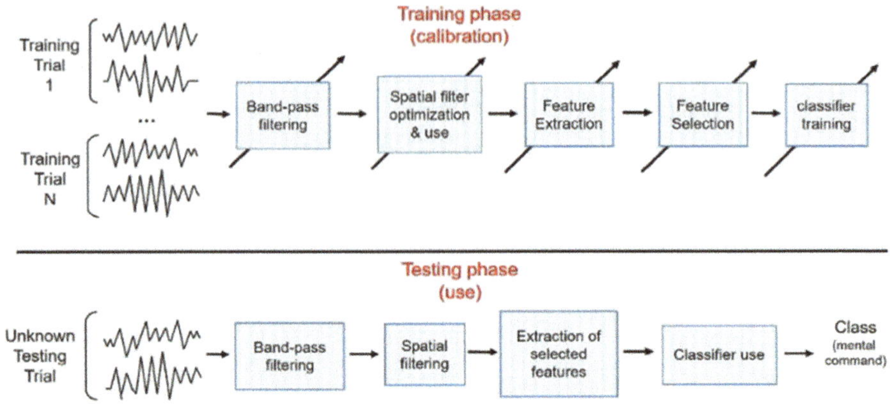

Fig. 8.5 Typical data classification process in EEG-based BCI system [15]

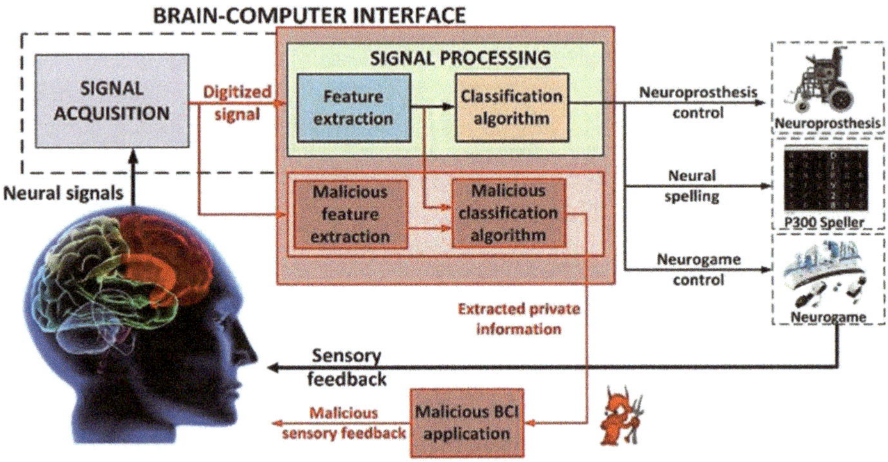

Fig. 8.6 The structure of the BCI system with AI (https://medium.com/@askwhy/brain-computer-interface)

In general, the RL algorithms has classified into model-based and model-free algorithms. In the case of model-free learning, the agent relies on some trial-and-error experience for action selection. In model-based learning, the agent deeds previously learned lessons. AI-based BCI system uses closed-loop brain-controlled interfaces. Iandolo et al. [16] provide an overview of the most common lower and upper neurorehabilitation devices. Bablani et al. [17] explained the various latest techniques for a brain-computer interface. Bockbrader et al. [18] explained the essential components of BCI for rehabilitation, discussed overview application of sensory restoration, and concluded the ethical issues associated with BCI technology. Tahernezhad-Javazm et al. [19] reviewed the experimental studies and evolutionary algorithms for the EEG-based brain-machine interface system.

8.3.4 Orthoses and Exoskeleton

The exoskeleton device provides the augments to the non-disabled wearer. An orthosis is a device used to assist a limb pathology person. Hsu et al. [20] gave a detailed overview of spinal, upper, and lower limb orthoses and concluded the necessity of robotic devices for rehabilitating patients with spinal cord injury and future orthosis trends. Cosmetic rehab will be significantly improved via complex autonomous and neuroscience technological innovation. While the full rehab procedure is time-consuming and more time-consuming, robots are the alternate and a complement to this one-on-one treatment. You will find just two options out there for upper limb rehab: over a single-side more easy apparatus, which can be two or one DOF, which might be utilized to coach unique performance or solitary articulation motions, as an instance, hand or elbow planar motions, and also across the flip hand multi-DOF robots which may train plasma and also more intricate motion. Within this specific classification, exoskeletons represent probably the most high-level robot since they induce maybe not just the ending effect or of their arm and hand, but likewise the whole kinematic series, in other words, supplying single-joint robotic help throughout movement implementation.

Upper limb exoskeletons are made correctly from an ergonomic and biomechanics perspective to perform engine features properly. Specifically, because exoskeletons are believed to do something in symbiosis using the individual operator, the kinematics is less pertinent than actuation. These problems have to be suitably examined while the non-ideal equivalence of individual joints into uncomplicated kinematic joints desires to correct exoskeleton measurements into individual anatomy dimensions. Also, three combined implementations ought to simply take into consideration the majority of the individual arm. It has been recognized that individual joints' actual body will not correspond to both the best rotational and curved joints if people confine. For example, toward the top of the nose, the shoulder intricate includes the glenohumeral, the sternoclavicular, the acromioclavicular, and the scapulothoracic joints. Thus the shoulder complex might be contemplated just as being a generalized round joint having a floating center.

Even with asserting technological breakthroughs from lower-limb prostheses along with exoskeletons, the widespread use of those wearable biomechatronic apparatus stays essentially reliant upon untethered ability resources. Electro-mechanical lower-limb prostheses and exoskeletons have customarily mandatory significant electric power levels to electricity onboard detectors, actuators, and microprocessors throughout human locomotion. Electric power was given through rechargeable lithium-polymer and lithium-ion. Contemplating the mass and geometric limits of biomimetic limb layouts the more limited power densities of batteries, and the substantial energy needs of jelqing programs have attracted roughly two well-known shortcomings with conventional passive apparatus: elevated limited and weight functioning durations. Most electro-mechanical lower-limb prostheses, along with exoskeletons, have demanded regular imports. Personal remarks suggested that the electricity knee's significant burden and battery lifespan would be

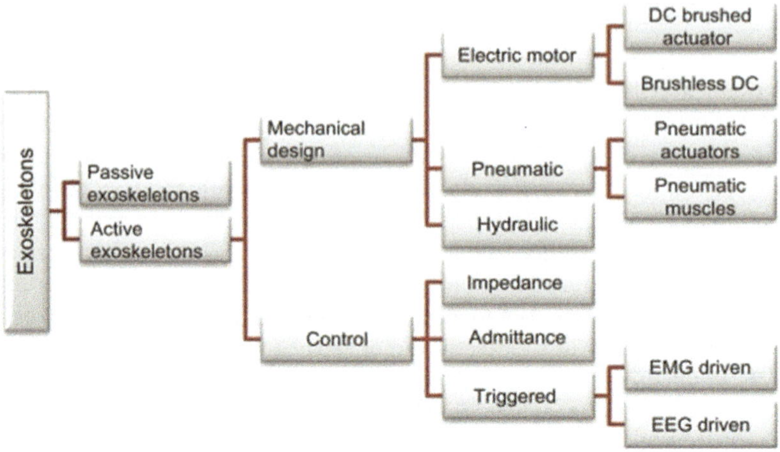

Fig. 8.7 The exoskeletons and its classification [21]

the critical deterrents to continuing utilization. Most motivated lower-limb exoskeletons have given 15 h of max performance. Thus, additional improvements in untethered strength resources for lower-limb biomechatronic apparatus are necessary. Biomechanical vitality harvesting signifies a promising way to solve the above openings. It will involve changing the differently dissipated mechanical vitality throughout the human locomotion to electric energy to recharge the onboard batteries. This vitality regeneration technological innovation can cut back the onboard battery or expand the functioning durations involving ethanol, allowing individuals to ambulate more time distances and possess greater freedom. Various investigations have lately contemplated integrating electrical power regeneration to lower-limb prostheses along with exoskeletons such as geriatrics and rehab sufferers (i.e., people who have a lower-limb amputation, stroke, and back trauma). To improve the closeness and following software of those wearable biomechatronic apparatus for medical uses, the purpose of the subsequent technical inspection was supposed to inspect the electro-mechanical style and optimization of lower-limb prostheses along with exoskeletons with electric power regeneration.

Figure 8.7 shows the exoskeletons and their classification.

Lyu et al. [22] discussed AI algorithms for autonomous control of knee exoskeleton. Benabid et al. [23] gave the demonstration proof for exoskeleton control using an epidural wireless brain-machine interface. Laschowski et al. [3] wrote the comprehensive review on exoskeletons with energy regeneration and lower-limb prostheses.

8.4 Conclusion

Technological innovations have given neurological disorder afflicted patient's mobility and the ability to perform routine tasks. Motorized wheelchairs have given such patient's mobility. The patient's parameters are monitored and analyzed continuously (via cloud-based scanners). The AI brain-computer interfaces, with appropriate driver interfaces, will allow even paralytic patients to walk.

References

1. Goleman, D., Boyatzis, R., & Mckee, A. (2019). Artificial intelligence an illustrated history. *Journal of Chemical Information and Modeling*. https://doi.org/10.1017/CBO9781107415324.004
2. Aggarwal, C. C. (2015). *Data classification algorithms and applications*. CRC Press Taylor & Francis Group.
3. Laschowski, B., McPhee, J., & Andrysek, J. (2019). Lower-limb prostheses and exoskeletons with energy regeneration: Mechatronic design and optimization review. *Journal of Mechanisms and Robotics, 11*(4), 1–43. https://doi.org/10.1115/1.4043460
4. Ngiam, K. Y., & Khor, I. W. (2019). Big data and machine learning algorithms for healthcare delivery. *The Lancet Oncology, 20*(5), e262–e273. https://doi.org/10.1016/S1470-2045(19)30149-4
5. Moritz, D. J., et al. (1997). Neurological and psychiatric predictors of mortality in patients with Alzheimer's disease in California. *Archives of Neurology, 54*(7), 878–885. https://doi.org/10.1001/archneur.1997.00550190066016
6. Anderson, L., et al. (2016). FDA regulation of neurological and physical medicine devices: Access to safe and effective neurotechnologies for all Americans. *Neuron, 92*(5), 943–948. https://doi.org/10.1016/j.neuron.2016.10.036
7. Islam, M. M., et al. (2019). Developing walking assistants for visually impaired people: A review. *IEEE Sensors Journal, 19*(8), 2814–2828. https://doi.org/10.1109/JSEN.2018.2890423
8. Kaur, P., & Garg, R. (2019). Camera and sensors-based assistive devices for visually impaired persons: A systematic review. *International Journal of Scientific and Technology Research, 8*(8), 622–641.
9. Meshram, V. V., et al. (2019). An astute assistive device for mobility and object recognition for visually impaired people. *IEEE Transactions on Human-Machine Systems, 49*(5), 449–460. https://doi.org/10.1109/THMS.2019.2931745
10. Zafari, F., Gkelias, A., & Leung, K. K. (2019). A survey of indoor localization systems and technologies. *IEEE Communication Surveys and Tutorials, 21*(3), 2568–2599. https://doi.org/10.1109/COMST.2019.2911558
11. Koubaa, A., et al. (2018). *Robot path planning and cooperation*. Springer International Publishing AG. https://doi.org/10.1353/sais.2002.0030
12. Takeda, K., Tanino, G., & Miyasaka, H. (2017). Review of devices used in neuromuscular electrical stimulation for stroke rehabilitation. *Medical Devices: Evidence and Research, 10*, 207–213. https://doi.org/10.2147/MDER.S123464
13. McCaughey, E. J., et al. (2016). Abdominal functional electrical stimulation to improve respiratory function after spinal cord injury: A systematic review and meta-analysis. *Spinal Cord, 54*(9), 628–639. https://doi.org/10.1038/sc.2016.31
14. Abdulkader, S. N., Atia, A., & Mostafa, M. S. M. (2015). Brain-computer interfacing: Applications and challenges. *Egyptian Informatics Journal: Ministry of Higher Education and Scientific Research, 16*(2), 213–230. https://doi.org/10.1016/j.eij.2015.06.002

15. Lotte, F., et al. (2018). A review of classification algorithms for EEG-based brain-computer interfaces: A 10-year update. *Journal of Neural Engineering, 15*(3), 2552. https://doi.org/10.1088/1741-2552/aab2f2
16. Iandolo, R., et al. (2019). Perspectives and challenges in robotic neurorehabilitation. *Applied Sciences, 9*(15), 3183. https://doi.org/10.3390/app9153183
17. Bablani, A., et al. (2019). Survey on brain-computer interface. *ACM Computing Surveys, 52*(1), 1–32. https://doi.org/10.1145/3297713
18. Bockbrader, M. A., et al. (2018). Brain-computer interfaces in rehabilitation medicine. *American Academy of Physical Medicine and Rehabilitation, 10*(9), S233–S243. https://doi.org/10.1016/j.pmrj.2018.05.028
19. Tahernezhad-Javazm, F., Azimirad, V., & Shoaran, M. (2018). A review and experimental study on the application of classifiers and evolutionary algorithms in EEG-based brain-machine interface systems. *Journal of Neural Engineering, 15*(2), 8063. https://doi.org/10.1088/1741-2552/aa8063
20. Hsu, J. D., Michael, J. W., & Fisk, J. R. (2008). *AAOS atlas of orthoses and assistive devices*. Mosby.
21. Frisoli, A. (2018). Exoskeletons for upper limb rehabilitation. In *Rehabilitation robotics*. Elsevier Ltd.. https://doi.org/10.1016/b978-0-12-811995-2.00006-0
22. Lyu, M., et al. (2019). Knee exoskeleton enhanced with artificial intelligence to provide assistance-as-needed. *Review of Scientific Instruments, 90*(9), 094101. https://doi.org/10.1063/1.5091660
23. Benabid, A. L., et al. (2019). An exoskeleton controlled by a wireless epidural brain-machine interface in a tetraplegic patient: A proof-of-concept demonstration. *The Lancet Neurology, 18*(12), 1112–1122. https://doi.org/10.1016/S1474-4422(19)30321-7
24. Anwar Lashari, S., et al. (2018). Application of data mining techniques for medical data classification: A review. *MATEC Web of Conferences, 150*, 1–6. https://doi.org/10.1051/matecconf/201815006003

Chapter 9
Enabling Speech Emotional Intelligence as a Service in Homecare Platforms

Panagiotis Stavrianos, Andrianos Pavlopoulos, and Ilias Maglogiannis

9.1 Introduction

The expeditious development of Artificial Intelligence technology (AI) has laid the foundations for the substantial advancement of Human-Computer Interaction (HCI) via machine intelligence, cognitive science, psychology and affective computing [1]. Affective computing is the scientific field that deals with research and development of special systems, techniques and devices that can identify, record, interpret, process and simulate various shades of human emotions. The specific field envisions a world where technologies respond to user frustration, boredom, or even help alleviate human suffering. Modern cognitive systems may be improved by incorporating such intelligence that involves the ability to perceive, assess, and influence the emotional state of a user. Especially in the case of homecare systems and platforms that remotely monitor the physical and mental health of individuals, the ability to continually sense emotion and associate it with a person's health status is of paramount importance. In this context, the emotional AI technology is anticipated to be a core component of future patient telemonitoring systems. Through the convergence of Cognitive Computing and AI, the Artificial Emotion Intelligence (Emotion AI) sets the goal of revealing and managing the emotion of users. In the latest years, emotion recognition has found a sheer amount of applications in assistive environments such as stress detection in medical-emergency cases [2], interactions with robots [3, 4], serious games [5, 6], and advance human-machine interfaces (HMI) for assisting older persons [7]. Advanced AI methods, such as deep learning could further enhance the technical innovation in the industry of Pervasive Health

P. Stavrianos · A. Pavlopoulos · I. Maglogiannis (✉)
Department of Digital Systems, University of Piraeus, Piraeus, Greece
e-mail: Imaglo@unipi.gr

M. S. Husain et al. (eds.), *Pervasive Healthcare*, EAI/Springer Innovations in Communication and Computing, https://doi.org/10.1007/978-3-030-77746-3_9

and Affective Computing [8–12] enabling emotion recognition in the machine—patient and doctor—patient interactions.

The strong relationship between emotions and human health has been recognized as early as the ancient times. Philosophers and scientists characterize emotions as key determinants of human health state and diseases. At the present time, the dynamic lifestyle leads to continuously appalling situations, accompanied by an escalating growth of stress, frustration, irritation and depression. The macroscopic existence of such continuous feelings leads to the deterioration of the physical functionalities of the human being, including appetite and sleep. In parallel, such feelings comprise the starting point associated with a weakened human immune system [13]. On the other hand, positive emotions play a considerable role in improving the physical and mental health. Both mental and physical health are influenced by self-esteem and self-efficacy, which can help in stressful situations and can prolong life by increasing the positive attitude and happiness [14]. In this context, the investigation and understanding of the relation between human emotions and health seems a good idea for application in the medical informatics domain and particularly in assistive and homecare environments.

Homecare and home telemonitoring are a focal point of emerging healthcare schemes, with proven benefits for both patients, caregivers and providers, including reduction of healthcare costs and improved patients' quality of life, especially in the case of older, disabled and chronic patients. Studies have evaluated solutions for remote monitoring of chronic patients based on technologies that allow daily symptom and vital signs monitoring, tailored to the needs of specific diseases, including cognitive and neurodegenerative diseases. Internet-based applications incorporate interactive monitoring systems that provide to the healthcare professional instant access to the Personal Health Records (PHRs) [15–17]. Through the assessment of the PHRs, healthcare professionals provide meaningful and personalized prescriptions, taking into great consideration the data analysis from the previous sessions. Through these applications, the available e-therapy models are differentiated and personalized through the interactivity with the patient, allowing the delivery of efficient preventive care. This approach allows the patient to actively engage in treatment in his environment, contributing to the reduction of his social anxiety. This issue comprises a considerable factor in medical cases where the patient lives alone or resides in isolated territories and immediate solutions need to be present.

The existence of relation between affective displays and specific audio and visual signals produced by individuals has been also explored in the literature [18–23]. Among the plethora of explicit means of expression, body and facial gestures are rendered as the main sources of emotion extraction. Although, speech constitutes one of the most natural, fastest and essential communication means of humans, it is not yet extensively exploited in the affective computing field. In this work, we will focus on this contemporary research field, namely, the speech emotion recognition (SER), that is the extraction of the emotional state of a speaker from his/her speech, which has been already reported to improve the performance of speech recognition systems [24]. Our goal is to incorporate SER-oriented methods in electronic healthcare management system and especially homecare and patient telemonitoring

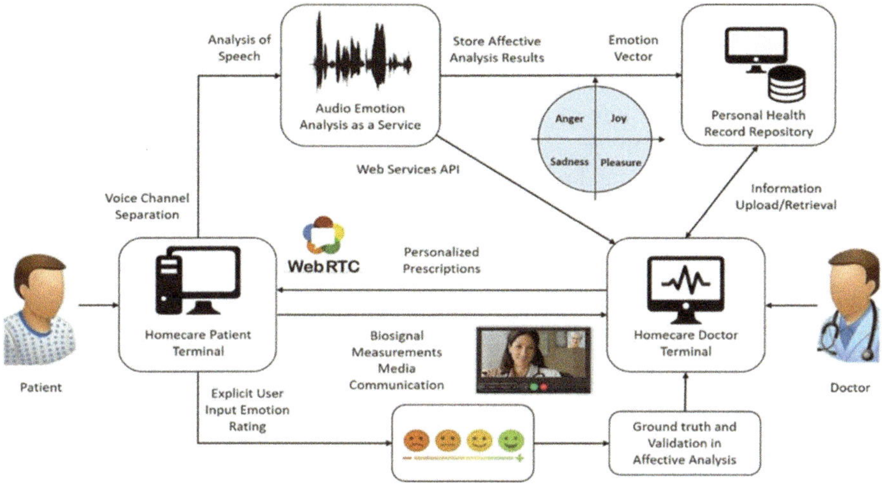

Fig. 9.1 Architecture and internal modules of the SER-enabled patient telemonitoring platform

platforms. More specifically in this paper, we describe the design and implementation principles of an emotion recognition module, which is integrated as a service with a patient telemonitoring platform, so as to form a holistic homecare management platform. The core of the homecare management platform is composed of an analytics-driven system with storage utilities and real-time processing of the speech utterances through the feedback of SER techniques. The overall architecture of the proposed holistic platform is illustrated in Fig. 9.1. The homecare management platform enables the planning of remote sessions through the respective terminal of each role, namely, the patient and doctor terminal. The terminal interactions entail the transmission of biosignal measurements and audiovisual information from the patient to the doctor. In a parallel channel, the audio-speech signal is separated with the aim of diverting this signal to the Audio Emotion Analysis as a service component where the SER is executed. The corresponding emotional states are delivered to the health professional for real-time monitoring, while the affective analysis results are stored in the personal health record along with the various biosignals for future access, decision-making, and assistive diagnosis. Furthermore, the patient has the ability of explicitly defining his current emotional state through ratings, providing additional validation to the speech emotion analysis. With a priori research on sound processing and existing SER systems (which is summarized in Sect. 9.2), the proposed work involves the integration of several machine learning algorithms from the conventional classification schemes to deep convolutional neural networks. The deployment of these algorithms is enabled in the audio emotion analysis as a service module, with the aim of providing results for comparison purposes and, thus, versatility in the adaptation of the service to the diverse environments. The integration of the classification schemes also involves the lifecycle of training phase through the interaction with the linked emotional speech databases (ESDs) and speech samples in the platform.

The remainder of this chapter is divided into four sections. In the following section, the related work is reviewed, highlighting recent advances and several challenges in speech processing and SER systems, depicting the motivation of our work. In Sect. 9.3, the architecture of the proposed framework is detailed, along with the experimental setup and the technical details of the proposed functionalities. Section 9.4 presents the experimental results, while Sect. 9.5 concludes the paper and presents future advances.

9.2 Background and Related Work

The necessity of explaining accurately the meaning of emotion is not a new problem. In the domain of psychology, researchers state that emotion is generally affected from both the emotional state and the behavioral intentions for an incident [25]. In a parallel manner, apart from clarifying a definition, it is believed that the segregation of emotions in clarified dimensions is feasible in order not to overlay them [26]. Thus, two categories of emotions are distinguished, namely, the *primary* (standard) and the *secondary* (produced) emotions. The former includes discrete classes of emotions, able to cause massive global changes to every living being through facial expressions, behavioral tendencies, etc. The latter comprise combinations of the primary emotions, which are perceived only by humans, emerging from cognitive procedures including estimation of perceptible conditions [27]. In the emotion recognition, primary emotions pose as a key factor as they are easily distinguishable and can be represented as an outcome of a direct sequence of events. The main characteristics of a primary emotion are (1) the independence of the human society and the living being, (2) the occurrence during the evolutionary process, (3) the expression through predetermined ways (e.g., particular pitch and energy in the voice), and (4) their appearance from the early years of the human being. On the other hand, secondary emotions can only be perceived from the human living beings and are mainly characterized from the fast, unintentional disorientation of thinking procedures and involuntary redirection of ongoing cognitive procedures such as planning, reasoning, and self-monitoring at the cognitive level without involving any modulation [18, 28].

As already stated body gestures, face expressions, and, more rarely, speech are utilized as the main sources of emotion [29, 30]. Regarding speech, digital signal processing (DSP) techniques are applied by consolidating psychological and linguistic analyses of emotion. Based on high levels of correlation found between the speech characteristics and various human gestures, researchers believe that the emotional state of the patient simultaneously triggers the production of both speech and gestures, sharing the same semantic meaning in different communication channels [19, 31]. Based on the triggering mechanisms from the emotional states, the production of the facial and speech characteristics is based on the nature of the human being. The characterization of an emotion is rather subjective across the different individuals, since emotion expressions in natural settings are frequently play-acted due to social requirements. In [32, 33], a comparison of the acted and natural reactions revealed differences in sound properties, such as articulation and pitch contour, indicating that measurable differences in the stimulus material between play-acting and authentic encoding condition exist. Among the existing approaches, SER has been studied with acted and natural samples of emotions. Although the test results deliver considerable accuracy with the training of acted samples, the efficiency of the system is degraded in the operation of the system in the wild. This issue is based on the strong emotional expressions of the acted samples [34, 35], while actual patients do not unveil intense emotion characteristics. Well-established machine learning techniques have been deployed in the existing SER approaches with the aim of emotion classification, such as support vector machines (SVM) [36], k-NN [37], artificial neural networks (ANNs) [38, 39], hidden Markov models (HMM) [40–42], and Gaussian mixture model (GMM) [43] classifiers. In general, it has been proved that every classifier delivers different performance characteristics [44]. For instance, HMM has been deployed as a SER classifier due to its dynamic time warping capabilities and high correlation of its algorithm structure with the production mechanism of speech signal. With the view of combining diverse advantages among the available classifiers, techniques with fusion of classifiers have been presented in [45, 46], introducing mean accuracy of 92.72%, outperforming the majority of base classifiers.

One of the main concerns in the design of SER systems is the selection of the most suitable sound features to be extracted from the speech. The acoustic variations, which are present by the existence of different utterances, speakers, speaking rhythms, and speaking rates, pose a paramount barrier as these properties directly correlate with the majority of the extracted features in SER. Thus, the conventional selection of a set of features gains substantial profit for the classification scheme. As depicted in Fig. 9.2, features can be generally grouped into four categories: (1) continuous features, (2) voice quality, (3) spectral-based speech, and (4) nonlinear features [47]. Most of the researchers firmly deem that the emotional state is substantially correlated with the categories of acoustic and voice quality features [48, 49]. Through the current state of the speaker, energy-related and pitch-related

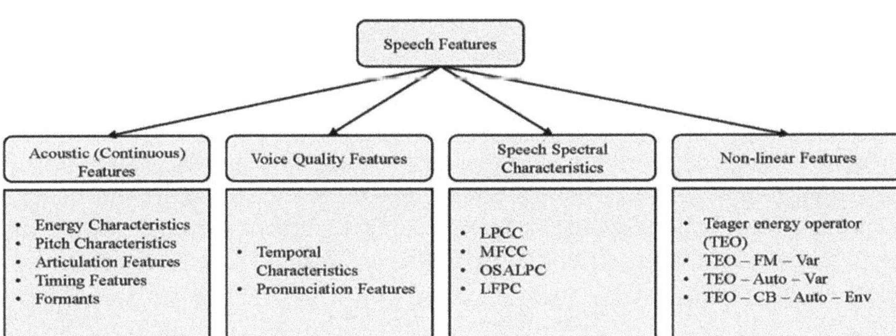

Fig. 9.2 Categorization of features in speech emotion recognition

features are significantly affected through the underlying mechanism of his articulation scheme and the vocal note correlation. In conjunction with these acoustic characteristics, the current emotional state is highly aligned with the pronunciation features of speech. Additionally, spectral characteristics of speech pose as time-independent features through the distribution of the spectral energy across the frequency plane. The extraction of spectral features is enabled through linear predictor coefficients (LPC), linear predictor cepstral coefficients (LPCC), Mel-frequency cepstral coefficients (MFCC), one-sided autocorrelation linear predictor coefficients (OSALPC), and log-frequency power coefficients (LFPC). On the fourth category, a set of features is representing the nonlinearities produced from the nonlinear air flow. The first feature of this category was introduced by Teager [50], referred to as Teager energy operator (TEO). Afterward, Zhou et al. [51] proposed additional TEO-based features in their study to categorize and recognize features of stress in the speech, namely, TEO-decomposed FM variation (TEO-FM-Var), normalized TEO autocorrelation envelope area (TEO-Auto-Env), and critical band-based TEO autocorrelation envelope area (TEO-CB-Auto-Env).

Only recently, deep learning methodologies and tools are introduced in SER, urged from the nonlinear boundaries of ANN functionality separating the emotional states. Deep neural networks (DNNs) were initially studied and outperformed the hybrid HMM-GMM classifier [52], enabling the major interest in applying similar approaches in SER applications. Consequently, substantial attention was given on DNN structures, such as deep long-short-term memory recurrent neural networks (LSTM-RNN) [53], deep convolutional neural networks (DCNN) [54, 55], and deep brief network (DBN) [56, 57]. As a combination, in [58], a hybrid DNN-HMM was compared with the HMM-GMM classifier, indicating higher accuracy results with a percentage of 91.67%.

Several approaches have been proposed with the aim of utilizing feature learning schemes for spectrograms generated from speech [54, 55, 59–61]. Based on the visual representation of the speech, this type of approach bypasses the traditional feature extraction engineering pipeline. The of time-frequency analysis and fast Fourier various methods that are deployed use mechanisms transform (FFT) for analyzing the audio and speech signals in 2D representation. These techniques achieve substantial results, in terms of accuracy for all classes compared to the conventional machine learning classifiers, on the grounds that spectrograms incorporate an abundant amount of information and characteristics of the voice signal. In Table 9.1, a summary of the surveyed works along with additional details on their design parameters is illustrated. In the evolution of speech-based emotion recognition systems for pervasive healthcare, there are specific challenges. Firstly, a lack of knowledge exists in detecting the speech features that enrich the actual information of the patient's emotional status. General prosodic aspects of speech, voice quality features (utterance-level statistics through pitch and intensity), and spectral features can be deployed in SER [43]. However, the acoustic variability in the diverse sentences, speaking styles, and rhythms significantly affect the contribution of the predetermined features of the SER system [8]. Another challenge in speech-based emotion recognition is the fact that there is an overlapping relationship between the

Table 9.1 Related works on SER algorithms with detailed information on the classification conditions

References	Type of data	Classification scheme	Features	Noise	Accuracy (%)
Wang et al. [36]	EMODB [62], CASIA [63], EESDB [64]	SVM, Naïve Bayes	MFCC, Fourier parameters, zero-crossing rate	Noiseless samples	93.62
Dellaert et al. [37]	In-house recordings	k-NN	Pitch-related	Noiseless samples	82.35
Rawat, Mishra [38]	Persian DB [38]	ANN	MFCC	Noiseless samples	93.42
Schuller et al. [42]	In-house recordings	HMM	Duration, pitch-related	Noiseless samples	91.1
Wu and Liang [46]	In-house recordings	GMM-ANN-SVM	MFCC, formant and pitch-related	Noiseless samples	92.72
Weninger et al. [53]	CHiME DB [65]	LSTM-RNN	MFCC, LFPC	Samples with noise	64
Zhu et al. [56]	DB of Chinese Academy of Sciences [35]	DBN-SVN	Pitch, formant, energy, zero-crossing rate, MFCC	Noiseless samples	95.6
Fayek et al. [55]	IEMOCAP DB	DCNN	Image of spectrogram	Samples with noise	64.83
Mao et al. [54]	SAVEE [66], EMODB [62], DES [67], MES [68]	DCNN	Image of spectrogram	–	80.1 noise 96 noiseless
Badshah et al. [69]	EMODB [62]	DCNN	Image of spectrogram	Noiseless samples	84.21

emotional states. This statement addresses the need of determining a set of demarcated important emotions to be initially classified. The clear majority of researchers agree with the "palette theory," stating that every emotion can be decomposed into primary emotions, namely, the *anger*, *disgust*, *fear*, *joy*, *sadness*, *and surprise*, also referred to as *archetypal emotions* [70, 71]. In parallel, many linguistic researchers have defined template repositories, hosting a variety of classified emotional samples [72, 73]. Equally important, a great limitation is entailed in the available ESDs [40, 41, 62, 67, 74]. Most of the ESDs are not available for public use, while there is a great limitation of introducing actuality in the emotional recorded samples. This statement is based on several physical factors, e.g., natural or acted [8, 75], incident of stimulation of the emotion [76, 77], professional or amateur actors [76], low quality and absence of significant speech features [47], etc. Thus, these issues introduce a deficiency in defining naturally stimulated and clear emotion samples, and, therefore, all available databases include the same interference in the recorded samples. Another important issue in SER is the division mechanism of the speech. Many approaches exploit techniques where the speech signal is divided into batches, in which local features are extracted, with the aim of constructing stationary samples of the signal. Other studies prefer the confrontation of the speech signal as a unified entity, with the relevant extraction of the global features [43]. The great advantage of global features constitutes the small subset of global features, facilitating the selection of features. On the other hand, global features can only be used in a classification scheme only to differentiate emotions with high severability. Thus, local features pose as a great selection for precision and distinguishing similar emotion characteristics [40].

The literature review revealed that none of the existing systems provided real-time analytics services [78]. In addition, regarding the pervasive healthcare field, the proposal of an integrated homecare management platform, with SER capabilities, is absent. Thus, a great deficiency exists in the development and the research of analytics-driven and real-time homecare management systems, where patients are emotionally assessed from a healthcare professional and provided with rehabilitation (especially, physical or occupational therapy). Especially, there is a great lack of unified patient telemonitoring platforms which will enable the transmission of useful information of the patient's current emotional state. The demand of such platforms is addressed on the grounds that the care delivery must be enhanced, and the patients need constant and personalized surveillance. This aim can be achieved through meticulous care planning. The diverse diagnoses of acute patients are often clearly defined, in contrast to rehabilitation patients that have considerable variability even within specific diagnostic categories. The examination of rehabilitation potential and their success for older patients is obscure and complicated, in the means of comorbidities [79], and demands management by health professionals in the exposed care settings [80].

9.3 Proposed Methodology

9.3.1 Audio Analysis

Conventional Classification Schemes

In the context of audio analysis, the open-access tool pyAudioAnalysis [81] is exploited for the deployment of sound feature extraction and the classification schemes. Thus, a segment classification functionality is provided, to enable the training and the exploitation of supervised models to a set of predefined classes. More specifically, we assess the performance of several classification schemes, such as k-NN, SVM, random forest (RF), extra tree (ET), and gradient boosting tree (GBT). Below, the main followed process of every classification scheme is analyzed. More specifically, in Fig. 9.3, the procedure of feature extraction is depicted. Since pattern recognition techniques are rarely independent from the problem domain, a proper selection of features significantly affects the classification performance. While many methods follow the ordinary procedure of dividing the speech signal into batches, from all of which a local feature vector is extracted, another

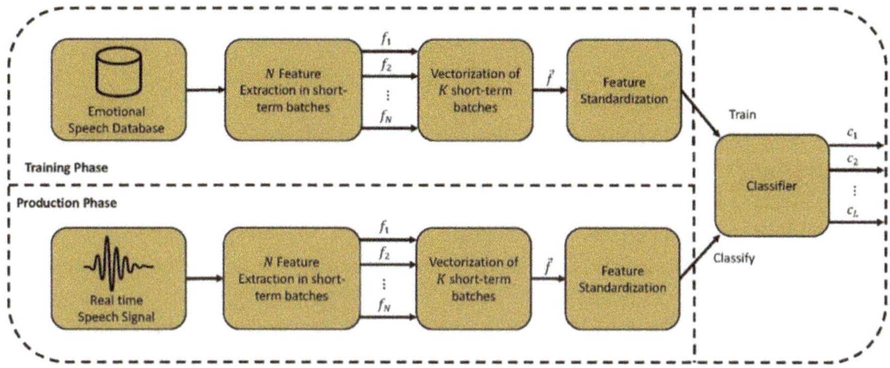

Fig. 9.3 Feature extraction algorithm in the conventional classification schemes for the training and the production phase

option is the extraction of global statistics from the whole speech utterance. In the deployment of the conventional classification schemes in our proposed framework, the procedure of feature extraction is analyzed below:

- *Short-term feature extraction*: In the short-term step of the feature extraction process, the input speech signal is divided into batches of predetermined length in the real-time recording of the user. Thus, the N features of each batch are computed, leading to a sequential computation of short-term vectors.
- *Mid-term feature extraction*: In the mid-term step of the feature extraction process, the short-term feature sequences are processed through the representation of their individual statistical characteristics (e.g., mean and standard deviation) over the mid-term batches. The mid-term batches are the combination of K short-term batches, all of which contribute to the extraction of the statistical characteristics of the features.

According to the literature [38, 47, 82–84], both the acoustic and the spectral features carry emotional information. In order to retain the complexity, the selection of the extracted features is based on selecting the most representative features from the two categories. Thus, the selected features are the zero-crossing rate, the energy, the spectral flux and the spectral roll-off of the spectrum, 13 MFC coefficients, and 12-element representation of the spectral energy through the chroma vector, along with their standard deviation. Regardless of the selected features, every feature choice represents a different aspect of the speech signal. Since none of them are measured in the same scale, they can include multiple dimensions. Normalization is commonly used in feature scaling with independent variables. The aim of normalization is to reach linearity and more robust relationship between the diverse features. In our methodology, the mid-term batches are normalized with the aim of diminishing the diverse unit ranges of the selected features as follows:

$$\overrightarrow{f_n} = \frac{\vec{f} - \text{mean}\left(\vec{f}\right)}{\text{std}\left(\vec{f}\right) + \varepsilon} \tag{9.1}$$

where $\vec{f} = \{f_1, f_2, \ldots, f_N\}$ denotes the feature vector, $\overrightarrow{f_n}$ the normalized feature vector, and mean and std estimates of the sample mean and sample standard deviation. Since the calculation of the mean and the standard deviation is enabled, each feature is normalized to zero mean and unit variance.

During the training phase, the training samples from the utilized ESDs are used as input in the feature extraction algorithm with the aim of fitting the parameters of the model through supervised learning. The validation phase is followed with the aim of monitoring the efficiency of the algorithm with the validation samples. In the training phase, we employ the statistical procedure of repeated random sub-sampling validation (Monte Carlo cross-validation) so as to preserve less-biased estimate of the model performance. Similarly, when the production phase is enabled, the trained classifier is employed in the framework with the real-time speech signal of the patient being analyzed with the same procedure of feature extraction. The classifier receives the standardized features and maps the current mid-term batch with the predicted class, according to the one with the highest probability over the *L* classes.

Convolutional Neural Network-Based Recognition

Due to their application on visual imagery, CNNs are vastly used in capturing and transforming high-level information from images [59, 61]. Since the spectrograms are two-dimensional visualization of audio frequency spectrum over time, CNNs can be also used for sound analysis. More specifically, a spectrogram is the visual representation of the distribution of the signal strength at the frequency domain for an examined waveform. While there is a significant effort in detecting the most suitable features for a specific classification in emotion recognition, in the case of CNNs, the only necessity is the extraction of the spectrogram. Thus, CNN-based classifiers are immutable to erroneous feature extraction. In addition, the computation of many acoustic parameters is computationally expensive and may be difficult to apply on a large scale or with limited resources. Therefore, it is highly pertinent to investigate the application of CNNs with the aim of alleviating the problem of feature extraction and designing SER systems with a simple pipeline and low latency. As designed to emulate the behavior of a visual cortex, CNNs mitigate the challenges posed by the other deep learning architectures by exploiting the strong spatially local correlation present in natural images. The corresponding approach is to feed the CNN with the relevant spectrogram of every computed window in order to train it efficiently. As a major advantage, the necessary features are significantly reduced to one, comprising only the spectrogram of the corresponding window being derived with fast Fourier transform (FFT).

The main tool used for the utilization of the convolutional neural networks is Keras [85]. The library of Keras provides the efficient building of CNNs through versatile and user-friendly methods. Due to the large number of experiments carried out in this paper, several computational resources were deemed as necessary. Computational experiments were conducted using GPU Nvidia TITAN X and 12 GB memory for the training of the diverse CNNs with an average time duration of training phase at 20 s/epoch. Table 9.2 lists various CNN architectures and their respective test accuracy. The respective architectures were trained with a predetermined window length of 0.5 s, frame overlap of 20%, batch size equal to 256 samples, and cross-entropy loss function. At the output of every CNN architecture, a softmax output layer of six units is followed by a maximum selection of the highest posterior probability as follows:

$$c_n = \underset{i=1,\dots,I}{\operatorname{argmax}} \left(y_n | \vec{x} \right) \tag{9.2}$$

where $I = 6$ denotes the number of output classes, c_n the predicted label of nth batch, x the input vector of spectrogram in the nth batch and y_n the output of the CNN architecture at the nth batch. From the results listed in the Table 9.2, the paramount advantage of network depth can be observed. The best results were obtained from the last experiment in Table 9.2 using three convolutional layers followed by a Max pooling layer as duplicate, with an ending of two fully connected layers and a dropout layer. In Fig. 9.4, the architecture of the best CNN scheme is depicted, along with the dimensions of the vectors, throughout the entire feedforward propagation of the signal. In general, the first experiments elaborate the existence of BatchNormalization technique and the potential contribution in the performance levels. Yet, the BatchNormalization layers revealed that the classification task delivers insufficient performance. In contrary to the BatchNormalization layer, the next experiments focused on the deflection of overfitting in the CNN through the

Table 9.2 Test accuracy for various CNN architectures. $C(m \times n \times k)$ denotes a spatial convolutional layer of m filters each of size $n \times k$. $C_{B,R}(m \times n \times k)$ denotes a spatial convolutional layer of m filters each of size $n \times k$ followed by BatchNorm and ReLUs. $FC(l)$ denotes a fully connected layer of l units. $FC_{B,R}(l)$ denotes a fully connected layer of l units followed by BatchNorm and ReLUs. $D(u)$ denotes a dropout regularization layer with a fraction of u. $P(f \times r)$ denotes a Max pooling layer with $(f \times r)$ dimensions. Best performance is marked and mentioned in the last entry

CNN architecture	Test accuracy (%)
$(C_{B,R}(64 \times 3 \times 3) - P(2 \times 2)) \times 2 - FC_{B,R}(2048) - D(0.5)$	0.6657
$(C_{B,R}(64 \times 3 \times 3) \times 2 - P(2 \times 2)) \times 2 - FC_{B,R}(2048) - D(0.4)$	0.84
$(C_R(64 \times 2 \times 2) \times 3 - P(2 \times 2) - D(0.6)) \times 2 - FC_{B,R}(4096) - D(0.6)$	0.901
$(C_R(128 \times 3 \times 3) \times 4 - P(2 \times 2) - D(0.6)) \times 2$ $(C_R(64 \times 2 \times 2) \times 4 - P(2 \times 2) - D(0.6)) \times 2 - FC_{B,R}(4096) - D(0.6)$	0.9014
$(C_R(64 \times 3 \times 3) - C(64 \times 3 \times 3) - P_{B,R}(2,2) - D(0.25)) \times 2$ $-FC_R(4096) - D(0.6)$	0.915
$(C_R(64 \times 3 \times 3) \times 2 - P_{B,R}(2,2) - D(0.6)) \times 2$ $-(FC_R(4096) - D(0.6)) \times 2$	0.916
$C_R(32 \times 3 \times 3) - C_R(32 \times 2 \times 2) \times 2 - P(2 \times 2) - D(0.25)$ $-C_R(64 \times 3 \times 3) - C_R(64 \times 2 \times 2) \times 2 - P(2 \times 2) - D(0.25)$ $-(FC_R(4096) - D(0.5)) \times 2$	0.925

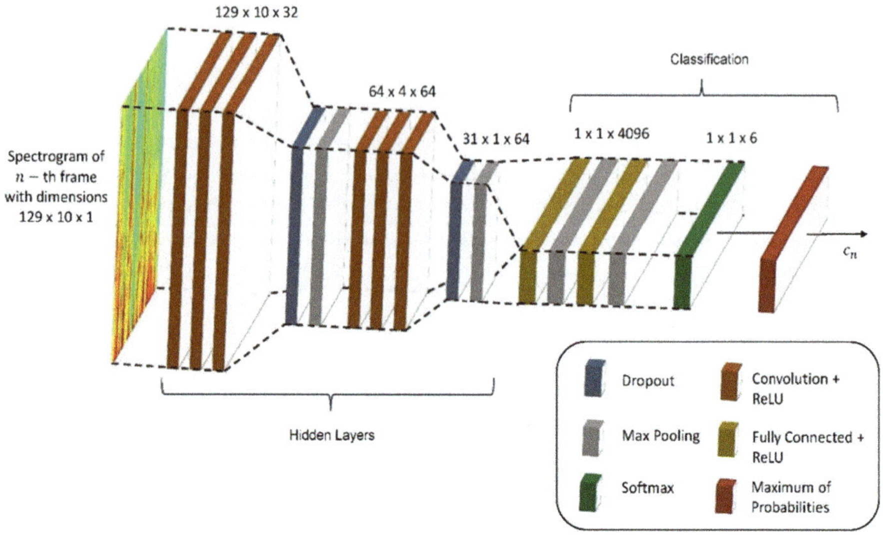

Fig. 9.4 Architecture of the proposed CNN for SER

addition of dropout layers. Furthermore, the results revealed that the number of filters, along with their kernel size, is negligible correlated with the performance of the CNN. As depicted, the dropout layers introduced adequate results and restricted the CNN from overfitting in a small number of epochs.

9.3.2 SER Integration in Homecare Platform

The SER module is integrated in the commercially available HeartAround homecare platform (www.heartaround.com) in a pilot staging. The specific platform is able to deliver superior remote monitoring and communication services through timely response and accurate recording of vital signs, lifestyle activities, and other patient critical information. Via its services, the homecare platform enhances compliance of the elderly population to their self-care commitments, providing peace of mind to them and their families while remaining minor intrusive and offering an excellent user experience. Our goal was the integration of the affective computing as a service module, which gives to the platform the ability to continually sense emotion and associate it with a person's health status. The emotion analysis is based on the six basic emotions identified by Ekman [86], and they are considered until today the basis of the affective computing field. The basic emotions are anger, disgust, fear, happiness, sadness, and surprise, while the module supports also a neutral emotional class. The specific service is based on the analysis of audio signals produced during the real-time WebRTC communication between the patients and the medical professionals or the caregivers. The affective service receives the patent's speech and provides a near-real-time assessment of his emotional state. Upon to the conclusion of the video conference session, the affective analysis results are stored in the patient's PHR, along with his biosignals and motion data. The two modes of operation are detailed in the following subsections.

Store in Personal Health Record

The efficient inclusion of affective analysis results through the Audio Emotion Analysis as a Service provides a plethora of advantages in the proposed homecare platform. First, the analysis of the emotional state is stored in the platform's embedded PHR with the aim of following up and improving the patient's condition. Hence, the data analysis of the current therapy and medical practice is monitored through each session. The patient's monitoring could lead to early interventions upon encountering deviation of the desired/normal emotional status. In this context, we focus on the delivery of the unified information, concerning the video conference session of the patient-doctor, by including the emotion vector probabilities. The summarization of the information in a final JSON file comprises a convenient tool for the final visualization through the aggregation of the data. Figure 9.5 depicts an exemplary instance of the JSON file schema, where the session emotional information is included after its finalization, along with the inclusion of necessary data for the subsequent retrieval. The doctor can query the records with the patient's name

Fig. 9.5 JSON schema of the stored session information in the PHR repository

Session Report JSON Format


```
{
    "patient_id": "126e4267-j46b-76d2-a438-92525419987"
    "patient_name": "James Aalen",
    "doctor_id": "766e2188-b97e-73p9-a197-08995108764",
    "emotion_vector": [{
            "timestamp": "1539775078",
            "happy_probability": 0.12,
            "neutral_probability": 0.23,
            "sad_probability": 0.3,
            "fear_probability": 0.14,
            "disgust_probability": 0.11
            "angry_probability": 0.1 },
           {
            "timestamp": "1539775079",
            "happy_probability": 0.10,
            "neutral_probability": 0.20,
            "sad_probability": 0.36,
            "fear_probability": 0.12,
            "disgust_probability": 0.12
            "angry_probability": 0.1 }],
    "dominant_emotion": "sad",
    "midterm_batch_duration_sec": 1,
    "call_creation_timestamp": "1539775078",
    "call_ending_timestamp": "1539775079",
    "session_id": "122g2555-z55n-58p9-a197-00142333458"
}
```

or ID and retrieve the relevant emotional findings of the accomplished sessions, along with medical history and other health data.

Near-Real-Time Operation

One of the biggest challenges of this work is the integration of affective speech analysis in the homecare telemonitoring platform with seamless and immediate time characteristics, in parallel with the transmission of the audiovisual content. Through the WebRTC framework (https://webrtc.org/), the audiovisual content is delivered, in addition to the doctor's terminal, to the Audio Emotion Analysis as a Service component for further processing. The meticulous overview of the real-time operation workflow is depicted in Fig. 9.6. Thus, the requirement of delivering speedily the SER results is essential. The emotion classification task requires the preprocessing of the speech utterances of the patient through his personal homecare terminal. The processing time of the affective speech analysis is a subject to the deployed classification techniques in the Audio Emotion Analysis as a Service. Among the different classification techniques, the time processing of the speech utterances is highly correlated with different aspects. More specifically, in the matter of the conventional classification schemes, the number of features comprises a substantial factor in the time complexity of the algorithm, exacerbating the challenge of feature engineering. From the aspect of the CNNs, the total time complexity of the convolutional layers is defined as follows [87]:

$$O\left(\sum_{i=1}^{l} n_{i-1} s_i^2 n_i m_i^2\right) \tag{9.3}$$

where i denotes the index of a convolutional layer, l the number of the convolutional layers, n_i the number of filters in the ith layer and n_{i-1} the number of input channels of the ith layer, s_i the spatial size of the filter, m_i the spatial size of the output feature map. The time complexity of the fully connected and the pooling layers are not included in the Eq. (9.3), while they require 5–10% computational time [87]. Thus, the CNNs provide substantial advantages in time complexity since it is depended only in the internal architecture. As shown in [87], the experimental results have shown the significance of the depth characteristic in the CNN for the improvement accuracy with the decrease of the width/filter sizes. On these terms, the time complexity of the CNN is limited with the appropriate design of the architecture, while it provides significantly enhanced performance compared to the conventional classification schemes.

The client side of the doctor's terminal receives the near-real-time results of the emotion classification task in a report with the format of a JSON file similar to the PHR storage file. This schema is presented in Fig. 9.7. In the real-time report, each class probability is listed with a mapping to the *session_id*, which characterizes uniquely the session of the patient-doctor. In this point, the real-time report needs to be consistent and informative without overloading the network of the services. As

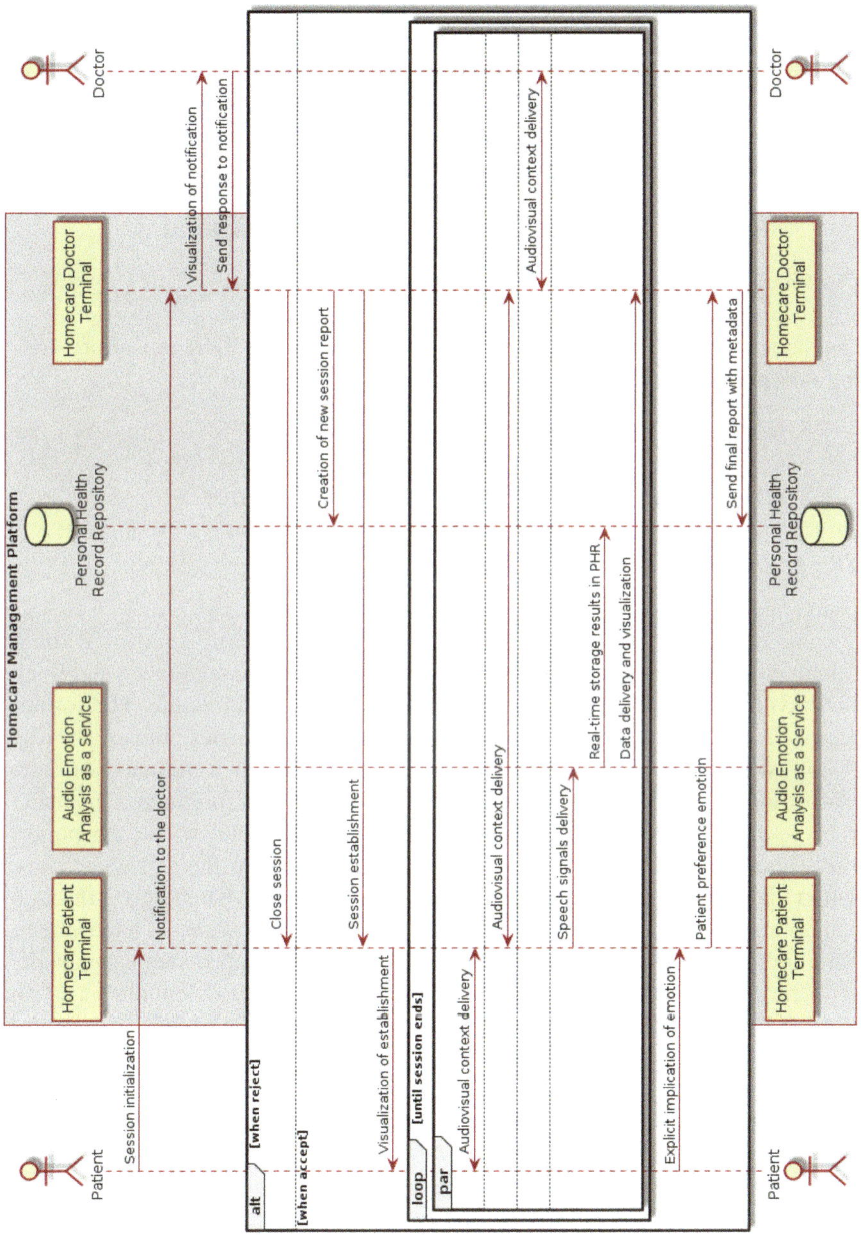

Fig. 9.6 Overall workflow of an established session through the homecare management platform

Real-time Report JSON Format


```
{
    "session_id": "122g2555-z55n-58p9-a197-00142333458"
    "emotion_vector": {
            "timestamp": "1539775078",
            "happy_probability": 0.12,
            "neutral_probability": 0.23,
            "sad_probability": 0.3,
            "fear_probability": 0.14,
            "disgust_probability": 0.11
            "angry_probability": 0.1
            {
}
```


Fig. 9.7 Real-time report of emotion classification results in JSON format

soon as the session finishes, a final report is delivered to the PHR repository concerning the specific session as described in the previous section.

9.4 Experimental Results: The System in Practice

9.4.1 Training Dataset Description

The Toronto emotional speech set (TESS), available from the University of Toronto [88], along with the Ryerson Audio-Visual Database of Emotional Speech and Song (RAVDESS) [89] is exploited for the training of the affective module. The former includes a set of 200 target words, which are spoken in the carrier phrase "Say the word" by two actresses (aged 26 and 64 years). The recordings were made with the aim of portraying each of seven emotions: *anger*, *disgust*, *fear*, *happiness*, *pleasant surprise*, *sadness*, and *neutral*. There are 2800 stimuli in total with each phrase (utterance) having an average time duration of 3.4 s. Both of the actresses speak English as their first language, are university-educated, and have undergone through musical training, while audiometric testing indicated that both actresses have thresholds within the normal range. The latter includes gender-balanced samples consisting of 24 professional actors, vocalizing lexically matched statements in a neutral North American accent. The database predominantly focused on speech utterances which are distinguished through the following emotions: *calm*, *happy*, *sad*, *angry*, *fearful*, *surprise*, and *disgust*. In order to be consistent with the several existing approaches on SER with the same databases, we select emotion classes to be *neutral*, *sad*, *happy*, *fear*, *disgust*, and *angry*.

A repeated random sub-sampling validation (Monte Carlo cross-validation) was deployed for the cross-validation scheme of the training stage of the classification algorithms. Samples of all speakers were used in the cross-validation subset for training the tuning parameters of the algorithms. Audio speech was analyzed using a mid-term window size of 0.5 s. As it is a standard practice in the field of automatic speech emotion recognition, results are reported using accuracy and to reflect imbalanced classes. Accuracy is reported for the average of repeated random sub-sampling validation with the output of the model during evaluation being the class with the highest-class probability.

9.4.2 *Classification Experiments*

Conventional Classification Schemes

In this section, experiment results are presented from the deployment of well-established classifiers such as SVM, k-NN, gradient boosting, random decision forest, and extremely randomized trees algorithms by modifying the short-term feature extraction window of the speech utterances and the parameters of each algorithm. In Fig. 9.8, the performance of the several algorithms is depicted as a function of the duration of the mid-term batch for the feature extraction, in terms of the accuracy and the F1 score. As it can be seen, the performance is maximized in various durations for the different algorithms. From a general overview of Fig. 9.8, performance is maximized for the mid-term batch of 0.5 s duration for a subset of the examined algorithms. A further examination is necessary in the parameters for selecting an appropriate mid-term batch duration with the aim of delivering an efficient trade-off between complexity and performance. Consequently, Table 9.3 depicts the experimental results of the classification algorithms, along with the parameters of each algorithm. Among the various durations presented, the performance of the algorithms presents a local or a global maximum for the mid-term duration of 0.5 s with optimal tuning parameters.

In Fig. 9.9, the classification results of the deployment of the SVM, k-NN, random decision forest, extremely randomized trees, and gradient boosting algorithms are depicted where test accuracy is plotted for several short-term frame overlaps as

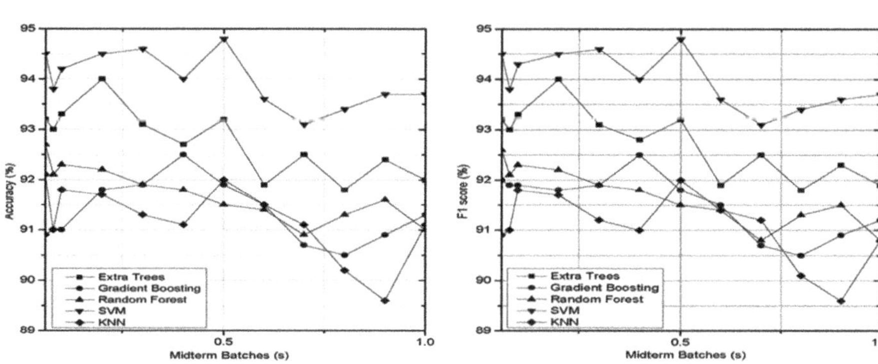

Fig. 9.8 Performance of the conventional classification algorithms as a function of the duration of the mid-term batch, in terms of test accuracy (left) and F1 score (right)

Table 9.3 Experimental results of the accuracy and the parameters of the conventional classification algorithms as a function of the mid-term batch

	Extra trees		Gradient boosting		Random forest		SVM		k-NN	
Batch (s)	Accuracy (%)	Number of trees	Accuracy (%)	Number of trees	Accuracy (%)	Number of trees	Accuracy (%)	*C*	Accuracy (%)	*k*
0.06	93.2	450	91.1	200	92.7	350	94.5	5	90.9	7
0.08	93	300	91	200	92.1	150	93.8	10	91	3
0.1	93.3	500	91	500	92.3	350	94.2	10	91.8	1
0.2	94	450	91.8	500	92.2	500	94.5	7	91.7	3
0.3	93.1	200	91.9	450	91.9	450	94.6	5	91.3	5
0.4	92.7	350	92.5	500	91.8	300	94	15	91.1	13
0.5	93.2	200	91.9	200	91.5	200	94.8	5	92	7
0.6	91.9	250	91.5	450	91.4	500	93.6	5	91.5	1
0.7	92.5	400	90.7	500	90.9	200	93.1	10	91.1	7
0.8	91.8	500	90.5	400	91.3	250	93.4	20	90.2	3
0.9	92.4	500	90.9	500	91.6	350	93.7	5	89.6	11
1	92	350	91.3	350	91	350	93.7	20	91.1	1
1.5	91.9	350	91.4	500	91	250	93	5	89.8	1
2	92.9	450	92.2	500	92.2	450	93.4	20	91.4	1
2.5	93.4	450	92.5	500	92.3	100	93.5	10	91.5	5

a function of each tuning parameter. In general, the results are deemed adequate, while the best performance is provided by setting the short-term frame overlap equal to 20%. In many cases, different short-term frame overlaps provide comparable performance with reduced cost complexity. As it can be seen, the accuracy is directly proportional to the short-term frame overlap, with levels above 90%. One of the main observations is that the SVM provides improved accuracy, even for small values of the tuning parameters, leading to reduced cost complexity. Also, the k-NN classifier delivers stable accuracy results, independently from the number of neighbors with suboptimal cost complexity. Similarly, the performance of the random decision forest, extremely randomized trees, and gradient boosting algorithms is sufficient with small cost complexity.

Table 9.4 depicts the confusion matrix of the best-trained SVM classifier architecture with a window length of 0.5 s and frame overlap of 20%. The model was able to perform predictions with accuracy above 91% for every emotion class. The neutral and sad emotions may be confused with the neutral emotion with a negligible negative predictive value. However, the performance of the best-trained SVM delivers adequate results. In general, Table 9.5 summarizes the best results from the experiment results through the deployment of SVM, k-NN, gradient boosting, random decision forest, and extremely randomized trees algorithms. In every classification algorithm, the best results are always firstly depicted on top, while suboptimal solutions listed below pertain to the time and cost complexity. For example, the random forest algorithm delivers an adequate performance with an accuracy of

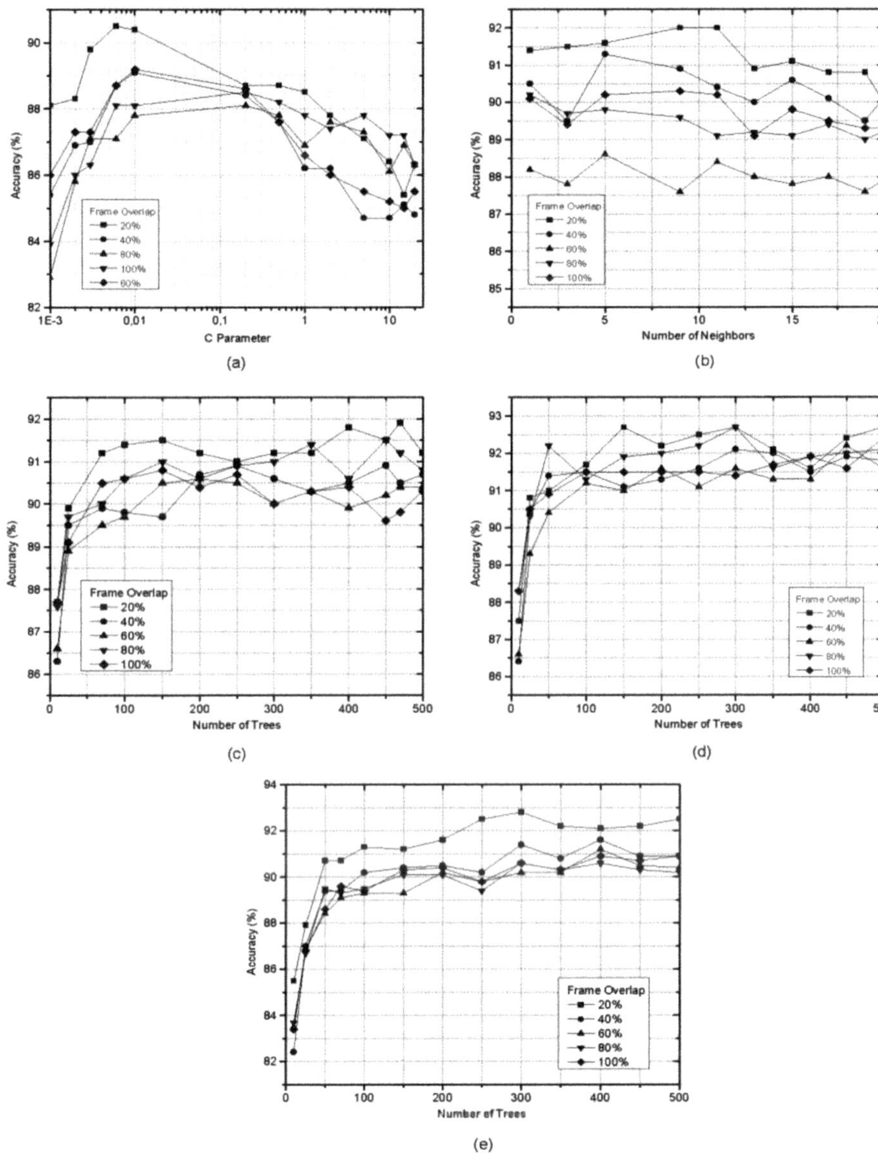

Fig. 9.9 Test accuracy of the conventional classification algorithms for several short-time frame overlaps as a function of the tuning parameter of each algorithm. From top, the performances of the (**a**) support vector machine, (**b**) k-nearest neighbors, (**c**) random decision forest, (**d**) extremely randomized trees, and (**e**) gradient boosting algorithm

Table 9.4 Confusion matrix for speech emotion recognition prediction using the SVM classifier

	Neutral	Sad	Happy	Fear	Disgust	Angry
Neutral	91.17	2.12	4.14	0.85	0.01	1.59
Sad	3.16	93.04	0.63	1.89	0.88	0.38
Happy	3.29	0.53	93.19	0.85	0.95	1.17
Fear	0.96	1.44	0.09	96.53	0.96	0
Disgust	0.42	1.28	0.42	1.14	94.42	0.28
Angry	0.91	1.03	1.60	0	0	96.44

Table 9.5 Summary of classification results of conventional algorithms

Classification algorithm	Parameters	Test accuracy (%)	Frame overlap (%)	
SVM	C	0.006	91.5	20
		0.006	89.2	40
k-NN	Number of trees	9	92	20
		5	91.2	40
Random forest		470	91.9	20
		100	91.5	20
		150	91	80
		70	90.5	100
Extra trees		150	92.7	20
		50	92.3	80
		100	91.7	20
Gradient boosting		300	92.4	20
		100	91.5	20
		50	90.7	20

91.9%, yet with 470 trees and 20% frame overlap, skyrocketing the time and cost complexity of the algorithm. A slightly lower performance is delivered with 100 trees, 91.5% accuracy, and 20% frame overlap.

Convolutional Neural Networks

In this section, experiment results are presented from the deployment of the convolutional neural network by modifying the short-term feature extraction window of the spectrograms. Figure 9.10a depicts the test accuracy in the training phase of the convolutional neural network for several short-term frame overlaps as a function of the 50 first training epochs. As depicted, the performance significantly deteriorates for lower values of 20% short-time frame overlap, while for higher values of 20%, the performance is stable. This can be justified, since small frame overlaps provide serendipity in the spectrogram samples and convergence is achieved with smaller training rate. However, the best performance of the CNN is equal to 92.5% as listed in Table 9.6. Similar characteristics are provided in Fig. 9.10b where the cross-entropy loss function is plotted as a function of the training epochs.

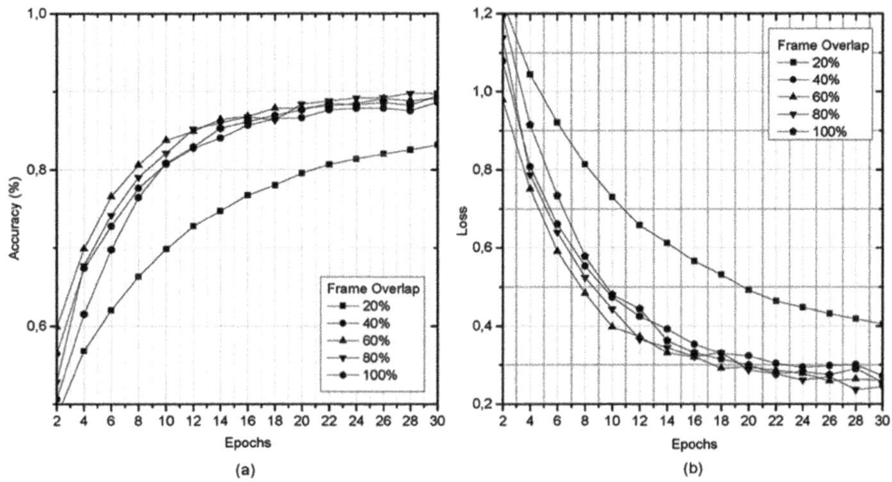

Fig. 9.10 Results from the deployment of the CNN for several short-time frame overlaps as a function of the epochs in the training phase. From left to right, (**a**) the test accuracy and (**b**) the loss function

Table 9.6 Confusion matrix for speech emotion recognition prediction using the CNN architecture

	Neutral	Sad	Happy	Fear	Disgust	Angry
Neutral	92.10	4.32	1.51	1.26	1.65	1.14
Sad	1.66	97.30	0.21	0.41	0.41	0
Happy	3.03	3.35	84.01	1.27	2.23	6.12
Fear	0.18	1.07	3.23	90.49	0.90	4.14
Disgust	1.62	2.28	2.02	1.05	90.30	2.72
Angry	1.06	1.33	0.91	0.85	1.70	94.14

Table 9.6 depicts the confusion matrix of the trained proposed model of CNN architecture with a window length of 0.5 s, frame overlap of 40%, batch size equal to 256 samples, and cross-entropy loss function. The model was able to perform predictions with accuracy above 76% for all class emotions. The happiness and fear emotions may be heavily confused with the angriness emotion which adversely affects the prediction performance. The confusion of happiness and fear with the angriness emotion is that the pitch and the energy of the voice utterances are at a comparable level. In comparison with the best-trained SVM classifier in Table 9.4, the CNN architecture delivers slightly decreased performance. This negligible difference is based on the fact that the SVM classifier includes a plethora of features, compared to the CNN architecture. However, the cost complexity of the SVM classifier is substantially increased than the complexity delivered from the CNN architecture.

9.5 Conclusions and Future Work

In this paper, we have presented the design and implementation of a proof-of-concept affective analysis service, which supports the continuous analysis of the speech utterances through SER techniques. This service is integrated to an existing homecare platform utilizing its video conference communication facility. Several classification techniques were trained with the TESS and RAVDESS datasets and evaluated for the prediction of six emotional states. In the first phase of the experiments, we trained the k-NN, SVM, RF, ET, and GBT classification algorithms with the speech utterances. The experimental results were satisfactory for all emotional states, compared to the existing approaches. In the next phase, we focused on the design of the deep convolutional neural networks, where we evaluated the performance of various architectures in terms of test accuracy. The training phase of the DCNN architectures was feasible with the spectrograms of the available datasets. The architecture with the optimum performance was deployed in the production phase of the homecare platform. Adequate results were achieved with significantly reduced time complexity, rendering the DCNN as a suitable classification technique for seamless time-restricted applications. During the initial testing of the service, the users perceived very well the new affective analysis functionality, and the general impression is that the value of the homecare platform is increased.

As a roadmap, investigation needs to be done to further improve the proposed homecare framework so that every emotion is recognized effectively in a robust manner. From the perspective of the conventional classification schemes, the feature selection engineering process is a major factor in the performance of the homecare platform. As for the DCNN, experiments on the size of the spectrograms are deemed necessary. In general, the future experiments will include more data with relatively complex models to improve the SER performance even further. On top of all, the involvement of facial characteristics in the classification task, in parallel with the speech utterances, needs to be included as it will improve the accuracy of emotional sensing. Additional work includes also the exploitation of other data types in the affective analysis module, such as the activity and lifestyle data, which are correlated with the affective status and can improve the emotional analysis.

References

1. Russel, S. J., & Norvig, P. (2016). *Artificial intelligence: a modern approach*. Pearson Education Limited.
2. Devillers, L., & Vidrascu, L. (2006). Real-life emotions detection with lexical and paralinguistic cues on human-human call center dialogs. In *Ninth international conference on spoken language processing*. ISCA.
3. Lee, C. C., Mower, E., Busso, C., Lee, S., & Narayanan, S. (2011). Emotion recognition using a hierarchical binary decision tree approach. *Speech Communication, 53*, 1162–1171.

4. Polzehl, T., Sundaram, S., Ketabdar, H., Wagner, M., & Metze, F. (2009). Emotion classification in children's speech using fusion of acoustic and linguistic features. In *Tenth annual conference of the international speech communication association*. ISCA.
5. Hibbeln, M., Jenkins, J. L., Schneider, C., Valacich, J. S., & Weinmann, M. (2017). How is your user feeling? Inferring emotion through human–computer interaction devices. *Group, 1000*, 248.
6. Kostoulas, T., Mporas, I., Kocsis, O., Ganchev, T., Katsaounos, N., Santamaria, J. J., Jimenez-Murcia, S., Fernandez-Aranda, F., & Fakotakis, N. (2012). Affective speech interface in serious games for supporting therapy of mental disorders. *Expert Systems with Applications, 39*, 11072–11079.
7. Tyagi, R., & Agarwal, A. (2018). Emotion detection using speech analysis. *Science, 3*, 18–20.
8. Zeng, Z., Pantic, M., Roisman, G. I., & Huang, T. S. (2009). A survey of affect recognition methods: Audio, visual, and spontaneous expressions. *IEEE Transactions on Pattern Analysis and Machine Intelligence, 31*, 39–58.
9. Zhang, Y., Gravina, R., Lu, H., Villari, M., & Fortino, G. (2018). PEA: Parallel electrocardiogram-based authentication for smart healthcare systems. *Journal of Network and Computer Applications, 117*, 10–16.
10. Iliadis, L. S., Maglogiannis, I., Papadopoulos, H., Karatzas, N., & Sioutas, S. (2012). *Artificial intelligence applications and innovations: AIAI 2012 international workshops: AIAB, AIeIA, CISE, COPA, IIVC, ISQL, MHDW, and WADTMB*. Springer.
11. Akbulut, F. P., & Akan, A. (2018). A smart wearable system for short-term cardiovascular risk assessment with emotional dynamics. *Measurement, 128*, 237–246.
12. Doukas, C., & Maglogiannis, I. (2008). Intelligent pervasive healthcare systems. *Advanced Computational Intelligence Paradigms in Healthcare, 3*, 95–115.
13. Bou-Ghazale, S. E., & Hansen, J. H. (2000). A comparative study of traditional and newly proposed features for recognition of speech under stress. *IEEE Transactions on Speech and Audio Processing, 8*, 429–442.
14. O'Leary, A. (1992). Self-efficacy and health: Behavioral and stress-physiological mediation. *Cognitive Therapy and Research, 16*, 229–245.
15. Broyles, D., Crichton, R., Jolliffe, B., & Dixon, B. E. (2016). Shared longitudinal health records for clinical and population health. *Health Information Exchange, 2016*, 149–162.
16. Yamin, C. K., Emani, S., Williams, D. H., Lipsitz, S. R., Karson, A. S., Wald, J. S., & Bates, D. W. (2011). The digital divide in adoption and use of a personal health record. *Archives of Internal Medicine, 171*, 568–574.
17. Doukas, C., & Maglogiannis, I. (2011). Managing wearable sensor data through cloud computing. In *IEEE third international conference on cloud computing technology and science (CloudCom)*. IEEE.
18. Sloman, A. (1999). Review of affective computing. *AI Magazine, 20*, 127.
19. Alfano, C. A., Bower, J., Cowie, J., Lau, S., & Simpson, R. J. (2017). Long-duration space exploration and emotional health: Recommendations for conceptualizing and evaluating risk. *Acta Astronautica, 142*, 289–299.
20. Fridlund, A. J. (2014). *Human facial expression: An evolutionary view*. Academic Press.
21. Caridakis, G., Karpouzis, K., Wallace, M., Kessous, L., & Amir, N. (2010). Multimodal user's affective state analysis in naturalistic interaction. *Journal on Multimodal User Interfaces, 3*, 49–66.
22. Doukas, C., & Maglogiannis, I. (2008). Enabling human status awareness in assistive environments based on advanced sound and motion data classification. In *Proceedings of the 1st international conference on PErvasive technologies related to assistive environments*. ACM.
23. Maglogiannis, I. G., Karpouzis, K., & Wallace, M. (2005). Image and signal processing for networked e-health applications. *Synthesis Lectures on Biomedical Engineering, 1*, 1–108.
24. Nicholson, J., Takahashi, K., & Nakatsu, R. (2000). Emotion recognition in speech using neural networks. *Neural Computing & Applications, 9*, 290–296.

25. Seidel, E. M., Habel, U., Kirschner, M., Gur, R. C., & Derntl, B. (2010). The impact of facial emotional expressions on behavioral tendencies in women and men. *Journal of Experimental Psychology: Human Perception and Performance, 36*, 500.
26. Schultz, D. P., & Schultz, S. E. (2016). Theories of personality. *Cengage Learning, 29*, 516.
27. Picard, R. W. (1995). Affective computing. M.I.T Media Laboratory Perceptual Computing Section Technical Report No. 321.
28. Simon, H. A. (1979). *Models of thought* (Vol. 2). Yale University Press.
29. Mansoorizadeh, M., & Charkari, N. M. (2009). Hybrid feature and decision level fusion of face and speech information for bimodal emotion recognition. In *IEEE computer conference CSICC*. IEEE.
30. Bejani, M., Gharavian, D., & Charkari, N. M. (2014). Audiovisual emotion recognition using ANOVA feature selection method and multi-classifier neural networks. *Neural Computing and Applications, 24*, 399–412.
31. Busso, C., & Narayanan, S. S. (2007). Interrelation between speech and facial gestures in emotional utterances: a single subject study. *IEEE Transactions on Audio, Speech and Language Processing, 15*, 2331–2347.
32. Jürgens, R., Grass, A., Drolet, M., & Fischer, J. (2015). Effect of acting experience on emotion expression and recognition in voice: non-actors provide better stimuli than expected. *Journal of Nonverbal Behavior, 39*, 195–214.
33. Jürgens, R., Hammerschmidt, K., & Fischer, J. (2011). Authentic and play-acted vocal emotion expressions reveal acoustic differences. *Frontiers in Psychology, 2*, 180.
34. Vogt, T., & André, E. (2005). Comparing feature sets for acted and spontaneous speech in view of automatic emotion recognition. In *IEEE international conference on multimedia and expo*. IEEE.
35. Datatang. (2015). *Chinese Academy of Sciences*. Retrieved September 10, 2018, from http://www.en.datatang.com/product.php?id=28
36. Wang, K., An, N., Li, B. N., Zhang, Y., & Li, L. (2015). Speech emotion recognition using Fourier parameters. *IEEE Transactions on Affective Computing, 6*, 69–75.
37. Dellaert, F., Polzin, T., & Waibel, A. (1996). Recognizing emotion in speech. In *Fourth international conference on spoken language processing*. IEEE.
38. Rawat, A., & Mishra, P. K. (2015). Emotion recognition through speech using neural network. *International Journal of Advanced Research in Computer Science and Software Engineering, 5*, 422–428.
39. Hamidi, M., & Mansoorizade, M. (2012). Emotion recognition from Persian speech with neural network. *International Journal of Artificial Intelligence Applications, 3*, 107.
40. Quan, C., & Ren, F. (2016). Weighted high-order hidden Markov models for compound emotions recognition in text. *Information Sciences, 329*, 581–596.
41. Nwe, T. L., Foo, S. W., & De Silva, L. C. (2003). Speech emotion recognition using hidden Markov models. *Speech Communication, 41*, 603–623.
42. Schuller, B., Rigoll, G., & Lang, M. (2003). Hidden Markov model-based speech emotion recognition. *IEEE International Conference on Acoustics, Speech, and Signal Processing, 2*, II.
43. Hu, H., Xu, M. X., & Wu, W. (2007). Fusion of global statistical and segmental spectral features for speech emotion recognition. In *Eighth annual conference of the international speech communication association*. IEEE.
44. Ververidis, D., & Kotropoulos, C. (2006). Emotional speech recognition: Resources, features, and methods. *Speech Communication, 48*, 1162–1181.
45. Schuller, B., Lang, M., & Rigoll, G. (2005). Robust acoustic speech emotion recognition by ensembles of classifiers. Tagungsband Fortschritte der Akustik-DAGA# 05, München.
46. Wu, C. H., & Liang, W. B. (2011). Emotion recognition of affective speech based on multiple classifiers using acoustic-prosodic information and semantic labels. *IEEE Transactions on Affective Computing, 2*, 10–21.
47. El Ayadi, M., Kamel, M. S., & Karray, F. (2011). Survey on speech emotion recognition: Features, classification schemes, and databases. *Pattern Recognition, 44*, 572–587.

48. Cowie, R., Douglas-Cowie, E., Tsapatsoulis, N., Votsis, G., Kollias, S., Fellenz, W., & Taylor, J. G. (2001). Emotion recognition in human-computer interaction. *IEEE Signal Processing Magazine, 18*, 32–80.
49. Argyle, M. (2013). *The psychology of happiness*. Routledge.
50. Teager, H. (1980). Some observations on oral air flow during phonation. *IEEE Transactions on Acoustics, Speech, and Signal Processing, 28*, 599–601.
51. Zhou, G., Hansen, J. H., & Kaiser, J. F. (2001). Nonlinear feature-based classification of speech under stress. *IEEE Transactions on Speech and Audio Processing, 9*, 201–216.
52. Hinton, G., Deng, L., Yu, D., Dahl, G. E., Mohamed, A. R., Jaitly, N., Senior, A., Vanhoucke, V., Nguyen, P., Sainath, T. N., & Kingsbury, B. (2012). Deep neural networks for acoustic modeling in speech recognition: The shared views of four research groups. *IEEE Signal Processing Magazine, 29*, 82–97.
53. Weninger, F., Geiger, J., Wöllmer, M., Schuller, B., & Rigoll, G. (2014). Feature enhancement by deep LSTM networks for ASR in reverberant multisource environments. *Computer Speech & Language, 28*, 888–902.
54. Mao, Q., Dong, M., Huang, Z., & Zhan, Y. (2014). Learning salient features for speech emotion recognition using convolutional neural networks. *IEEE Transactions on Multimedia, 16*, 2203–2213.
55. Fayek, H. M., Lech, M., & Cavedon, L. (2017). Evaluating deep learning architectures for speech emotion recognition. *Neural Networks, 92*, 60–68.
56. Zhu, L., Chen, L., Zhao, D., Zhou, J., & Zhang, W. (2017). Emotion recognition from Chinese speech for smart affective services using a combination of SVM and DBN. *Sensors, 17*, 1694.
57. Sangeetha, J., & Jayasankar, T. (2019). Emotion speech recognition based on adaptive fractional deep belief network and reinforcement learning. *Cognitive Informatics and Soft Computing, 2019*, 165–174.
58. Li, L., Zhao, Y., Jiang, D., Zhang, Y., Wang, F., Gonzalez, I., Valentin, E., & Sahli, H. (2013). Hybrid deep neural network--hidden Markov model (DNN-HMM) based speech emotion recognition. In *Humaine association conference on affective computing and intelligent interaction (ACII)*. ACII.
59. Uzair, M., Shafait, F., Ghanem, B., & Mian, A. (2018). Representation learning with deep extreme learning machines for efficient image set classification. *Neural Computing and Applications, 30*, 1211–1223.
60. Lim, W., Jang, D., & Lee, T. (2016). Speech emotion recognition using convolutional and recurrent neural networks. In *IEEE signal and information processing association annual summit and conference*. IEEE.
61. Mu, N., Xu, X., Zhang, X., & Zhang, H. (2018). Salient object detection using a covariance-based CNN model in low-contrast images. *Neural Computing and Applications, 29*, 181–192.
62. Burkhardt, F., Paeschke, A., Rolfes, M., Sendlmeier, W. F., & Weiss, B. (2005). A database of German emotional speech. In *Ninth European conference on speech communication and technology*. ISCA.
63. Tao, J. H., Liu, F., Zhang, M., & Jia, H. B. (2008). Design of speech corpus for mandarin text to speech. In *The Blizzard challenge workshop*. IEEE.
64. Wang, K. X., Zhang, Q. L., & Liao, S. Y. (2014). A database of elderly emotional speech. In *Proc. int. symp. signal process*. Biomed. Eng Informat.
65. Vincent, E., Watanabe, S., Barker, J., & Marxer, R. (2016). *The 4th CHiME speech separation and recognition challenge*. CHiME.
66. Haq, S., Jackson, P. J., & Edge, J. (2009). Speaker-dependent audio-visual emotion recognition. *AVSP, 2009*, 53–58.
67. Engberg, I. S., Hansen, A. V., Andersen, O., & Dalsgaard, P. (1997). Design, recording and verification of a Danish emotional speech database. In *Fifth european conference on speech communication and technology*. ISCA.
68. Mao, X., & Chen, L. (2010). Speech emotion recognition based on parametric filter and fractal dimension. *IEICE Transactions on Information and Systems, 93*, 2324–2326.

69. Badshah, A. M., Ahmad, J., Rahim, N., & Baik, S. W. (2017). Speech emotion recognition from spectrograms with deep convolutional neural network. In *International conference on platform technology and service*. IEEE.
70. Chandrasekar, P., Chapaneri, S., & Jayaswal, D. (2014). Automatic speech emotion recognition: A survey. In *IEEE international conference on circuits, systems, communication and information technology applications* (pp. 341–346). IEEE.
71. Pervaiz, M., & Khan, T. A. (2016). Emotion recognition from speech using prosodic and linguistic features. *Emotion, 7*, 84.
72. O'Connor, J. D., & Arnold, G. F. (2004). *Intonation of colloquial English*. РГБ.
73. Schubiger, M. (1958). *English intonation, its form and function*. M. Niemeyer Verlag.
74. Hozjan, V., Kacic, Z., Moreno, A., Bonafonte, A., & Nogueiras, A. (2002). *Interface databases: Design and collection of a multilingual emotional speech database*. LREC.
75. Campbell, N. (2000). Databases of emotional speech. In *ISCA tutorial and research workshop (ITRW) on speech and emotion*. ISCA.
76. Lee, C. M., & Narayanan, S. S. (2005). Towards detecting emotions in spoken dialogs. *IEEE Transactions on Speech and Audio Processing, 13*, 293–303.
77. Breazeal, C., & Aryananda, L. (2002). Recognition of affective communicative intent in robot-directed speech. *Autonomous Robots, 12*, 83–104.
78. Zhu, M., Zhang, Z., Hirdes, J. P., & Stolee, P. (2007). Using machine learning algorithms to guide rehabilitation planning for home care clients. *BMC Medical Informatics and Decision Making, 7*, 41.
79. Wells, J. L., Seabrook, J. A., Stolee, P., Borrie, M. J., & Knoefel, F. (2003). State of the art in geriatric rehabilitation. Part I: Review of frailty and comprehensive geriatric assessment. *Archives of Physical Medicine and Rehabilitation, 84*, 890–897.
80. Coleman, E. A. (2003). Falling through the cracks: Challenges and opportunities for improving transitional care for persons with continuous complex care needs. *Journal of the American Geriatrics Society, 51*, 549–555.
81. Giannakopoulos, T. (2015). Pyaudioanalysis: An open-source python library for audio signal analysis. *PLoS One, 10*, e0144610.
82. Beeke, S., Wilkinson, R., & Maxim, J. (2009). Prosody as a compensatory strategy in the conversations of people with agrammatism. *Clinical Linguistics & Phonetics, 23*, 133–155.
83. Borchert, M., & Dusterhoft, A. (2005). Emotions in speech-experiments with prosody and quality features in speech for use in categorical and dimensional emotion recognition environments. In *IEEE International conference on natural language processing and knowledge engineering*. IEEE.
84. Li, X., Tao, J., Johnson, M. T., Soltis, J., Savage, A., Leong, K. M., & Newman, J. D. (2007). Stress and emotion classification using jitter and shimmer features. In *IEEE international conference on acoustics, speech and signal processing*. IEEE.
85. Chollet, F. (2015). *Keras: Deep learning library for theano and tensorflow*. Keras.
86. Ekman, P. (1970). Universal facial expressions of emotions. *California Mental Health Research Digest, 8*(4), 151–158.
87. He, K., & Sun, J. (2015). Convolutional neural networks at constrained time cost. In *Proceedings of the IEEE conference on computer vision and pattern recognition* (pp. 5353–5360). IEEE.
88. Dupuis, K., & Pichora-Fuller, M. K. (2010). *Toronto emotional speech set (TESS)*. University of Toronto.
89. Livingstone, S. R., & Russo, F. A. (2018). The Ryerson Audio-Visual Database of Emotional Speech and Song (RAVDESS): A dynamic, multimodal set of facial and vocal expressions in North American English. *PLoS One, 13*(5), e0196391.

Chapter 10
A Study of the Impact of Covid-19 Using a Sieve Approach

Brijesh Kumar Bhardwaj and Kavita Srivastava

10.1 Introduction

Displaying viral illnesses, for example, COVID-19, is critical in deciding their conceivable future effect. Exhibiting the spread and the effect of such an infection can be particularly critical in understanding its impact [1]. Conventional techniques to measure the effects of such diseases can not depict exact models [2], modern thinking could be the best approach to finding extraordinary farsighted models [3]. In this paper, the scholars present a machine learning plan, a sieve chart, to show the spread of the disease, which predicts the maximal number of people who became infected per zone in each time unit, the maximal number of people who recovered per region in each time unit, and the maximal number of passing through a particular region in each time unit. The sieve diagram has been chosen for its straightforwardness in contrast with different examples, because the creators wished to test the chance of utilizing basic strategies, because of the limited preparation time related to such techniques, on the grounds the results achieved are significant when demonstrating illnesses, owing to the as-quick as-possible prerequisite for models with sufficient execution. Modeling should be possible based on existing information, utilizing factual investigations. However, with regard to amazingly complex models, factual investigation can neglect to appreciate the complexities contained in the dissected information [4]. More unpredictable calculations, in particular, machine calculations, and particularly machine learning calculations, can be utilized to "learn" the overall pattern; yet, the complexities of the information bring about better models ([5]). Artificial intelligence (AI) calculations have become increasingly appropriate

B. K. Bhardwaj (✉)
Department of MCA, DR R M L Avadh University, Ayodhya, India

K. Srivastava
Department of Computer Science, SRMU, Lucknow, India

M. S. Husain et al. (eds.), *Pervasive Healthcare*, EAI/Springer Innovations in Communication and Computing, https://doi.org/10.1007/978-3-030-77746-3_10

in different parts of medical fields and industrial domains. The models consider burying the impacts of different information boundaries that probably would not have been contemplated if customary demonstrating techniques had been utilized [6]. This capacity to consider hard-to-watch complexities put away inside information ought to lend itself well, when utilized in an endeavor of relapsing an unpredictable model, for example, the spread of COVID-19. As of now, existing models of COVID-19 spread have reasonably weak results or have not used real time data.

10.2 Machine Learning

Machine learning is the result of the combination of computer science and statistics. Programming designs bases on building machines that tackle explicit issues, and endeavors to perceive if issues are plausible using any and all means. The essential technique that statistics uses on an extremely fundamental level is data derivation, showing hypotheses and assessing steadfastness of the models. The concept of machine learning is incorporating the fundamentals of computer science and statistics upto some degree yet not completely dependent on both. Although computer science centers around programming of PCs, machine learning observes the issue of getting PCs to re-program themselves at whatever point they are introduced to new data subject to some basic learning approaches. Machine learning attempts to elevate the system to a genuine level by giving the data essential to a machine to get ready and change sensibly when introduced to new data. This is known as "preparing." It revolves around isolating information from essentially huge amounts of information; furthermore, a while later it recognizes and perceives concealed models using distinctive authentic measures to improve its ability to unravel new data and produce more practical results. Obviously, any limits can be "tuned" toward the starting levels for better benefit. It is the basis of automated thinking. It is implausible to design any machine to have a partner with knowledge, similar to language or vision, to arrive without a moment's delay. That task would have been practically difficult to fathom. Also, a framework cannot be considered totally intuitive on the off chance that it falls short on the capacity to take in and improve on its past presentations.

10.3 COVID-19 and Medical Science

Under current circumstances, without immunization, the world is asked to implement some of the significant moderation measures to resolve and control COVID-19 [7, 8]. In view of the learning from worldwide developments, the Indian government at first declared to maintain social distancing (1 m separation), which has to be followed every day by all individuals. Under these conditions, a slow increase in COVID-19 cases has been observed; because of that, the state and local government have placed limitations on parties. There are still groups of people in India who do not realize the gravity of COVID-19, that is, Indian residents are acting like the inhabitants of Italy, where it more casualties accumulated than in China [9]. This is the time when Indians should take action to reduce mortality, as India is in the third phase of COVID-19 spread, which is spread via networks. To accomplish this, we have a few techniques that have been implemented by some countries and are quite effective.

Indian government announced that segregation by the general public is attainable for nations such as the USA or European countries; however, not all Indians are in favor of this condition, because of their cash-related business issues. To conquer these problems, the government ought to ensure provision of their essential necessities, which are all concerned with cashflow. Henceforth, cash shortfall will be a significant issue for the legislature to implement this sort of plan, so that the administration can solicit compensation for affected area laborers (both government and private), and government should provide essentials like food items through the public distribution system. These sorts of activities will induce individuals to follow the social distancing and self-isolation from the general public.

After avoiding social contacts, the government needs to smooth the working conditions for civil servants, and for them, the government should provide proper protective equipment (such as hand wash, sanitizers, masks). Consequently, the government ought to have regulate the use of hand wash and liquid sanitizers entering in any office or campus, as scientists announced that hand washing is a basic protection against COVID-19 [10]. The administration authorities ought to analyze the circumstances cautiously and consider additional procedures for safety. They ought to give certainty to individuals; at that point, on those individuals who have been infected will come to medical clinic, where they have to remain for 14 days in isolation. In the event that the management discloses their identity, individuals will dread for the disconnection of isolation. When the government increases individuals' assistance and strengthens their psyche, everybody can comply with the administration rules, and then it will be easy to eliminate COVID-19.

At the same time, the government ought to give proper clinical facilities to every individual who has been infected; more than that, the medical clinics must be provided with all the necessities for a crisis and essential comforts (such as beds). Henceforth, appropriate measures will ensure that we can accommodate all the patients while they are in the emergency clinic. The groups of infected people must be isolated from the all the other patients in the emergency clinic; in particular special wards ought to be assigned to COVID-19 patients. This seclusion step will assist with controlling the spread in medical clinics; subsequently, they ought to be worried about it, in light of the fact that in the clinic most people are already weak. Furthermore, the adjusting specialist and attendant's wellbeing status must be checked every now and again, and they have to take all the preventive measures before taking care of the patients [11, 12]. On account of the absence of specialists, the government can use house specialists; consequently, they can ask help from retired specialists. The top government authorities needs to manage all the circumstances and should settle on choices productively in the crisis. Positively, COVID-19 has become a great danger for India; notwithstanding, because of the government's knowledge, it will end soon. The previously mentioned procedures to battle with Covid-19 and safe the life and jobs of Indians is proving ineffecient, and progression of annihilation in India is continued. Because all nations have been following comparable techniques at the arbitrary stage, and these have ended their terrible experience. These clear paths are useful for Indians to eliminate COVID-19 during the early phase.

10.4 Discussion with Sieve Diagram

A sieve diagram shows the frequencies in a two-manner possibility table comparable with anticipated frequencies under autonomy, and features the example of the relationship between the line and segment factors. In a sieve diagram, the region of every square shape corresponds to the normal recurrence, whereas the observed recurrence appears by the quantity of squares in every square shape. A favorable position of frequencies can be controlled by the force of concealing. Cells whose normal recurrence is more noteworthy than the observed recurrence appear less extreme than those cells where the observed recurrence is more prominent than the normal recurrence. Deviations from autonomy can likewise be effectively controlled by shading, utilizing one for positive deviations and the other for negative deviations. There are two impediments to a sieve diagram. To start with, it does not require apart from these two factors. Second, the request for the classes affects the example of affiliation with the end goal that an unexpected result of classifications can prompt an alternative understanding. An example of these sorts of plots (Fig. 10.1), is shown in the appendix to this chapter. Sieve diagrams are very valuable as an opening stage in light of the fact that these sorts of plots show the observed frequencies comparable with the normal frequencies. The zone of every square shape in the diagram corresponds to the normal recurrence, as it is built with the end goal that the widths are relative to the absolute recurrence in every section and the statures correspond to the complete recurrence in each column. Figure 10.1 is a sieve diagram of information from Kanggle.com. Observed frequencies appear by the quantity of squares in every square shape, and the distinction between observed and expected frequencies (pneumonia, pregnancy, chronic obstructive pulmonary disease (COPD), asthma, immunosuppression, hypertension, weight and much more) appears through the density of the concealing. The tones in which one speak reflects positive and negative deviations from freedom. To make the plot accessible to all readers, including isually challenged, cordial red and blue printer agreeable tones were picked. Orange indicates positive deviations from autonomy, and purple indicates negative deviations from freedom.

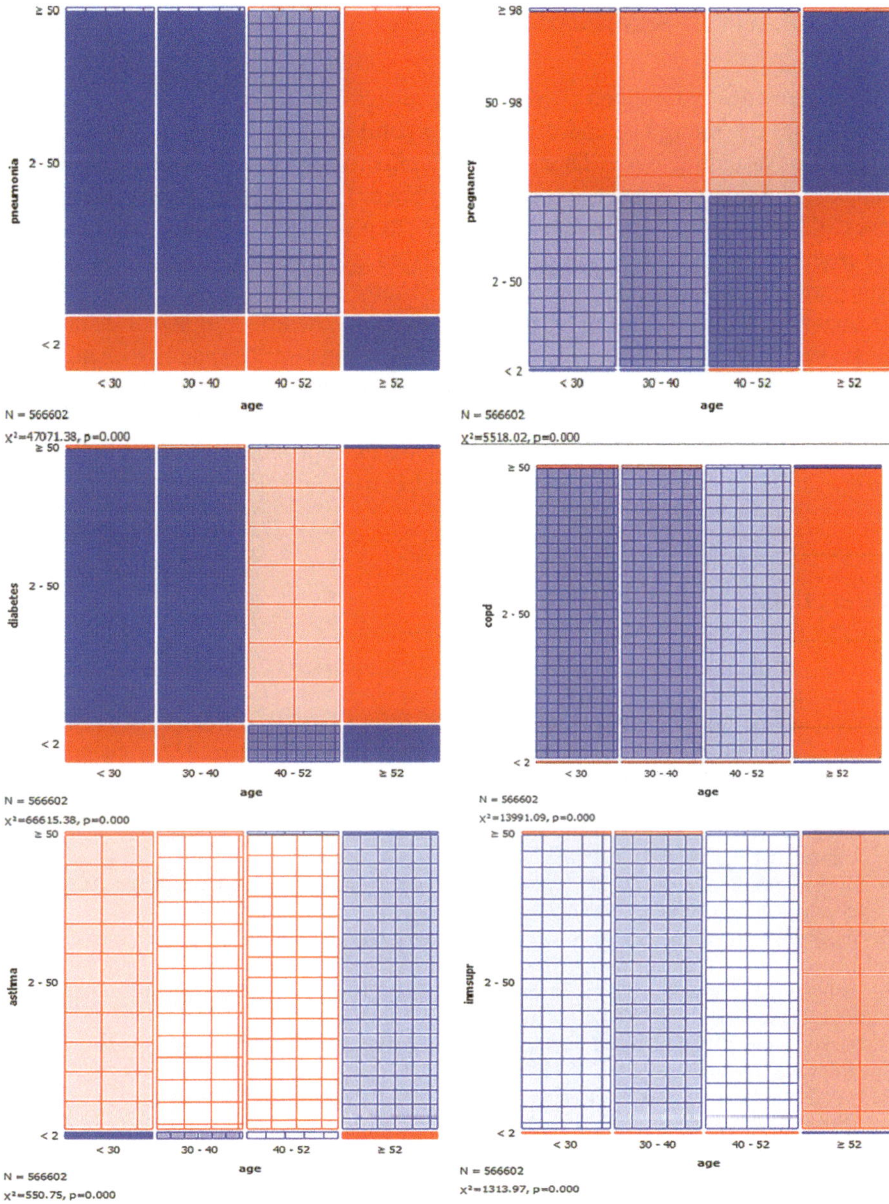

Fig. 10.1 Sieve diagram of COVID-19 instances corresponding with age

10.5 Observed Significance

This examination introduced a thorough investigation of the COVID-19 crisis in India. Cases are rising fast and they need forceful control methodologies from the administrative unit of India. There are more effective symptems in a person which relates to the different aspects covered up patient (patient type, pneumonia, pregnancy, COPD, asthma, immunosuppression, hypertension, obesity, and tobacco) and research contributions have been addressed exhaustively. They are identified with introducing the development patterns of infected cases in India, forecasts for the quantity of infected cases for the next few days, the effect of social distancing on the residents of India, the effect of mass functions on the quantity of infected cases in India, network examination, and mining of examples of patients experiencing COVID-19, and dissecting the procedures for increasing lockdown in India. The current examination compares different disease examples against age to introduce the investigation and the outcomes of Sieve approach.

References

1. Hamet, P., & Tremblay, J. (Apr. 2017). Artificial intelligence in medicine. *Metabolism, 69*, S36–S40.
2. Jamshidi, M., Lalbakhsh, A., Mohamadzade, B., Siahkamari, H., & Mousavi, S. M. H. (Oct. 2019). A novel neural-based approach for design of microstrip filters. *AEU - International Journal of Electronics and Communications, 110*. Art. no. 152847.
3. Kolker, E., Özdemir, V., & Kolker, E. (2016). How healthcare can refocus on its super-customers (patients, n = 1) and customers (doctors and nurses) by leveraging lessons from Amazon, Uber, and Watson. *Omics: a Journal of Integrative Biology, 20*(6), 33–329.
4. Mintz, Y., & Brodie, R. (2019). Introduction to artificial intelligence in medicine. *Minimally Invasive Therapy & Allied Technologies, 28*(2), 73–81.
5. Murdoch, T. B., & Detsky, A. S. (2013). The inevitable application of big data to healthcare. *Journal of the American Medical Association, 309*(13), 1351–1352.
6. Parikh, R. B., Obermeyer, Z., & Navathe, A. S. (Feb. 2019). Regulation of predictive analytics in medicine. *Science, 363*(6429), 810–812.
7. Becker. (Jun. 2019). Artificial intelligence in medicine: What is it doing for us today? *Health Policy and Technology, 8*(2), 198–205.
8. Huang, C., Wang, Y., Li, X., Ren, L., Zhao, J., Hu, Y., Zhang, L., Fan, G., Xu, J., Gu, X., & Cheng, Z. (2020). Clinical features of patients infected with 2019 novel coronavirus in Wuhan, China. *Lancet, 395*(10223), 497–506.
9. Wong, K. T., Antonio, G. E., Hui, D. S., Lee, N., Yuen, E. H., Wu, A., Leung, C. B., Rainer, T. H., Cameron, P., Chung, S. S., & Sung, J. J. (2003). Severe acute respiratory syndrome: Radiographic appearances and pattern of progression in 138 patients. *Radiology, 228*(2), 401–406.
10. Narin, A., Kaya, C. & Pamuk, Z. (2020). Automatic detection of coronavirus disease (COVID-19) using X-ray images and deep convolutional neural networks, arXiv, 2020 preprint arXiv:2003.10849.

11. Schork, N. J. (2019). Artificial intelligence and personalized medicine. In *Precision medicine in Cancer therapy* (pp. 265–283). Springer.
12. Al-Turjman, F., Nawaz, M. H., & Ulusar, U. D. (Jan. 2020). Intelligence in the internet of medical things era: A systematic review of current and future trends. *Computer Communications, 150*, 644–660.

Chapter 11
A Comparative Study on Data Mining Approach Using Machine Learning Techniques: Prediction Perspective

Anshul Mishra, M. H. Khan, Waris Khan, Mohammad Zunnun Khan, and Nikhil Kumar Srivastava

11.1 Introduction

It is clear that we are living in an era of data annihilation, an evidence of this phenomenon that a large amount of data is constantly being generated at unprecedented and ever-increasing scales. With an enormous amount of data stored in databases and data warehouses, it is increasingly important to develop powerful tools for the analysis of such data mining's interesting knowledge from it. Data mining is a process of inferring knowledge from such huge data. It is obvious that some important data should be separated from them by putting them together and then through any approach. A commission of data mining is contributing in a variety of areas such as medical, economics, computer science, etc. Both data mining and machine learning approaches are capable of performing a particular task simultaneously. Files, documents, and record items are used at a much higher level to keep information in different areas. The machine learning-based approaches are best to utilize these data in

A. Mishra (✉)
Department of IT, BBAU, Lucknow, India

M. H. Khan
Department of Computer Science & Engineering, Institute of Engineering and Technology, AKTU, Lucknow, India
e-mail: M.h.khan@ietlucknow.ac.in

W. Khan
Department of Computer Application, Integral University, Lucknow, India

M. Z. Khan
Department of Computer Science and Engineering, Integral University, Lucknow, Uttar Pradesh, India

N. K. Srivastava
City Collage of Management & Technology, Lucknow, India

M. S. Husain et al. (eds.), *Pervasive Healthcare*, EAI/Springer Innovations in Communication and Computing, https://doi.org/10.1007/978-3-030-77746-3_11

better ways. Machine learning performs a special kind of prediction that separates data from large-scale data from usage. The development of information and technology has led to a large amount of database and large data being used, which has led to the birth of many types of issues. Machine learning approach is used to correct these problems. This paper analyzes their impact using various approaches to machine learning. Many types of algorithms can be used to analyze how and which type of cancer can be treated. Complete analysis of machine learning and using its parameters make the concept of data mining more effective, and the appropriate data is collected and used in a particular perimeter. Data mining has a classification, regression, and clustering approach. Based on these approaches, grouping is used. Machine learning is a special way of demonstrating this foundation. This research paper has also shown which algorithm is most important for data mining.

11.2 Background

A new idea was implemented to prevent breast cancer. Breast cancer is a slow-growing disease in world-level environment. There are various approaches and methods available for curing BCD cases. Modern technology and medicine are working as a powerful tool to reduce the tumor efficiency. The experts and researchers discussed on how to prevent the disease and assess the patients' health status. A literature review has done in two phases. The first phase focuses on data mining, machine learning, algorithms, and its behavior. The second phase focuses on cancer and its prediction techniques. The main objective is to observe a specific evaluation process for various segments.

Kalapanidas et al. [1] explained about noise sensitivity with various algorithms (05 Algorithms) and mainly focused on prediction problems and one classification problem. They also used four artificial datasets and presented prediction in graphics, in which up and down curves are hard to be separated. Er in [2] develops a model for complete prediction of student's valuation in a specific course. Prediction algorithms (Naïves Bayes, K*, and C4.5) are evaluated in this research paper. Evaluation of the above-mentioned techniques uses the following terms accuracy, sensitivity, and precision. Vijayarani and Muthulakshmi [3] compared Lazy and Bayesian (Bayesian Network and Naïve Bayes) classifiers for text mining problems. In text mining concepts, these algorithms have played an important role for accuracy measurement. Observation and evaluations are considered in Table 11.1.

11.3 Breast Cancer

Cancer is a critical disease in medical perspective. Breast cancer is increasingly developed in the cell of the breast. Breast It occurred in both men and women. Mostly breast cancer is found in women's cells. Researchers and the government provide a special support to prevent this kind of disease. A number of experts have

Table 11.1 Breast cancer review

Expert/year	Techniques/model/method/ approach	Outcomes
Breast cancer		
Crisóstomo et al. [4]	Extensive literature	Glucose dysmetabolism, insulin resistance, and changes in adipokine secretion
Cole [5]	Methods to measure HER2 levels	Improve the quantitation and reliability of cancer biomarkers
Hwa et al. [6]	Logistic regression Model uses to measure lymph node	Logistic regression model can improve the predictive sensitivity
Assiri and Kamel [7]	Calculate the predictive value of serum levels of Leptin, resistin, and visfatin	Obesity is responsible for cancer
Gromski et al. [8]	Variable selection approaches	Comparative study between modern feature selection and classification approaches
Sivakami [9]	DT-SVM hybrid model	Prediction of breast cancer
Salama [10]	Multi-classifiers	Different evaluation at various datasets
Dumitru [11]	Naive Bayesian classification	Prediction of recurrent events in BC
Katsis [12]	Artificial immune recognition systems	Prediction
Ahmed Iqbal Pritom et al. [13]	Classification and feature selection technique	Predicting breast recurrence
Ming et al. [14]	Machine learning techniques	Compare with the BCRAT and BOADICEA models
Phase 2 data mining algorithms machine learning BC		
Fort and Lambert Lacroix [15]	Classification	Bioinformatic
Kotsiantis [16]	Machine learning approach	Review on classification
Liu et al. [17]	Multiple regression analysis	Evaluation of digital mammograms
Zhang et al. [18]	Neural and genetic algorithm-based feature selection	Feature selection
Liao [19]	Examined various approaches	Data mining techniques at various levels
Idowu and Obafemi [20]	Predictive model for the classification	Risk of kidney stone
Saba et al. [21]	Multi-layer classifiers	Prediction disease
Hiba et al. [22]	Machine learning algorithms	For breast cancer risk prediction
Ahmed Iqbal et al. [13]	Classification	Prediction BC
Gayathri Devi [23]	Data mining methods	Breast cancer prediction system

initiated to understanding the problem. During the growth of breast cancer, changes convert to such types of symptoms as redness, thickness, shape change, peeling, and scaling. Doctors predict this cancer based on these symptoms with cells changing abnormally.

The changed cell continuously divides into more cells. In order for researchers to identify various factors such as hormonal, life style, and environment issues that support to the increase of its negative impacts, various segment tests (biopsy, blood cell counts, blood chemistry, bone scans, breast cancer index, chest x-ray, and EndoPredict test) are used to diagnose the cancer theory at early stages. According to the WHO, 1.2 million women are affected with this disease. In the case of breast cancer disease, the tumor plays an important role in the effective measurement of the disease. At present all the existing techniques and related machine learning theories are the are not fully capable to predict the disease accurately. The latest machine learning technology is incapably being used for predicting the disease and also provides significant complete descriptions about the problem. At present all exiting techniques, machine learning theory are the most affections to any prediction. It has been elaborated that 250 types of variances are found in cancer category. Tumor sensitivity depends on the stage's category (stage 0, 1, 2, 3). Stages 0 and 1 indicate the size of tumor. Breast cancer is known as a ductal carcinoma in situ which indicates that the tumor cell is increasing. Stage 2 highlights the increased size of lymph nodes. Stage 3 attacks the lymph nodes and muscles. Stage 3 have to decide the complications at various stages and its affected factors are as mentioned below:

Tumor (< 2 cm)	Tumor (< 5 cm)	Tumor (> 5 cm)
Spared to 4.9 lymph nodes	Cluster in lymph nodes	Lymph nodes near the underarms

This approach is to predict cancer symptoms at an early stage. Cancer is highly a critical disease. There are various contributing factors of cancer. Some of the significant factors are age, BMI, glucose, insulin, HOMA, leptin, adiponectin, resistin, and MCP-1.

11.4 Data Mining Approaches

Data mining is an important technique that applies to large and complex databases. This is to take out the irregularity and find the masked example. A data mining method is quite a computational problem. The industry use data mining approaches and theories for data recognition. Also, this is the motivation behind why data mining has turned out to be such a significant aspect of study, as data mining has extensive applications. Hence, it is a promising field for the present scenario. It has dragged in a lot of considerations in the data business, because of the wide availability of large measures of data requirement for transforming the data and learning. Along these outlines, we use data and learning for applications and predict market investigation. This is the motivation behind why data mining is known as information disclosure from data. The goal of this comparative study of algorithms and utilized data mining techniques is shown in Fig. 11.1.

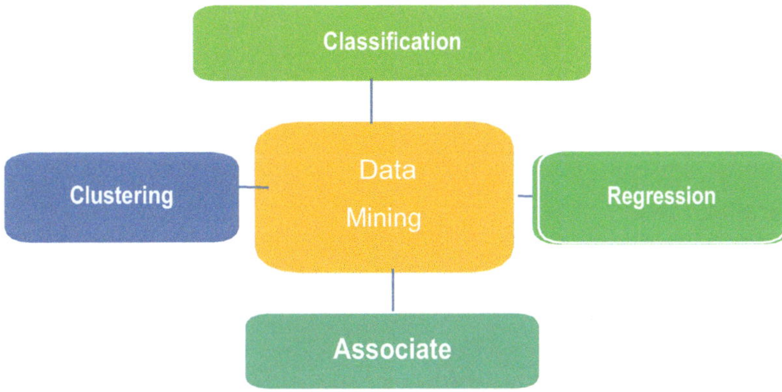

Fig. 11.1 Data mining approach

It is relevant to contemplate about concept of data mining before proceeding to the classification concepts. In this perspective, classification is applied in this assessing or prediction of breast cancer symptoms.

11.4.1 Classification

According to the expert's name, classification is a bond based on some time of training sets, whereas interaction is defined as a rule governed by algorithms. In the society of computer science with continuous changes, there are numerous examples of cancer dataset. In order to conduct an empirical examination of the classification with structured and unstructured datasets, a large dataset has great challenges in front of classification approaches. A similar view is expressed by machine learning approach within the conceptual framework of prediction concepts. There may be combinations of different factors for high-risk evaluation in classification approaches, but it is vital to include the resistance perspective in classification concept. In the empirical parading, attention of cancer dataset is paid in two segments. The first category denotes the dataset, and the second is its category. Classification algorithm has a significant role for data mining concepts. With a starting point in a critical discussion of the classification toward achieving and analyzing cancer datasets, data mining experts accept a significant relationship with two contexts. The classification has involved two steps of process. The Data mining and classification algorithms are providing effective results in various domains [25, 26]. These ML techniques have been quite effectively used by many researchers for computer aided diagnosis and cancer prediction [22–24].

Learning Steps

Classification models are used to develop a classifier using with trained datasets. These datasets predict the accurate result.

Classification Steps

To predict the class-level datasets and check the accuracy of the classifications.

11.5 Basic Algorithms for Cancer Detection

Various research works have been presented to diagnose symptoms of cancer with accuracy. The cancer diagnosis system uses various algorithms for detection theory. Its system is based on the historical records and test value. Data mining approaches (classification) are used for various types of algorithms. These algorithms include the various parameters and factors, which target to the objective of predictions. In this section, we have described the detail of each Machine learning Algorithm on the basis of its parameter and domain structure.

- Bayes Net

  Bayes net algorithms are discussed by Duda and Hart, in 1973. The style of that algorithm depends on the classification node (see Fig. 11.2). Every node will be connected to only parent nodes. No other connections are allowed in Bayes net algorithms. Naive Bayes do play an important key factor as an effective classifier. It provides two types of benefits for a classification domain. First, it is easy to develop the structure with a given priority. Second, the classification process is very efficient.

- Logistic

  Logistic regression is the best approach in terms of prediction with machine learning and data mining. The approach is depending on the binary classification values 0 and 1. Logistic regression methods are applied in two perspectives: **first** is "local declaring of parameters," and **second** is "global declaring of parameters." So,

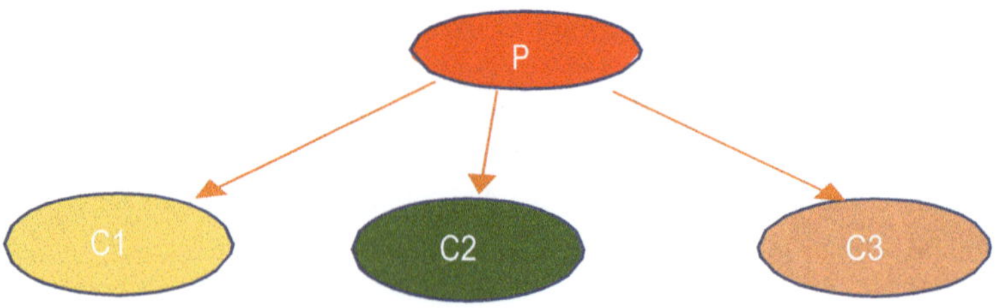

Fig. 11.2 Structure of Bayes net

they work in two segments as local and global. Logistic regression calculates the coefficient of function from the dataset. Logistic regression can be divided according to the situation in data mining such as binomial, ordinal, or multinomial. Binomial or binary logistic regression deals with various conditions in which the observed outcome for a dependent variable can have only two possible types, "0" and "1."

11.5.1 Data Interpretations

The data have been taken from [13] mentioned reference for analysis and predicting the symptoms of breast cancer. The data presented here were collected as part of a larger cancer 56 HCC patients. These attributes are used in age, BMI, glucose, insulin, HOMA, leptin, adiponectin, resistin, and MCP-1. The present interpretations are an attempt to quantify the predictions of cancer. Its major objective is to provide a specific descriptive analysis of dataset. In the following analysis, the first and last objective is to predict breast cancer. A brief interpretation of the research setting and methods is demonstrating it in order. Basically, two types of algorithms (**Logistic**, **Bayes Net**) are used in this prediction terminology (Fig 11.3). Classification of recurrence and non-recurrence samples of 56 HCC patients has been taken by the Decision Classification Tree algorithm in the training data set.

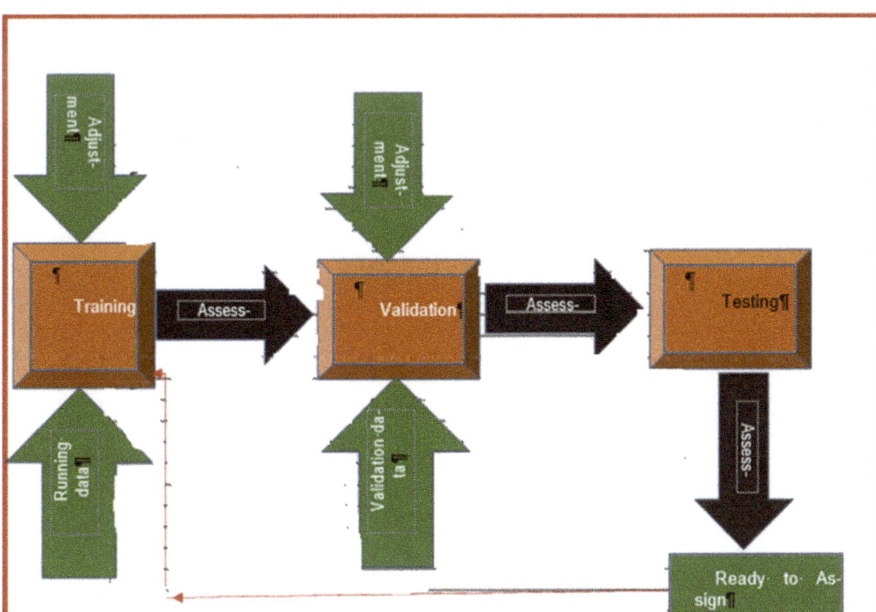

Fig. 11.3 Steps of data evaluation in machine learning approach

11.5.2 Dataset

The topic of training and tested dataset has gained increasing attention to evaluating data mining concepts. Trained and tested dataset is based on the neural network and machine learning approach that is applied from linear and nonlinear transformation to the input data. Trained and tested dataset is a subset of computing dataset which is applied to model prediction. A dataset can be applied to all types of area, images, voice, or some combinations. It also provides some help to solve a complex problem or issue, so that it can quantify the accurate issues for taking the decisions.

11.6 Experimental Results

The paper presents a comparative analysis of the algorithms. Bayes net and logistic algorithms are the most often used algorithms for prediction with classification methods. The Bayes net and logistic algorithm are the most used algorithms for data mining approaches. They give appropriate path and accuracy level in terms of predicting the issues. Combining it with classification algorithm leads to several accuracy levels and its various errors. A method can be used to solve breast cancer prediction at an early stage and find a problem with various attributes. This method examines all the possible cases, 286 instances, and 10 attributes of the patient, usually starting from one specific solution and seeking to broaden it with every step. If it is determined that one of the following steps leads to a dead end, the algorithm Bayes net and logistic algorithm provide two f-measure values using these algorithms.

In this experiment the medical data related to breast cancer is considered because breast cancer is one of the leading causes of death in women. The experiments are conducted using Weka tool. In this study Bayes net and logistic algorithm are chosen to predict cancer tissues from datasets because it delivers accuracy from examining the issues. After applying with an intension to find out the f-measure value, it may lead to the best accuracy for various datasets of the same domain. Various experiments are conducted in one breast cancer dataset. Further, to analyze the importance of accuracy with 286 instances and 10 attributes are presented in Table 11.2. The data is collected from UCI machine learning repository, which is publicly available.

All information (Table 11.3 [Bayesian Network], Table 11.4 [Logistics]) concerning the predictive performance of the resulting two model can be extracted from the breast cancer dataset. It means that the built classifier (Bayes net and logistics algorithms) classifies simultaneously the instance correctly (72.028%, 68.8811%). The labels on the test set are supposed to be the actual correct classification. Performance is computed by asking the classifier to give its best guess about the classification for each instance in the test set. Then the predicted classifications are compared to the actual classifications to determine accuracy.

Table 11.2 Bayesian network tabular data for Prediction

Table 2 Baye Net Attributes Table for Predictions
Relation: breast-cancer
Instances: 286
Attributes: 10
Class->age
Class->menopause
Class->tumor-size
Class->inv-nodes
Class->node-caps
Class->deg-malig
Class->breast
Class->breast-quad
Class->irradiat
Test mode: 10-fold cross-validation

Table 11.3 Bayesian Network Computation table

Correctly classified instances	206	72.028%
Incorrectly classified instances	80	27.972%
Mean absolute error	0.3297	
Root mean squared error	0.4566	
Relative absolute error	78.7898%	
Root relative squared error	99.9047%	

Table 11.4 Logistic Computation table

Correctly classified instances	197	68.8811%
Incorrectly classified instances	89	31.1189%
Mean absolute error	0.37	
Root mean squared error	0.4631	
Relative absolute error	88.4196%	
Root relative squared error	101.3094%	

Root-mean-square error (RMSE) is the standard deviation of the residuals (prediction errors). Residuals are covering the distance from the accuracy values. Root-mean-square error is a quantification of residual's area. The table (Table 11.3 Bayesian Network, Table 11.4 Logistics) tells that how focused the data is around the accuracy. Root-mean-square error is commonly used in data mining and regression prediction analysis to verify experimental results.

In table (Table 11.5 Bayesian Network, Table 11.6 Logistics), Precision indicates the positive predictive values of relevant instances. And Recall indicates the sensitive observations of relevant instances that have been retrieved in two forms (no-recurrence events and recurrence events). Precision and Recall are totally dependent on attributes and instances.

11.7 Discussion and Conclusion

In this quantification for predictions, the present various quantitative values including ten attributes are associated with breast cancer. f-Measure scores (mentioned in Tables 11.5 and 11.6) can be used to identify prediction rate. Present time, Precision, and Recall can complement and improve evaluation of cancer dataset with new insights. The algorithm (logistics, Bayes net) can realize all ten directions while seeing its predictions in accuracy with two classification algorithms. In the comparative study between them, we found that Bayes net algorithms predict more reliably and accurately in terms of the disease. The prediction graph has been given in Figs. 11.4 and 11.5. Basically the graph has given the comparative study between recurrence events^{Logistic} and recurrence events$^{\text{Bayes Net}}$. In this graph X denoted the False$^{\text{Positive Rate}}$ and Y denoted the True$^{\text{Positive Rate}}$. After implementing the logistics and Bayes net algorithm, the prediction value of breast cancer symptoms is very high and low in recurrence events. The coordinates of the points through which the values pass, from the starting position to the final position, are used directly in Figs. 11.4 and 11.5 and show the false$^{\text{positive rate}}$ and True$^{\text{Positive Rate}}$. The prediction values major between 0 and 1 are the coordinates of the maze points. The results in the research described hereby show that logistics and Bayes net algorithm can be used effectively in data mining, as it will find the best prediction for the disease. Also, our experiments showed that algorithms significantly improve accuracy of predictions over baseline models, and we found that the Bayes net algorithm is more reliable for prediction at an early stage (Fig. 11.5).

Table 11.5 Bayesian Network Observation Data table

Precision	Recall	f-Measure	MCC	No-recurrence events
0.779	0.841	0.809	0.295	
Precision	Recall	f-measure	MCC	Recurrence events
0.536	0.435	0.481	0.295	

Table 11.6 LogisticsObservations Table 11.1

Precision	Recall	f-Measure	MCC	No-recurrence events
0.752	0.831	**0.790**	**0.202**	
Precision	Recall	f-measure	MCC	Recurrence events
0.469	**0.353**	**0.403**	**0.202**	

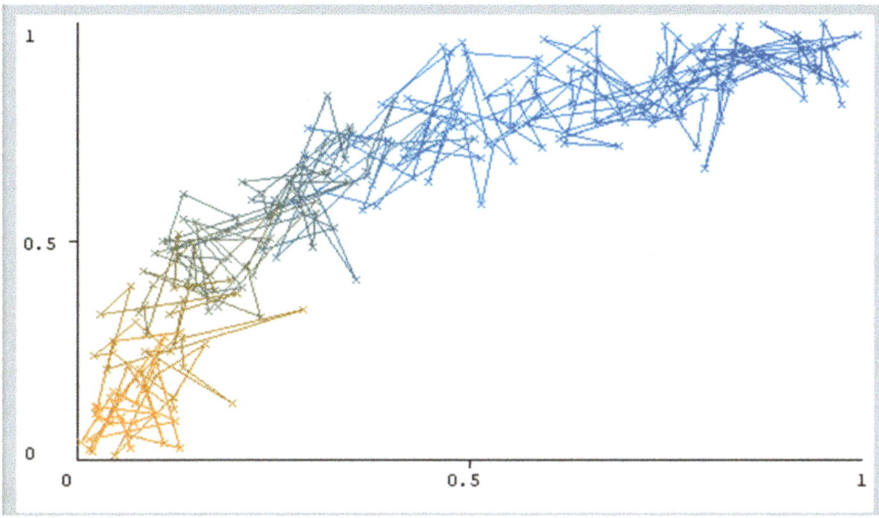

Fig. 11.4 Recurrence events$^{\text{Bayes net}}$ ith X and Y

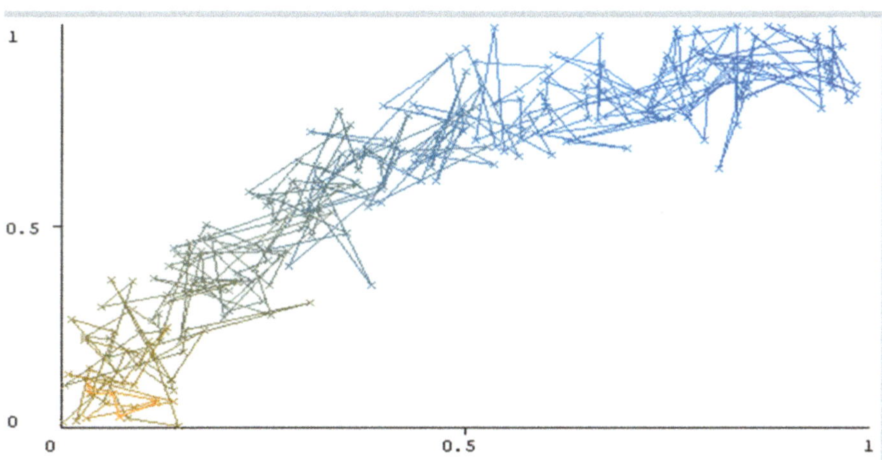

Fig. 11.5 Recurrence events^{Logistics} with X and Y

References

1. Kalapanidas, E., et al. (2003). Machine learning algorithms: A study on noise sensitivity. In *First Balkan Conference in Informatics* (pp. 356–365).
2. Er, E. (2012). Identifying at-risk students using machine learning techniques: A case study with IS 100. *International Journal of Machine Learning and Computing, 2*(4), 279.
3. Vijayarani, S., & Muthulakshmi, M. (2013). Comparative analysis of Bayes and lazy classification algorithms. *International Journal of Advanced Research in Computer and Communication Engineering, 2*(8), 3118–3124.

4. Crisóstomo, J., et al. (2016). Hyperresistinemia and metabolic dysregulation: The close cross-talk in obese breast cancer. *Endocrine, 53*(2), 433–442.
5. Cole, K. D., He, H. J., & Wang, L. (2013). Breast cancer biomarker measurements and standards. *Proteomics – Clinical Applications, 7*(1–2), 17–29.
6. Hwa, H. L., et al. (2008). Prediction of breast cancer and lymph node metastatic status with tumors markers using logistic regression models. *Journal of Evaluation in Clinical Practice, 14*(2), 275–280.
7. Assiri, A. M., & Kamel, H. F. (2015). Evaluation of diagnostic and predictive value of serum adipokines: Leptin, resistin and visfatin in postmenopausal breast cancer. *Obesity Research & Clinical Practice, 10*(4), 442–453.
8. Gromski, P. S., et al. (2014). A comparative investigation of modern feature selection and classification approaches for the analysis of mass spectrometry data. *Analytica Chimica Acta, 829*, 1–8.
9. Sivakami, K. (2015). Mining big data: Breast Cancer prediction using DT-SVM hybrid model. *International Journal of Scientific Engineering and Applied Science (IJSEAS), 1*(5), 418–429.
10. Salama, G. I., Abdelhalim, M. B., & Zeid, M. A. (2012). Breast cancer diagnosis on three different datasets using multi-classifiers. *Breast Cancer (WDBC), 32*.
11. Dumitru, D. (2009). Prediction of recurrent events in breast cancer using the naive Bayesian classification. In *Annals of the University of Craiova-Mathematics and Computer Science Series* (pp. 92–96).
12. Katsis, C. D., Gkogkou, I., Papadopulos, C. A., Goletsis, Y., Boufounou, P. V., & Stylios, G. (2013). Using artificial immune recognition systems in order to detect early breast cancer. *International Journal of Intelligent Systems and Applications, 5*(2), 34.
13. Ahmed Iqbal, P., Munshi, M. A. R., AnzarusSabab, S., & Shihab, S. (2016). Predicting breast cancer recurrence using effective classification and feature selection technique. In *Computer and Information Technology (ICCIT), 19th International Conference on* (pp. 310–314). IEEE.
14. Ming, C., et al. (2019). Machine learning techniques for personalized breast cancer risk prediction: Comparison with the BCRAT and BOADICEA models. *Breast Cancer Research, 21*.
15. Fort, G., & Lambert Lacroix, S. (2005). *Classification using partial least squares with penalized logistic regression*. Bioinformatics-Oxford.
16. Kotsiantis, S. B. (2007). Supervised machine learning: A review of classification techniques. *Informatica, 31*, 249–268.
17. Liu, C.-C., Tsai, C.-Y., Liu, J., Yu, C.-Y., & Yu, S.-S. (2012). A pectoral muscle segmentation algorithm for digital mammograms using Otsu thresholding and multiple regression analysis. *Computers and Mathematics with Applications, 64*, 1100–1107.
18. Zhang, P., Verma, B., & Kumar, K. (2005). Neural vs. statistical classifier in conjunction with genetic algorithm-based feature selection. *Pattern Recognition Letters, 26*, 909–919.
19. Liao, S.-H. (2012). Data mining techniques and applications – A decade review from 2000 to 2011. *Expert Systems with Applications, 39*, 11303–11311.
20. IdowuP., A., & Obafemi (2019). Model for predicting the risk of kidney stone using data mining techniques. https://doi.org/10.5120/ijca2019918404
21. Saba, B., Qamar, U., Khan, F. H., & Naseem, L. (2016). HMV: A medical decision support framework using multi-layer classifiers for disease prediction. *Journal of Computational Science, 13*, 10–25.
22. Hiba, A., Mousannif, H., Al Moatassime, H., & Noel, T. (2016). Using machine learning algorithms for breast Cancer risk prediction and diagnosis. *Procedia Computer Science, 83*, 1064–1069.
23. Gayathri Devi, S. (2011). Breast Cancer prediction system using feature selection and data mining methods. *International Journal of Advanced Research in Computer Science*. https://archive.ics.uci.edu/ml/datasets.php
24. Dalamaga, M., et al. (2013). "Serum resistin: A biomarker of breast cancer in postmenopausal women?", association with clinicopathological characteristics, tumor markers, inflammatory and metabolic parameters. *Clinical Biochemistry, 46*(7–8), 584–590.

25. Khan, M. Z., Husain, M. S., & Shoaib, M. (2020). Introduction to email, web, and message forensics. In *Critical concepts, standards, and techniques in cyber forensics* (pp. 174–186). IGI Global.
26. Suaib, M., Akbar, M., & Husain, M. S. (2020). Digital forensics and data mining. In *Critical concepts, standards, and techniques in cyber forensics* (pp. 240–247). IGI Global.

Chapter 12
Indoor Air-Quality Monitoring Systems: A Comprehensive Review of Different IAQM Systems

Rasha Shakir AbdulWahhab, Karan Jetly, and Shqran Shakir

12.1 Introduction

Air pollutants with the growth of other pollutions such as vehicles, industries, and others have a significant effect on human health. Such noteworthy influences on human health will eradicate policies, work establishments, and human development. Responding to the challenges of pollution eradication, researchers made considerable efforts to deepen employing advanced technologies such as wireless sensor networks (WSN) and the Internet of Things (IoT) to cultivate the fruits of a healthy environment.

Air pollution is becoming a significant problem nowadays, attributing to 5.5 million people deaths globally due to the air's high pollutants [1, 2]. This study aims at furnishing empirical available methodology about understating and monitoring air pollution's impact on human development. The large population wishes to improve the living atmosphere and take a respective action of any abnormal changes in their places. Several studies show that understanding air pollution's impact will help humans change their attitude and impose healthy daily routine activities to improve air quality [3]. Therefore, this study sheds some light on health development by showing the contribution of various techniques to develop economical air pollution monitoring system.

R. S. AbdulWahhab (✉) · K. Jetly
Information Technology Department, University of Technology and Applied Sciences, Suhar, Sultanate of Oman
e-mail: rashas.soh@cas.edu.om; karan.soh@cas.edu.om

S. Shakir
Information Technology Department, University of Technology and Applied Sciences, Shinas, Sultanate of Oman
e-mail: shqran.almansoory@hct.edu.om

M. S. Husain et al. (eds.), *Pervasive Healthcare*, EAI/Springer Innovations in Communication and Computing, https://doi.org/10.1007/978-3-030-77746-3_12

Humans in the indoor environment are exposed about two to five times to contamination due to indoor air pollutants. According to the US Environmental Protection Agency, humans who live indoor are exposed to about 80% to 90% of indoor toxin levels than outdoor toxin levels. Indoor toxin levels give off from concentrated pollutants emitted by furnishings and the daily activities of humans. Clean air can protect humans from the hazards of some diseases such as cough, asthma, sore eyes, and even death. Therefore, there is a need to furnish and understand the available methodology for protecting humans from these diseases' risks. Recently, several new techniques have been worked out for the possibility of monitoring pollutant levels in the air to increase air-quality efficiency. The rapid development of IoT technology and Wi-Fi communication technologies has helped researchers use these technologies to establish smart air-quality monitoring systems capable of measuring pollutant concentrations in the air.

This research paper's primary domain is to contribute to the literature by highlighting approaches, technologies, and methodology that had been published over the last few years. This paper aims at furnishing comprehensive study about indoor air-quality monitoring systems (IAQMs). In the meantime, we highlight inclusively and deeply some of the literature about IAQMs. The review has been organized with an overview and a brief discussion of understanding theories and empirical studies applied by the researchers to collect, study, and analyze IAQMs and identify their strengths and weaknesses. Thereafter, air pollution definition and its types are presented in Sect. 12.2. Some well-known IAQM categories are discussed in Sect. 12.3. While Sect. 12.4 aims to present the main reasons to start developing IAQMs, section 12.5 discussed the main requirements of IAQMs. Sections 12.6 and 12.7 briefly outline the available approaches and architecture that can help researchers plan the measures for a pollution-free environment. This paper in Sect. 12.8 also provides well-known awareness about IAQM's domains, followed by some concluding remarks in Sect. 12.9.

12.2 Air Pollutant Types

Air pollution means the contaminants resulting from either human activities or caused by natural events such as a fire. Air pollutants, regardless of their origin, can be characterized into two types. The primary pollutants are the first category, while the secondary pollutants are of the other type.

Definition 1 Primary pollutants: Pollutants by this type are generated by natural or human activities such as nitric oxide (NO), ammonia (NH_3), sulfur dioxide (SO_2), carbon monoxide (CO), volcanic organic compound (VOC), and nitrogen dioxide (NO_2). These types of pollutants have a high health impact.

Definition 2 Secondary pollutants: The interaction between the primary pollutants generates the pollutants of this type, such as particulates (PM2.5 and PM10), ozone (O_3), sulfur trioxide (SO_3), and ammonium (NH_4).

The presence and the concentration of pollutants in the environment are variable. Some of them have a short-term impact, while the other has a long-term effect. Both of them affect human health, ecosystem, and cultural heritage.

12.3 Air Pollution Monitoring System Categories

To build a new air's pollutant monitoring system requires knowing the main available types that were widely used in this arena. Without empirical investigation, understanding the new system's functioning remains inadequate to make decisions about human health requirements. Generally speaking, the main types are [4, 5] are:

1. Outdoor air pollution systems can detect Nox, SO_2, O_3, CO, and particulate matters (PM2.5 and PM10). Additionally, the outdoor pollution system is related to environmental factors like temperature, humidity, etc. [4]. Deployment and maintenance with outdoor systems should be average.
2. Indoor air pollution monitoring systems are able to detect nitrogen oxides, sulfur dioxide (SO_2), ozone (O_3), carbon monoxide (CO), CO_2, CH_4, and smoke. Indoor air pollution is generated in small areas inside homes, laboratories, workplaces, offices, and closed areas, such as underground shopping centers and subway stations [5]. Such system must ensure that maintenance and deployment in their designed remain smooth and user-friendly [6].
3. Industrial environment air pollution monitoring systems can detect air pollutants and hazardous gases in the broad area exposed to these dangerous materials.

12.4 Reasons for Developing IAQM System

According to the Environmental Protection Agency of the United States (EPA), humans who live indoors are exposed to about 100 times of indoor air contaminants more than the outside air. Children or elderly people spend about to 80–90% of their life in a closed area, so breathing in particles' pollution can be significantly harmful to their health. Indoor pollutants are easily transmitted to the human body, causing different diseases such as asthma, eye irritation, lung and throat irritation, and trouble breathing compared to outdoor pollutants. This section aims to furnish the main reasons for developing a system able to monitor indoor air pollutants. A study of this nature permits identifying important reasons and, therefore, can be used as measures for future planning. These reasons include:

- Bad air quality has a very harmful effect on the health of human beings. Its effects can range from the risks of diseases to rising temperatures. Actually, because of air pollution, people are at high risk of disease and premature death.
- In the United States, the Environmental Protection Agency (EPA) noted that indoor pollutants are higher than outdoor pollutant levels. According to the EPA,

rapid growth of pollutants in the air ranked among the top five environmental risks declines human's health [7].
- People need to understand the determinants of indoor air pollution. Such information will help them reduce suffering from different diseases.
- Daily routine activities of the people, as well as industrial processes, increase rates of indoor air pollutants. Supporting people about the relationship between daily routine activities and the pollution level provides many environmental benefits.
- Pollution driven by climate changes, population density, and transportation is increasing at alarming rates. Monitoring and improving the living atmosphere will reduce air pollution's influence on human beings, animals, and plants.
- Helps the society facilitate access to valuable information and lower their lack of awareness to make them prepared for the new changes that might degrade their indoor places' activities.
- Monitoring air pollution levels can raise awareness between the societies, and they can become more vigilant toward safeguarding their environment.

12.5 Requirements of IAQM System

The population wishes to improve the living atmosphere and take a respective action of any abnormal changes in their places. To protect humans who spend their lives indoors or outdoors requires new monitoring systems to avoid the possible risk of bad air; for instance, individuals who spend about 12 hours working with chemical emissions greatly impact their health without even feeling it. Undoubtedly, measuring and monitoring online air pollutant levels will increase individuals' capability to enhance their lifestyle. The emphasis on understanding IAQM's requirements is essential for building a competitive monitoring system powered by new technologies. Below are a few key points that must be taken into account when we begin to design a new IAQM system:

- Performance: IAQM must be capable of detecting most of the air pollutants such as CO_2, nitrogen oxides, ozone (O_3), carbon monoxide (CO), sulfur dioxide (SO_2), volatile and semi-volatile organic compounds, smoke, CH_4, humidity, particulate matters, temperature, and microorganism [6].
- Reliability: IAQM must give reliable results and inform users of the variations in the air-quality level.
- Usability: IAQM needs to have a good communication infrastructure to increase the accessibility of IAQM system from any place. Most of the researchers proposed to provide air parameters in real time either with a convenient web interface for users [1, 8], Android mobile application [9], desktop application, or by cloud viewing platform [10].

- Serviceability: IAQM needs to be simple to use and to suit the needs of users. Most researchers stated that IAQM in the indoor environment must be easily operated, efficient in loading data, and have an intuitive sense of pollution levels.
- Configuration and installation: Installation and configuration must not be complicated; users must not have a professional experience to install IAQM systems [7].
- Maintaining historical data: Most professional IAQM systems must have a unit used to record historical data for data consulting purposes.

Within many of these studies, IAQMs have to be adaptable and user-friendly for monitoring air pollutants. Therefore, understanding the system requirement of IAQMs is essential to develop a system that lives up to its promise to address indoor pollutants.

12.6 Fundamentals of Data Mining Methods for Environmental Pollution Controls

In recent years, the methodology of data mining has been employed in environmental monitoring systems as an instrument for the automatic process of collecting, analyzing, and discovering valuable information.

Definition 3 Data mining is an automated method in which large data repositories collect, analyze, and discover useful information to observe hidden patterns and hidden information [11–13].

According to [14] data mining provides detailed information about the hidden patterns, showing how relationships among data are established. It draws on machine learning concepts, artificial intelligence, database systems, and statistics. Data mining has successfully applied in different applications, including manufacturing, banking, health, and many other sectors [2, 13, 14]. Data mining tasks are widely.

used in countries where economic expansion and growth in their number of industries are highly noticed [2]. Under this circumstance, the use of the data mining forecasting model is one of the most popular practices in environmental protection work. It has been used to determine pollutants in the air. This paper will highlight several works with different approaches to ecological trend analysis capabilities, drawing on existing literature works.

In recent years, environmental scientists have proposed a wide range of various researches to protect human health from the most significant number of environmentally related illnesses. Most of these studies are undertaken either to forecast air pollution concentrations, such as carbon monoxide (CO), or to predict some future course of action.

Definition 4 Forecast air pollutant is an approach which provides an advanced air pollutant information to control public health in which the concentration of air pollutants will be predicted automatically. Such an approach can be used to reduce the risks of environmental health as long as possible.

Area of forecast air pollutant has been examined by various research methodologies that are commonly employed to predict air pollutant concentration in the air. This study is furnishing detailed information about prediction based on machine learning and prediction based on numerical forecast models for air contamination's prediction, underpinning an understanding of the researchers.

Definition 5 Machine learning is an automated process that acquires patterns or knowledge from data and thus learns to solve problems. The main broad areas with this approach are neural network (NN) and evolutionary algorithms (EAs).

As a methodological tool, NN and GA are widely used to solve the problems of many applications, such as biological applications that have gained considerable attention. For this benefit, there is a significant interest in employing these two broad areas to predict pollutant air levels in recent years [11, 12].

Multiple linear equation (DME) is the used model in [15] to forecast PM2.5 in Santiago. This linear model proved that overfitting issues related to nonlinear models such as ANNs are solved. This research paper has shown that a multiple equation approach is a competitive method comparable to ANN and SARIMAX.

Niska et al. carried out [16] an approach for optimizing NN models using GAs for forecasting 1 day later of the air-quality level at the traffic station in Helsinki such as nitrogen dioxide (NO_2). The researchers suggest using GAs to avoid the time consumed in developing the construction of a multilayer perception module. The results show that GAs are helpful and can be considered an excellent approach to handling NN construction's real problems. Thus, it results in a smaller cost of air-quality forecasting due to the smaller amount of measurement requirements required in NN's design.

Similar work was carried out by Feng et al. [17], who employed multi-artificial neural network (ANN) to detect the concentration of ozone in Beijing. The data in this model are classified into its corresponding categories using support vector machine (SVM). Additionally, the genetic algorithm (GA) was applied to tune the backpropagation neural network (BPNN) for forecasting ozone concentration. The proposed model was examined using the collected records of Aug. 2009, and the predictive capability of the proposed model was significant. The study in this research paper suggested applying the developed model forecast ozone concentration in Beijing.

Another work was carried out by [18] et al. to forecast carbon emission in China. Using the apriorism algorithm, the affected variables of carbon emissions have been obtained in the proposed model. A firefly algorithm has also been used to generate the grey model GM (1,N) 's coefficients and get the carbon emission value. To optimize the gray coefficient and search for the best parameters, firefly algorithm has been used. The authors have proven that their proposed methodology obtained good results compared to other methods.

Credit for the development of environmental monitoring and early-warning systems goes to [19]. Yang integrates a new hybrid model to forecast six primary air pollutant data recorded in China. In this study, several methods were used to compare the proposed study's performance, including the model's accuracy and stability. In the end, the obtained results have a significant impact on the result accuracy compared to the other models.

The related ideas discussed in Kurt et al. [8] include developing a web-based system for 10 districts in Istanbul. This study provides detailed information about forecasting air pollutants' levels. In the meanwhile, all the predicted data has been published using their proposed website. In order to predict pollutant levels, their system was composed of three central units. These units include different modules, including data collection, forecasting, and a website. The pollutant levels have been predicted for the next 3 days by using a neural network model. Satisfactory prediction results were obtained from this study.

Wu and et al. [20] identified the linkage between BRICS countries' GDP, energy consumption, urban population, and CO_2 emissions. Their study was based on the grey model to forecast CO_2 emissions based on GDP and energy consumption. Authors' conclusion in reducing CO_2 emissions was this study's finding for BRICS countries, like Brazil, to improve their energy efficiency. In the end, the conclusion brought by this study that different energy conservation policies should be adopted by Brazil while India and China can use more renewable energy to reduce CO_2 emissions.

The study in [21] aims at forecasting energy consumption and GHG emissions of the organization manufacturing pig iron in India. Such analysis sheds some light on understanding the current and upcoming patterns of these indicators. One of the significant features of this study is to compare actual and forecast values of energy consumption and GHG emissions using ARIMA models. The finest-fitted model for forecasting energy consumption and GHG emission was ARIMA (1,0,0) × (0,1,1) and ARIMA (0,1,4) × (0,1,1), respectively.

12.7 IAQM System Architecture

Air pollution is becoming a more severe problem day by day due to population, climate changes, industry, and transportation. Recently, intensive attempts were made to develop systems that could monitor air pollutants, resulting in researchers and innovators capable of providing an essential picture of the damage contaminations done to the human. Remarkably, a set of researchers' monographs recently introduced the possibilities of using new technologies (i.e., WSN and IoT) to improve these systems' capabilities. In the next subsections, we will present the existing works that have extended these systems' infrastructure.

12.7.1 WSN-Based Architecture

The rapid development of wireless communication systems in every aspect and its applications are growing every day and open up new doors for researchers to deploy such new technology for developing air-quality monitoring systems. Additionally, in line with the need to protect human health from various diseases, the development of WSN-based monitoring air-quality systems has received considerable attention in recent years. To carry out such a system requires reliable sensors to be integrated with WSN to detect and monitor pollutant air parameters such as O_3 (ozone), NO_2 (nitrogen dioxide), and CO concentrations (carbon monoxide) [22–24]. The sensed data are processed and communicated to the end beneficiary. The data are perceived from the sensing nodes that are sharing information wirelessly among each other. In short, three important components were used to build the architecture of the WSN-based monitoring system (see Fig. 12.1):

- First, end-user device (sensor or source) emphasis on sensing data and facilitate communicate with each other.
- Second, sink node emphasis to gather data and pass them to the middleware.
- Third, middleware emphasis on processing data before delivering them to the end-users.

Several reviewed research papers have already addressed this emerging vision of WSN-based air-quality monitoring. These research papers typically explain the

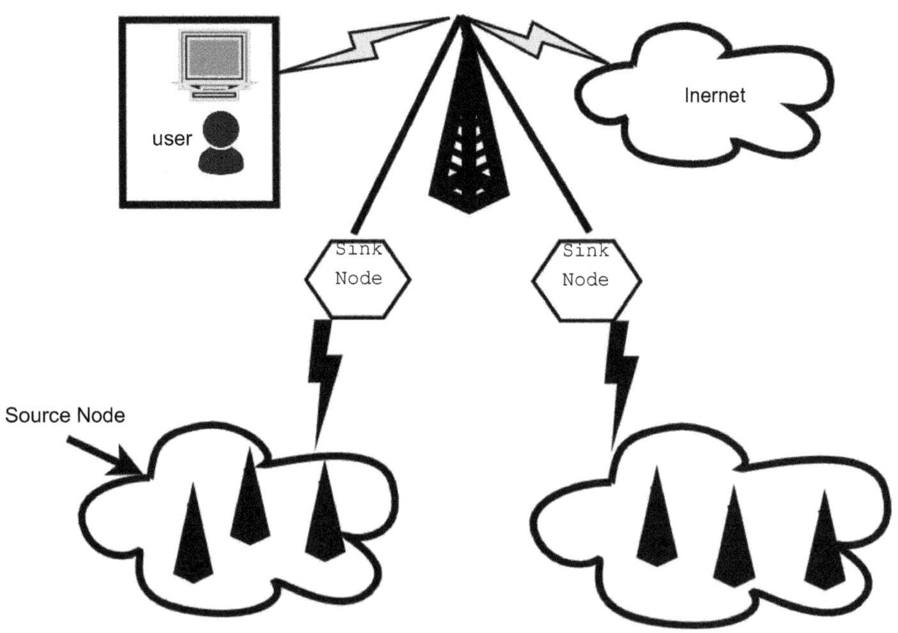

Fig. 12.1 WSN-based monitoring system architecture

needs, architectures, and new directions of WSN-based pollution monitoring models for different applications. Hence, this section aims to discuss current works of literature on WSN technologies in air pollution control processes.

One of the previous experiments in [3] was also proposed to develop WSN-based monitoring systems in order to receive and record sensed data. The impact of using WSN platform in their study is to create a micro-scaled monitoring system to detect pollutants in the air. Among other things, the authors have successfully tested their system in a crowded zone of population and vehicles. The authors showed that through MySQL software, their system could store many data in a database.

Meanwhile, a study in Pengpeng develops a web-based indoor monitoring system. In this study, WSN technology with a set of sensors was used to improve environmental monitoring. Closely related to the study in [3], all the sensed data are stored in an organized collection of data. Making such information available enhances the capabilities of accessing sensed data via the web. The proposed system can maintain a fair workplace for people by monitoring the indoor environment in real time and long term.

Air pollutant monitoring system (APOLLO) introduced by Choi et al. [25] was used to detect CO, NO_2, VOC, PM, and CO_2. WSN technology was used as a platform for transmitting the sensed data in order to achieve their study objectives. The proposed system is equipped with economic sensors to control and monitor air pollutants. Meanwhile, the authors in their study discussed all the related issues of WSN-based hardware and software. Through their experiments and evaluation, gas sensors' characteristics with their practical consequences for air pollution have been determined.

WSN technology was used by another earlier study described in [26] to collect the data and view it to the public through a desktop application. The proposed environmental parameter monitoring system is equipped with individual sensor nodes. The proposed sensors can transfer the sensed data to a coordinator node in a preassigned Zigbee wireless channel. The GUI using Java NetBeans was developed as an interface that logged and monitored sensor data collected from different sensor nodes. The coordinator node is manufactured using GSM-based mobile data networks to communicate with remote machines.

Closely related to the above study is the work proposed in Mughal et al. [27] which proposed WSN-based system for observing indoor ecological at home. The authors discussed the framework that controls the indoor environment and identified air toxins including light, temperature, pressure, and humidity. The rise of the smart sensors helped authors gather air-quality information about the level of humidity, temperature, pressure, illumination, and (CO_2), benzene (C_6H_6), and oxygen (O_2) gases. The sensed parameters are gathered for information analysis and decision-making. Several indoor plants toward decreasing pollution in the atmosphere are proposed in this study. This study's main objectives was to adjust the indoor atmosphere, position a nurturing plant system, upgrade sensors that screen the plants, and install the communication infrastructure to increase accessibility by using a notification scheme.

12.7.2 IOT-Based Architecture

IoT or the Internet of things is about billions of connected objects worldwide. These related objects can exchange information as a sender and receiver. People and businesses will stay connected for producing more meaningful results.

Definition 6 IoT [28] is defined as interconnection of sensor nodes and controller devices that can exchange information using unique identifiers. This is made possible with the unifying framework that consists of ubiquitous computing, data analytic and information representation, and cloud computing.

As an emerging technology with its wide variety of applications, it plays a major role in our lifestyles. Researchers nowadays are working to exploit IoT's full potential to improve the indoor monitoring system's technologies. As we know, poor IAQ one of the significant reasons for severe medical health issues, and IAQM applications can significantly help control IAQ and health.

Internet of Things (IoT) technology is widely used to monitor and measure air pollution levels over the last few years. IoT is considered another opportunity for the existing systems to monitor air quality due to rapid growth in digital technology and its capability to solve current systems' problems [29, 30]. IoT plays an essential role in creating, acquiring, and transmitting data in which the physical devices are connected and interacted to reach the common goals of IoT.

IoT-based monitoring system comprises of set smart sensors to collect an online air information, managing, and processing all air information in the IoT cloud, thereby contributing to the increase of the productivity of IAQM systems. Generally speaking, IoT-based monitoring system should be designed to consist three different layers mainly sensing, network, and application layer (see Fig. 12.2).

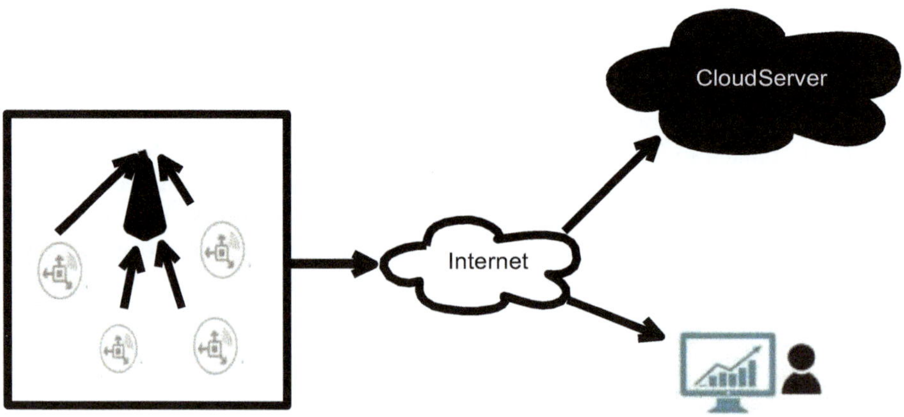

Fig. 12.2 IoT based monitoring system architecture

With the recent improvements and developments in technologies like the Internet of Things (IoT) and sensor network, it is now possible to develop smart, small, cost-effective air-quality monitoring systems to enhance the IAQ and improve individual.

well-being level of life. For endorsing modernization, building effective air-quality monitoring systems is necessary to support users in assessing how contaminated the air is. The most significant challenges faced by most air-quality monitoring systems are how the user can understand and interpret the sensed data's value. Building such a system will facilitate notifying users in real time without displaying complicated numerical values. Therefore, in recent years, several models have taken IoT technology with IAQM systems to enhance the indoor work environment. IoT technology and building a real-time air monitoring application are all essential components of the new version of IAQM that need to be used to protect the ecosystem environment. This section emphasizes researchers' efforts in this field while identifying the goals and future challenges.

In [31], IoT and big data approaches have proposed for online air monitoring systems to detect CO_2 concentration. In this study, CO_2 concentration has identified to measure and control buildings' ventilation systems. At the same time, the study in [32] proposed a IoT-based layered intelligent indoor environment monitoring system. The proposed system is made of different layers that would collect, transport, and process data. The proposed system is capable of monitoring in real time a set of environmental parameters including temperature, humidity, formaldehyde, and volatile contents through using various sensors including SHT31, MiCS-VZ-89TE, CCS811, SMD1013, ZE08-CH20, and iAQ-Core C. A mobile and a PC application are proposed for enabling the users to monitor indoor conditions in real time.

In [7] presents a solution to monitor the CO_2 level in real time based on IoT technology. The reason for selecting CO_2 in their study are:

- CO_2 is produced by people and combustion equipment and can be easily measured.
- Health professionals can be supported to perform clinical analysis based on data of CO_2 levels.
- High concentrations of other pollutants can be known by monitoring CO_2 levels.

Moreover, a web portal or a smartphone application is proposed in their system to facilitate access to the sensed data. Furthermore, in their study, the authors mentioned that the proposed system costs around USD 41.88 and can be considered a low-cost solution for improved living environments. The finding shows that the obtained results are promising and contribute to IoT-based CO_2 monitoring systems significantly.

Marques et al. in [33] proposed to develop IAQ system. It is an IoT-based IAQ system for monitoring indoor air quality where Arduino, ESP8266, and XBee sensors and technologies have been used. The advantages of using these sensors come from their capabilities to communicate, process, and collect data. Users can access sensed data in real time from different sites, either their website or mobile application. Their study has identified different environmental parameters, including carbon dioxide, temperature, monoxide, humidity, and luminosity. Their plan's objective is to employ their system to automatically support the building's managers to know the level of air pollutants. The user can view sensed data from the PHP-built IAQ web portal. The sensed data are displayed as numerical values or in the form of a graph. An alert manager built into the IAQ web alerts the user if some environmental parameter crosses a threshold value.

The study's idea in [34] is to develop a tiny air-quality monitoring system that uses an intuitive color LED display and provides air-quality data in real time. Additionally, the proposed system can combine the information collected from different air-quality systems on the World Wide Web and give relevant air-quality information. The system includes various low-cost sensors measuring data about concentration levels of PM, VOC, CO, temperature, and humidity. Hence, unlike costly professional devices to measure air quality, the proposed system making an economical indoor air-quality monitoring system is possible for homes, factories, etc.

A "smart air" system was developed in [35] to control IAQ and efficiently communicate online data. To store and transmit data precisely to the cloud, smart air integrates IoT sensor network in its architecture. Cloud computing-based web server is improving IAQ capabilities to visualize real-time data effectively. It could also issue alerts to the users using an installed mobile application to minimize risk and reduce air pollution. Smart air contains different sensors to collect dust, gases, temperature, humidity, etc.

12.8 IAQM's Domain

A variety of work has been done to study the issues related to the pollutants' level in the small and closed area, resulting in various health issues caused by these pollutants. The research study, such as this by [36], proposed a system to control air pollution and protect subway ridership. The critical reason for presenting such an application is to ensure passengers' safety, health, and comfort level. Responding to such a need, the authors developed a web-based information system to monitor crowded subways to identify pollutants' level through collecting the appropriate values including temperature, humidity, CO, CO_2, and particulate matter levels. This work's findings show the efficiency and effectiveness of a web-based system for monitoring and controlling the pollution levels in the subway stations.

While in [37], a study aims to assess the indoor air quality in the office building located in Delhi, India. The study's main idea was to evaluate CO_2 and PM2.5 levels in four different locations equipped with air-conditioner device. This study's findings proved the concentration of CO_2 and PM2.5 was higher than the 12 standard levels of CO_2 and PM2.5.

A new device called home pollution embedded system (HOPES) is proposed in [38]. This device was used to improve the well-being and style of life at home. The device can alert users through messages if foul smell, gas leakages, or combustion are detected. HOPES is a real-time device where IOT was used to upload historical data and monitor IAQ from everywhere. The research paper's finding confirms the accuracy of the device to give hints about concentration levels of indoor pollutants. In [39], several methods were used to measure the effects of air pollution in schools. This study's objectives are to identify the main IAQ's factors that may lead to sick building syndrome, including age and number of occupants, their activities, building design, outdoor pollution concentration, and ventilation. In this respect, this paper made a remarkable IAQ monitoring system that covers three major areas, i.e., environmental measurements, building and ventilation parameters, and occupant questionnaire.

In the research paper [40], they developed and deployed a WSN-based system in two rooms in NDUM (National Defense University, Malaysia). The sensors measured CO_2, humidity, and temperature and transmitted data to a central computer. It was observed that the CO_2 concentration increased due to poor ventilation. An IQ test was given to students, and some of the students were seated under air-conditioning, and some without it, the students with air conditioning performed better than other students. Thus, it is concluded that classroom air pollution obviously influences students' concentration in the class.

12.9 Conclusion

Air pollution is a dangerous threat to the whole ecosystem and humans. Air pollutants directly or indirectly affect the environment and the living organisms. Environmental protection systems are more often employed in industrialized countries because of industrialization, urbanization, and population growth. The field of monitoring air pollution is just the beginning. Recently, it has been noticed that air pollutants have been increased to the hazard level, and many discoveries are waiting to be made. There are sufficient research papers that solved many air pollution problems by integrating new technologies in the environmental monitoring management system, helping researchers and developers do something that has never been known. We must keep in mind that this study is based on other research findings stated in monitoring air pollution for several years.

This study is not unique in its empirical literature but different in presenting the available worldwide systems. Researchers used a wide range of methodological tools such IoT and big data to control the quality of the air in real time at indoor and outdoor pollution systems. The usefulness of such technologies can play a significant role in data storage and retrieve a relational database. Integrating IoT with big data technologies in one system adds an empirical value to research in various fields, increasing the efficiency of health ecosystem management and enhancing plans for developing such systems.

Additionally, this paper highlights the WSN technological model's primary challenges with their complexities since it was integrated with the air pollution monitoring system. However, this technology has its challenges, particularly in deciding between cost, spatial coverage, and accuracy. It is worth noticing that some problems and experiences need more attention in this area, as well as some features of the existing systems can be manifested when there is a plan to develop a new version of IAQM.

Generally speaking, the main aims of this research paper are:

- This research paper will help researchers understand the restriction of air pollutants' emissions and allow the stakeholder to take prompt strategic measures to protect people's lives from decadence.
- This paper will help researchers find the literature discussing the leading technologies and strategies for regularly monitoring indoor environmental data and identifying the primary pollutants' measures.
- This paper will help researchers find the literature that is discussing, analyzing, and monitoring air pollution levels in real time.

As a sound methodology, the above challenges should be addressed when a good air monitoring system has to be developed. We believe that all these challenges can help scientists improve the current system's stability and significantly reduce the system's cost.

Currently, much of the air pollution research has been undertaken by China and the United States, while this has been significantly fewer for other countries, particularly in the Middle East. Therefore, further research needs to be carried out in areas that suffer elevated levels of emissions.

References

1. Chen, P., & Lu, Z. (2013). A web-based indoor environment monitoring system using wireless sensor networks. In *Published in: 2013 international conference on computational and information sciences*. https://doi.org/10.1109/ICCIS.2013.529
2. AbdulWahhab, R. S. (April 2019). Air quality system using IoT for indoor environmental monitoring. In *ICCTA 2019: Proceedings of the 2019 5th International Conference on Computer and Technology Applications* (pp. 184–188). https://doi.org/10.1145/3323933.3324088
3. Liu, J.-H., Chen, Y.-F., Lin, T.-S., Lai, D.-W., Wen, T.-H., Sun, C.-H., Juang, J.-Y., & Jiang, J.-A. (2011). Developed urban air quality monitoring system based on wireless sensor networks. In *Fifth International Conference on Sensing Technology* (pp. 549–554).
4. Ang, L.-M., & Seng, K. P. (2016). Big sensor data applications in urban environments. *Big Data Research, 4*, 1–12. https://doi.org/10.1016/j.bdr.2015.12.003

5. Idrees, Z., & Zheng, L. (2019). Low cost air pollution monitoring systems: A review of the protocols and the enabling technologies. *Journal of Industrial Information Integration*. https://doi.org/10.1016/j.jii.2019.100123
6. Idrees, Z., Zou, Z., & Zheng, L. (2018). Edge computing based IoT architecture for low cost air pollution monitoring systems: A comprehensive system analysis, design considerations and development. *Sensors, 18*(9), 3021. https://doi.org/10.3390/s18093021
7. Marques, G., Ferreira, C. R., & Pitarma, R. (2019). Indoor air quality assessment using a CO2 Monitoring system based on internet of things. *Journal of Medical Systems, 43*, 67.
8. Kurt, A., Gulbagci, B., Karaca, F., & Alagha, O. (2008 Jul). An online air pollution forecasting sys- tem using neural networks. *Environment International, 34*(5), 592–598. https://doi.org/10.1016/j.envint.2007.12.020
9. Hojaiji, H., Goldstein, O., King, C. E., Sarrafzadeh, M., & Jerrett, M. (2017). Design and calibration of a wearable and wireless research grade air quality monitoring system for real-time data collection. In *Global Humanitarian Technology Conference (GHTC), 2017 IEEE* (pp. 1–10). IEEE.
10. Tien, S.-C., Lin, R., Lee, T.-Y., Lee, R.-G., & Huang, S.-Y. (2014). Development and implementation of wireless multigas concentration cloud system. *ISRN Sensor Networks, 2014*, 1–11.
11. Bruce, R. (2011). *Statistical and machine-learning data mining: Techniques for better predictive modeling and analysis of big data* (2nd ed.). CRC Press.
12. Kelleher, J. D., Namee, B. M., & D'Arcy, A. (2015). *Fundamentals of machine learning for predictive data analytics: Algorithms, worked examples, and case studies*. The MIT Press.
13. Tan, P.-N., Steinbach, M., & Kumar, V. (2013). *Introduction to data mining: Pearson new international edition* (1st ed.). Pearson.
14. Han, J., Kamber, M., & Simon, J. P. (2012). *Data mining concepts and techniques* (3rd ed.). Elsevier.
15. Moisan, S., Herrera, R., & Clements, A. (2018). A dynamic multiple equation approach for forecasting PM2.5 pollution in Santiago, Chile. *International Journal of Forecasting, 34*(4), 566–581. https://doi.org/10.1016/j.ijforecast.2018.03.007
16. Niska, H., Hiltunen, T., Karppinen, A., Ruuskanen, J., & Kolehmainen, M. (2004). Evolving the neural network model for forecasting air pollution time series. *Engineering Applications of Artificial Intelligence, 17*(2), 159–167. https://doi.org/10.1016/j.engappai.2004.02.002
17. Feng, Y., Zhang, W., Sun, D., & Zhang, L. (2011). Ozone concentration forecast method based on genetic algorithm optimized back propagation neural networks and support vector machine data classification. *Atmospheric Environment, 45*, 1979–1985.
18. Ma, X., Wang, Y., & Wang, C. (2017). Low-carbon development of China's thermal power industry based on an international comparison: Review, analysis and forecast. *Renewable and Sustainable Energy Reviews, 80*, 942–970.
19. Yang, Z., & Wang, J. (2017). A new air quality monitoring and early warning system: Air quality assessment and air pollutant concentration prediction. *Environmental Research, 158*, 105–117. https://doi.org/10.1016/j.envres.2017.06.002
20. Wu, L., et al. (2014). Modelling and forecasting CO2 emissions in the BRICS (Brazil, Russia, India, China, and South Africa) countries using a novel multi-variable grey model. *Energy*. https://doi.org/10.1016/j.energy.2014.11.052
21. Sen, P., Roy, M., & Pal, P. (2016). Application of ARIMA for forecasting energy consumption and GHG emission: A case study of an Indian pig iron manufacturing organization. *Energy, 116*, 1031–1038. https://doi.org/10.1016/j.energy.2016.10.068
22. Nograles, A. H., Agbay, C. P. D., Flores, I. S. L., Manuel, L., & Salonga, J. B. C. (2014). Low cost internet based wireless sensor network for air pollution monitoring using Zigbee module. In *Proc. fourth Int. Conf. Digital information technology and applications* (pp. 310–314).
23. Anjaneyulu, Y., Jayakumar, I., Bindu, V. H., et al. (2007). Real time remote monitoring of air pollutants and their online transmission to the web using internet protocol. *Environmental Monitoring and Assessment, 124*, 371.

24. Liu, J.-H., Chen, Y.-F., Lin, T.-S., Lai, D.-W., Wen, T.-H., Sun, C.-H., Juang, J.-Y., & Jiang, J.-A. (2011). Developed urban air quality monitoring system based on wireless sensor networks. In *Proc. Fifth Int. Conf. Sensing technology* (pp. 549–554).
25. Choi, S., Kim, N., Cha, H., & Ha, R. (2009). Micro sensor node for air pollutant monitoring: Hardware and software issues. *Sensors, 9*(10), 7970–7987. https://doi.org/10.3390/s91007970
26. Girish, S. V., Prakash, R., Swetha, S. N. H., Pareek, G., Senthil Kumar, T., & Balaji Ganesh, A. (2015). A network model of GUI-based implementation of sensor node for indoor air quality monitoring. In *Advances in intelligent systems and computing* (pp. 209–217). Springer International Publishing.
27. Mughal, S., Razaque, F., Malani, M., Hassan, M. R., Hussain, S., & Nazir, A. (2019). Context-aware indoor environment monitoring and plant prediction using wireless sensor network. In M. Miraz, P. Excell, A. Ware, S. Soomro, & M. Ali (Eds.), *Emerging Technologies in Computing. iCETiC 2019. Lecture Notes of the Institute for Computer Sciences, Social Informatics and Telecommunications Engineering* (Vol. 285). Springer.
28. Bessis, N., & Dobre, C. (January 2014). *Big data and internet of things: A roadmap for smart environments*. Springer International Publishing.
29. Nait Malek, Y., Kharbouch, A., El Khoukhi, H., Bakhouya, M., Deflorio, V., Elouadghiri, D., Latre, S., & Blondia, C. (2017). On the use of IoT and big data Technologies for Real-time Monitoring and Data Processing in the 7th international conference on current and future trends of information and communication Technologies in Healthcare (ICTH 2017). *Procedia Computer Science, 113*, 429–434.
30. Atzori, L., et al. (2010). The internet of things: A survey. *Computer Networks, 54*(15), 2787–2805.
31. Malek, Y. N., Kharbouch, A., Khoukhi, H. E., Bakhouya, M., Florio, V. D., Ouadghiri, D. E., & Blondia, C. (2017). On the use of IoT and big data Technologies for Real- time monitoring and data processing. *Procedia Computer Science, 113*, 429–434. https://doi.org/10.1016/j.procs.2017.08.281
32. Zhang, H., & Liu, P. (2019). Intelligent indoor environment monitoring system based on IoT and cloud platform. In K. Deng, Z. Yu, S. Patnaik, & J. Wang (Eds.), *Recent developments in mechatronics and intelligent robotics. ICMIR 2018. Advances in intelligent systems and computing* (Vol. 856). Springer.
33. Gonçalo, M., & Pitarma, R. (2016). An indoor monitoring system for ambient assisted living based on internet of things architecture. *International Journal of Environmental Research and Public Health, 13*, 1152.
34. Kang, J., & Hwang, K.-I. (2016). A comprehensive real-time indoor air-quality level indicator. *Sustainability, 8*, 881.
35. Jo, J., Jo, B., Kim, J., Kim, S., & Han, W. (2020). Development of an IoT-based indoor air quality monitoring platform. *Journal of Sensors, 2020*, 8749764.
36. Choi, G. H., Choi, G. S., & Jang, J. H. (2009). Web information Systems for Monitoring and Control of indoor air quality at Subway stations. *Lecture Notes in Computer Science*, 195–204.
37. Gupta, A., Goyal, R., Kulshreshtha, P., & Jain, A. (2020). Environmental monitoring of PM2.5 and CO2 in indoor office spaces of Delhi, India. In A. Sharma, R. Goyal, & R. Mittal (Eds.), *Indoor environmental quality. Lecture notes in civil engineering*. Springer. https://doi.org/10.1007/978-981-15-1334-3
38. Gugliermetti, L., & Astiaso Garcia, D. (2017). A cheap and third-age-friendly home device for monitoring indoor air quality. *International journal of Environmental Science and Technology, 15*(1), 185–198. https://doi.org/10.1007/s13762-017

39. Shelestov, A., Sumilo, L., Lavreniuk, M., Vasiliev, V., Bulanaya, T., Gomilko, I., & Skakun, S. (2018). Indoor and outdoor air quality monitoring on the base of intelligent sensors for Smart City. In *Recent developments in data science and intelligent analysis of information* (pp. 134–145). Springer.
40. Wang, S., Chew, S., Jusoh, M., Khairunissa, A., Leong, K., & Azid, A. (2017). WSN based indoor air quality monitoring in classrooms. In *AIP Conference Proceedings* (Vol. 1808, article 020063).

Chapter 13
Computer-Based Techniques for Detecting the Neurological Disorders

Mohd. Suhaib Kidwai and Mohd. Maroof Siddiqui

13.1 Introduction

Millions of people around the world are affected by various neurological disorders. These disorders lead to difficulty in daily activities and often lead to the medical assistance for prolonged period of time. Neurological disorders like epilepsy affect the muscular functions of the body and may lead to fatal injuries because of the loss of control over the body during the epileptic fits. Similarly, Alzheimer's disease is found mostly in elderly people and leads to memory loss. Bruxism is another such neurological disorder which leads to clenching of the teeth during sleep or while the patient is awake.

13.1.1 Significance of EEG in the Detection of Neurological Disorders

Doctors and clinicians use various methods to detect the neurological disorders. These methods include analyzing the EEG signal patterns or observing the symptoms of the patient. But analyzing the EEG patterns is not an easy task as EEG signals are highly spontaneous and chaotic and they vary at a very fast pace.

M. S. Kidwai (✉)
Department of Electronics and Communication Engineering, Integral University, Lucknow, India

M. M. Siddiqui
College of Engineering, Dhofar University, Salalah, Oman

M. S. Husain et al. (eds.), *Pervasive Healthcare*, EAI/Springer Innovations in Communication and Computing, https://doi.org/10.1007/978-3-030-77746-3_13

13.1.2 Significance of the Computer-Assisted Algorithm in Detection of Neurological Disorders

The computer-assisted algorithms play a vital role in efficiently detecting disorders, and such algorithms also reduces the involvement of medical professionals as they can be handled by a person with basic understanding of the computers. The person can be given a short training after which he can work on the computer-assisted technique for obtaining results from the patients. This will give more time to medical professionals to deal with curing and treatment of disease rather that detecting it.

This chapter talks about a novel computer-assisted method for the detection of neurological disorders based on the phenomena of recurrences that are generally found in EEG signals of the patients with neurological disorders. The method discussed in this chapter is new and different from the other existing computer-assisted methods in various ways.

Firstly, it has used the mathematical concept of recurrence as its basis for detection of disorders. This property of recurrence has not been used till now in detection of disorders. Various related works have used various analysis approaches of EEG signals like discrete wavelet transforms and other parameters like laminarity, etc. for getting the information from the EEG signals, but recurrence has never been used till now.

Secondly, this technique is a single-feature technique, i.e., a single parameter has been calculated, and all the analysis and detection have been done by using that single parameter. In all the relevant works, more than one feature has to be extracted from the EEG signals in order to detect disorders. The increase in number of features or parameters complicates the entire procedure, so this method has simplicity as one of its most appealing factors. This factor has been a very appealing and innovative part as it has the potential of revolutionizing the entire concept of algorithm designing that are based on single feature for detection of neurological disorders.

The computer-assisted algorithm which has been discussed in this chapter involves source programs whose coding has been done in MATLAB. To quantify the recurrence, a parameter called "coupling index (ρπ)" has been used. The disorders are detected on the basis of the value of coupling index.

The use of machine learning classifiers has been done to classify the values of coupling index for the various neurological disorders. The machine learning models are trained and tested by taking values of "coupling index (ρπ)" as an input, and the Python platform is used for testing and training of various machine learning classifiers. Once the models are trained and tested with the known patients, it had led to the setting of the range of coupling index for the patients with epilepsy, Alzheimer's disease, and bruxism. Thus this computer-assisted technique acts as an easy test for detecting neurological disorders, and further it classifies the patients of epilepsy, Alzheimer's, and bruxism, which will help in more focused treatment of patients. Moreover its results can be downloaded and shared on various e platforms which will provide flexibility in remote patient monitoring.

This method has been implemented on the real-time EEG datasets of patient's having epilepsy, Alzheimer's, and bruxism and had yielded significant results. The various sources from where data has been taken are as follows:

(a) UCI machine learning repository [1].
(b) physionet.org [2].

Further, this chapter is divided in a way that initially talks about the neurological disorders, followed by its prevalence in India. Then it has been explained how the seizures can prove useful in detecting neurological disorders. Then subsequently the chapter talks about the concept of recurrences, the computer-assisted algorithm, and finally the novel technique that has been developed. Further the results and conclusions are included.

The main objectives of this chapter are:

- To give basic idea of neurological disorders.
- Significance of EEG signals in detection of neurological disorders.
- To give the idea of recurrence and its occurrence in EEG signals.
- To give the idea of computer-assisted algorithms.
- Finally to discuss about the novel algorithm and compare its results with the other latest and relevant works.

13.2 Neurological Disorders

Neurological disorders are the diseases that affect the nervous system. They affect the brain and its activities. Their affects are also seen on the spinal cord, autonomous nervous system, and various motor functions like muscular movements. There are various neurological disorders. Of them, few can be genetic and few can be due to the factors like ageing, etc.

A report on dementia by the WHO states that in most of the patients this occurs because of the Alzheimer's disease [3] (Fig. 13.1).

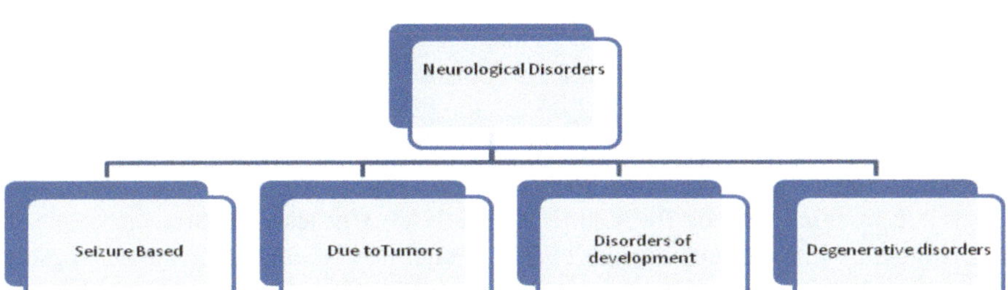

Fig. 13.1 Classification of neurological disorders

13.3 Prevalence of Neurological Disorders in India

The National Institute of Neurological Disorders and Stroke reported that there exist more than 600 neurological disorders, and around 50 million Americans are affected with some type of neurological disorders each year [4, 5].

The cases of neurological disorders in India are increasing day by day. The prevalence rate (the proportion of the population that has a specific neurological disorder at a specified point of time or over the specified period of time) of neurological disorders in India is 2394 and ranged from 967 to 4070 per 100,000 population. This prevalence rate is even more in rural India, as compared to urban population [6].

Among all the neurological disorders, the most common disorder found was headache. Seizure-based neurological disorders like epilepsy and Alzheimer's disease were also among the commonly found disorders in India [7].

Another study was also conducted by the National Institute of Mental Health and Neurosciences among the urban and rural population of Bangalore district. The highest prevalence rate was of headache (1119) followed by epilepsy (883) [7].

Similar prevalence rate-based survey carried out at Malda district also concluded that PR of epilepsy was considerable (305), followed by vertigo (24.45), mental retardation (42.90), paralytic poliomyelitis (53.63), movement disorders (26.81), and spinal cord disorders (21).

There are many studies carried out by international, national, and private organizations that unanimously show that occurrence of neurological disorders in India are on the rise.

13.4 Seizures as Biomarkers of Neurological Disorders

All the activities in the body are controlled by the brain. So, any changes in the brain activity can be used to study the changes or disorders in the body. The changes in the brain activity can be observed by recording and analyzing the bioelectrical signals that are developed in the brain. The bioelectrical signals from the brain are recorded using the EEG (electroencephalogram) machine. This machine has various electrodes which record the biosignals from the brain and feed it to the processing and display unit that displays the signals. From various studies it is evident that various disorders like epilepsy manifest themselves in seizures and these seizures can be visualized (using a EEG machine) as the repeating or synchronized values of EEG signal states [8–10].

So, if the EEG signals recorded from the brain show high degree of repetition or recurrence in signal values for significant interval of times, it shows the onset of seizures. Since the seizures are the common characteristics of many neurological disorders, they are used as the biomarkers for studying and detecting neurological disorders [11].

13.5 Introduction to Coupling

Coupling is the phenomenon that has been observed in two physical entities or systems when they are in tandem with each other, in some, or the other way. There exists some kind of synchronization between the various physical systems that interact with each other. Sometimes, two or more than two systems seem to be chaotic and random, but it is possible that they are coupled or synchronized in a specific interval of time.

There are many real-world examples of two or more than two systems coupled together. For example, the symphony has so many musicians playing different instruments, but all are coupled and synchronized in such a way that a beautiful music is created.

The coupling is also found in biological systems. All the activities happening inside the human body are synchronized with each other. This synchronism is maintained in the bioelectrical signal generated in the brain and is transmitted to various parts and organs of the body. This also establishes the fact that there is a pattern of EEG signals for all the normal activities and any changes in the EEG states indicate that there is something wrong in the human biological system. That's why the EEG signals and their synchronization patterns are used to detect various neurological disorders. Moreover, these patterns can also be monitored during the surgery of patients or during the process like deciding the depth of anesthesia that is to be given to the patient. This is because when the heart is working normally, then the synchronization between the ECG and EEG signals has a specific coupling or synchronization pattern. Using this pattern as a reference, it is possible to monitor whether the heart is working normally during the surgery of a patient. If any problem comes during surgery or during the anesthesia dispensing, it can be observed by the changes in synchronism between ECG and EEG signals. This way it becomes easier to decide the dose of anesthesia or for monitoring the patient during the entire surgery [12].

13.6 Significance of Detection of Coupling in Biomedical System

Biological systems are profoundly mind boggling, and so are signals which are taken from them. This is particularly valid for the cardiovascular framework and brain. A huge measure of exertion has been made as of late to create time-based examination for diagnostic purposes, i.e., to discover approaches to decide the physiological state by investigation of the complex biological signals [13].

Furthermore, synchronization-related marvels coupled with complex frameworks have been found to happen, in physical, yet additionally in numerous natural frameworks, e.g., the cardio-respiratory cooperation and neural signals. Proportions of intricacy have been built up that recognize standard, chaotic, and arbitrary practices and can attempt to foresee a respiratory failure or a seizure-based neurological issue [14]. It has been accounted for that multifaceted nature of heart and brain information can recognize a sick subject from a healthy one, and thus it can be used for detecting disorders.

13.7 Computer-Based Techniques for Detection of Neurological Disorders by Using EEG Signals

Analyzing the patterns of EEG signals and detecting neurological disorders is a very challenging task and requires highly skilled neurophysiologists. The problem in analyzing EEG signals is because:

- EEG signals are highly spontaneous.
- Though the expert neurologists can analyze and study the EEG signal patterns by looking at them, it is a time-consuming and a tedious process.

Therefore, computer-aided detection is very useful for the neurophysiologists in interpreting the EEG.

The computer-aided design (CAD)-based techniques are generally the algorithms that are made for extracting out the features for analyzing the EEG data and then classifying the EEG data on the basis of extracted features, so as to find out the disorders. The feature extraction process is all about obtaining the useful information from the recorded EEG data. This process can be actualized in frequency, time, and time-frequency domains. The time space and frequency area are utilized for signal preparing when the EEG is thought to be a stable and unchanged signal. Then again, when the EEG signal is considered highly varying, at that point the time-frequency domain is utilized.

Once the features are extracted and processed, they are analyzed and processed using classifiers like k-nearest neighbors, random forest, etc. These classifiers classify the data based on different approaches that compare the values of the features that are extracted from recorded EEG signals. The diagrammatic representation of a general structure of computer-based seizure detection is given in Fig. 13.2.

13.8 Recurrence-Based and Machine Learning-Assisted Computer-Based Method for Detection of Neurological Disorder

Poincare firstly observed the phenomenon of recurrence in physical systems. He concluded through his studies that after certain time interval the trajectory of any random system traverses the same path again in phase space.

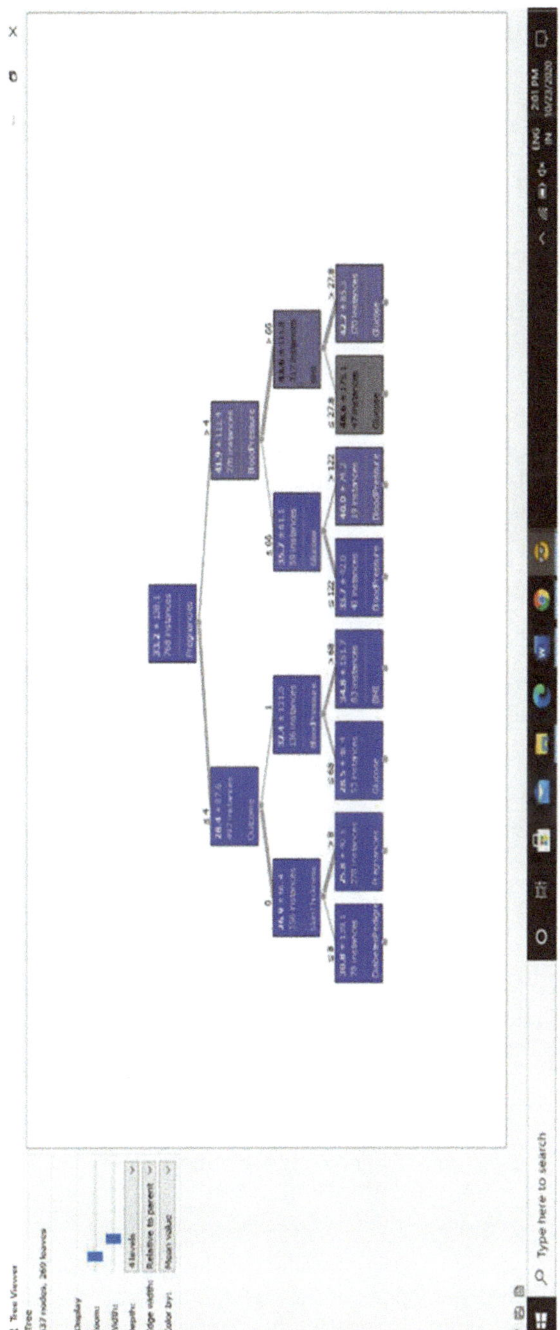

Fig. 13.2 Block diagram of computer-based seizure detection system

This phenomenon has also been reported in EEG signals by various scientists [15, 16].

The recurrence in EEG signals increases during seizures. These seizures are the indicators of various neurological disorders.

13.8.1 Recurrences

They can be briefly categorized as given below:

- Recurrence Matrix: The elements of this matrix are the difference of signal values of same signal series, taken at different instants. The elements of the recurrence matrix are found out by using the following formula:

ee classifier has been used, and the $\varepsilon = 10\%$ of the maximum value of the signal over a given interval of time.

x_i, x_j are the *i*th and *j*th sample of the same signal series, and *Rij* is the recurrence matrix. Θ represents Heaviside function.

- Cross- Recurrence Matrix: The elements of this matrix are the differences in signal instants of two different time series. The elements of cross-recurrence matrix are found out by using the following formula:

$$CR_{ij} = \Theta\left(\varepsilon - \| x_i - y_j \|\right) \tag{13.1}$$

xi, *yj* are two different samples of time series, among which the recurrence, i.e., CR*ij*, has to be determined.

- Joint Recurrence Matrix: t is the product of recurrence matrix of two time series. It is represented as.

$$JR_{ij}^{xy} = R_{ij}^{x} * R_{ij}^{y}. \tag{13.2}$$

- Order Recurrence Matrix: The elements of this matrix are found out firstly by finding the order patterns.

Order patterns are represented by $\pi x(t)$ and $\pi y(t)$, corresponding to two different time series $x(t)$ and $y(t)$**:**

$$\pi_x(t) = 1, \text{if } x(t) > x(t+k) \text{otherwise } 0 \tag{13.3}$$

$$\pi_y(t) = 1, \text{if } y(t) > y(t+k) \text{otherwise } 0 \tag{13.4}$$

Here, *k* refers to the integer values of the signal instants.

Once the order pattern matrix is formed, they both are compared to find the order recurrence matrix which is represented by following formula:

$$\mathrm{ORP}(t,\tau)=1, \pi_x(t)=\pi_y(t+\tau) \\ 0, \text{otherwise} \tag{13.5}$$

τ = nearest neighbor values.

Recurrence-based analysis is simple to apply and is applicable easily on larger datasets [17].

13.9 The Novel Computer-Assisted Algorithm for Detection of Neurological Disorders

The phenomenon of recurrence in EEG signals is the crux of this algorithm. This is a computer-aided algorithm, i.e., it uses coding on a specific computer language, and the EEG signals are recorded, visualized, and analyzed on computer though this algorithm follows the basic framework that is somewhat similar to the existing computer-based disorders detecting algorithm, yet it differs from them on the basis of domain in which it works, the features used for detecting the disorders, the classifiers used, and above all the approach that is being followed to detect the seizure-based neurological disorders. The proposed method is basically the time domain analysis of EEG signals, and hence it has simplicity and all the other advantages that a time domain analysis offers. Moreover, the disadvantages of time domain methods like difficulty in analyzing larger datasets have been removed by carefully selecting a feature, on the basis of which seizure detection has been done. The generalized block diagram of the algorithm is given below for better understanding:

Each and every block of Fig. 13.3 has been defined below:

(a) Data acquisition: The signals from the human brain are recorded using EEG machine, and they are used as input for the programs developed by using the algorithm discussed here in this chapter. For this work EEG data of normal subjects and the subjects having epilepsy, Alzheimer's disease, and bruxism are taken from online sources: UCI machine learning repository ("UCIMachine Learning Repository: EEG
(b) Database Data Set," [1]) and physionet.org [2].

   Moreover, few of the datasets for this work have also been obtained from the Integral Institute of Medical Science and Research.

   The EEG dataset used in this work is pre-processed, i.e., the EEG signals used for this work are already filtered and de-noised.

   The EEG of ten subjects is taken for the entire work, i.e., ten subjects having epilepsy, Alzheimer's disease, and bruxism. For comparison of results, the EEG data of ten normal subjects are taken who are having no neurological disorders.

   Data from 27 channels of an EEG machine is taken into consideration for detecting all the disorders, and 6000 samples of EEG time series are considered.

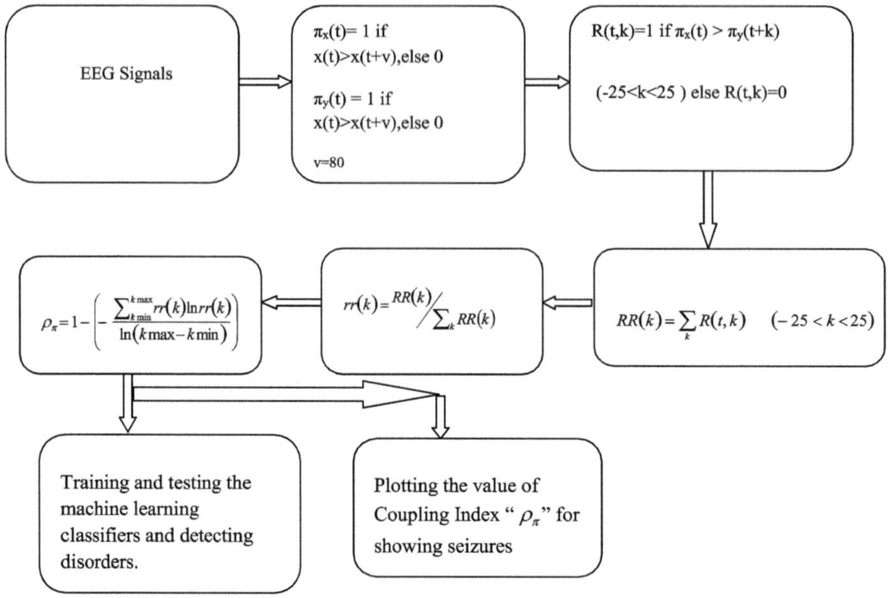

Fig. 13.3 Block representation of the novel computer-based technique

(c) Feature extraction: The second and third block represent the process of feature extraction for detection of seizures. This algorithm uses the EEG data of two EEG channels at a time for calculations.

Out of the many features that can be extracted from EEG signals, this algorithm uses the recurrence rate (R.R) as the feature to classify the seizure and non-seizure instants of the EEG signals. Here, the matrix of the values of recurrence rate is obtained using the matrices of order patterns pi x (π_x) and pie y (π_y).

pie x(π_x) is the array of ones and zeroes that is found by comparing EEG sample values taken from a channel of an EEG machine and named as "x." The values of a channel are compared with each other as shown in the second block.

For example, the xth signal value is compared with $(x + v)^{th}$ signal value of the EEG signal from a single channel.

If the xth signal value is greater than or equal to the $(x + v)^{th}$ signal value, then.

"1" will be assigned to the matrix referred to as pie x(π_x), and if xth signal value is less than the (x + v)th signal value, then a "0" will be assigned to the pie x(π_x) matrix. Similarly pie y (π_y) matrix is also found.

"*v*" is the number of EEG states that will be skipped while comparing the signal values of same channel of EEG machine. This skipping is done because EEG signals are highly chaotic and their values are in microvolts and milivolts, the values adjacent to a specific signal values are difficult to differentiate, and their isn't much difference between them, so comparing them with each other does not hold any significance.

In this work, the value of "*k*" is taken as 80, i.e., the first sample is compared with 81st sample of EEG signal.

The arrays of pie x(π_x) and pie y (π_y) are further compared to find out the recurrence matrix as follows:

$$\begin{aligned} &R(t,k) = 1 \, if \; \pi x(t) = \pi y(t+k) \\ &0, \text{ otherwise} \end{aligned} \tag{13.6}$$

Here "*k*" is the number of values of EEG signals taken from any channel named as "y" and compared with a EEG signal value from channel "*x*."

In this case the value of "*k*" is 50, i.e., any signal instant of channel "*x*" will be compared by 25 values of channel *y* before the instant of signal *x* and 25 values after it.

Finally, the matrix of rate of recurrence and matrix of its averaged value is found out. This is done by using the following formulas:

$$RR(k) = \sum_k R(t,k) \tag{13.7}$$

$$rr(k) = {RR(k)} \Big/ {\sum_k RR(k)} \tag{13.8}$$

Finding the Recurrence Quantification Parameter Once the feature called recurrence rate is extracted, it is used to find out a parameter called "coupling index (ρ_π)." The formula for coupling index is as follows:

$$\rho_x = 1 - \left(- \frac{\sum_{k\min}^{k\max} rr(k) \ln rr(k)}{\ln(k\max - k\min)} \right) \tag{13.9}$$

where $0 < \rho_\pi < 1$

The coupling index quantifies the recurrence, i.e., it determines the strength of the coupling between the EEG signals taken from a subject.

The value near to 1 shows a strong coupling, and the strength of coupling decreases if the value is near to 0.

$\rho\pi = 1$ means perfect or complete coupling between the signals or systems. $\rho\pi = 0$ means the signals or the systems are not coupled or synchronized at all.

Since the key feature of EEG signals during seizures is the coupling between them, so with the "coupling index ($\rho\pi$)" values, it is easier to find out the onset of seizure and hence it is possible to detect seizure-based neurological disorders.

Further, the values of coupling index can also be plotted by using PLOT command of MATLAB, which will provide the visualization of onset of seizures in patients having neurological disorders.

Classification of Values of Coupling Index While the graphs of coupling index gives the visualization of coupling between the EEG signals, the values of coupling index are fed to machine learning classifier models, so as to detect the neurological disorders based on the range of coupling index values.

The dataset of coupling index of various known patients of Alzheimer's disease, epilepsy, and bruxism has been prepared by repeatedly finding the values using the steps that are mentioned above.

Then this dataset has been divided into training and testing data using the standard 80:20 ratio, i.e., 80% of the dataset is taken as training data and 20% as testing data.

Then various machine learning models like KNN (k-nearest neighbor), SVN (support vector machine), etc. have been trained and re-trained to get the range of coupling index, on the basis of which the patients having epilepsy, Alzheimer's disease, and bruxism can be determined. Meanwhile, by feeding the dataset of the coupling index of normal patients along with the patients of disorders, the range for the normal people is also determined.

The algorithm discussed in this chapter is based on the fact that seizures are found in EEG signals (that are developed in various regions of the brain) of patients suffering from epilepsy, Alzheimer's disease, and bruxism.

These seizures are studied and analyzed here by using the concept of recurrences in EEG states that is found in the patients of neurological disorders.

The codes for the algorithm are written using MATLAB 2013a, and Python is used for classification purposes.

To implement the algorithms, programs and sub-programs are written by using various software and languages. The coding has been done by using MATLAB. It is an elite language for specialized processing. It incorporates calculation, representation, and programming in a simple to-utilize condition where issues and arrangements are communicated in natural numerical documentation.

It consolidates a work area condition tuned for iterative examination and configuration measures with a programming language that communicates lattice and cluster arithmetic straightforwardly.

Similarly, python language has been used here, for result comparison and analysis. Python is generally used in computer-based seizure detection techniques because it is user-friendly, multipurpose, and a high-level language.

13.9.1 Features

Extraction of feature and arrangement are the two basic techniques for a seizure recognition framework. Since an EEG signal is an excess discrete-time succession, it is important to dispense with its repetition, and this handling step is known as extracting of a feature. To discover an ideal element extraction strategy, various time-based, frequency-based, and time-frequency-based strategies are accessible. A portion of the usually utilized features in time domain are variance, averaged power, and so on. Power spectral density is generally preferred in frequency-based approach.

In time-frequency area, the features used are standard deviation, skewness, kurtosis, mean frequency, peak frequency, etc. [18].

13.9.2 Machine Learning Models that Can be Used with Computer-Assisted Algorithms

Classifiers are the models that classify the dataset on the basis of certain differences between the features that are extracted from the raw data.

In AI or machine learning and measurements (i.e., stats), classification is a directed learning approach in which the PC program gains from the information input given to it (likewise called as preparing information) and afterward utilizes this figuring out how to order novel perception (otherwise called testing information). This informational collection may just be bi-class (like distinguishing whether the individual is grown up or not or that the ink is blue or dark), or it might be multi-class as well. A few instances of arrangement issues are biometric identification, document classification, etc.

Various types of classifiers are:

Naive Bayes Classifier

It is a classification technique that is based on Bayes' theorem. This classifier accepts that the nearness of a specific element in a class is random to the nearness of some other element. Regardless of whether these highlights rely upon one another or upon the presence of different highlights, these properties freely add to the likelihood. This classifier is particularly useful for very large datasets.

Nearest Neighbor

This classifier algorithm takes a new data value and compares it with the nearest labeled or already classified data value. Once the raw data value is compared, it is labeled as those datasets which have the nearest value to it. The "k" is the number of neighbors compared with the data.

Logistic Regression (Predictive Learning Model)

It is a factual strategy for investigating an informational index where there is at least one autonomous factor that decides a result. The result is estimated with a variable that has only two possible outcomes.

Decision Trees

Decision tree classifies the data as a tree structure. It separates an informational index into smaller, subsets while simultaneously a related choice or decision tree is created. The choice tree has a leaf hub and a choice hub. A choice hub is additionally grouped into at least two hubs, while the leaf hub speaks to an arrangement or choice. Choice trees can deal with both straight-out and mathematical information.

Random Forest

They are classification strategies that work by building a large number of choice trees at preparing time and yielding the class that is the method of the classes (characterization) or mean forecast (relapse) of the individual trees.

Neural Network

It comprises of primary elements called neurons in several stages. These units or neurons take an input value and convert it into some form of yield. Every unit takes information, applies a (frequently non-linear) capacity to it, and afterward gives the yield to the following layer. The non-linear function which is applied to the input at each stage is generally tuned during training phase so as to give a proper neural network that can classify the data under consideration.

For better understanding, the pseudo-codes of the algorithm are given as follows:

Pseudocode of the Main Program

```
Start;
Take EEG signals from EEG machine (two EEG channels at a time);
Comparison of EEG signal values of two channels individually;
if (x(t)>x(t+v)) {pie x=1;}else{pie x=0} Resultant order pattern
matrix pie x; Comparison of EEG values of channel y; If(y(t)>y(t+v))
{pie y=1;}else{pie y=0}; Resultant Order Pattern Matrix pie y;
Comparison of pie x matrix with pie y matrix;
if(pie x > pie (y+k) where -25<k<25 ) {R(t,k)=1;}else{R(t,k)=0};
Resultant Recurrence Matrix R (t, k);
Calculating Recurrence Rate;
Calculation of Normalized recurrence rate; Calculating
"Coupling Index";
Using machine learning classifiers on coupling index dataset; Plot
(Graph of Coupling Index);
Switch (Detection Of Disorders)
{0<coupling index<0.15 => Normal; If Not Normal
{
if (0.16<Coupling Index<.40) {Bruxism} else { if (.41<Coupling
Index<.80)
{Alzheimer} else {if (.81<Coupling index<1) Epilepsy; Function
[piex, piey] =order_ pattern (x ,y, N, v)
pie x=zeros(1,N-v); piey= zeros(1,N-v); for i=1:N-v,
if y(i)<y(i+v) piey(i)=0; else
```

Pseudocode of Sub-program for Finding Order Patterns

```
Function [piex, piey] =order _pattern (x ,y, N, v) pie
x=zeros(1, N-v);
pie y= zeros(1, N-v); for i=1:N-v,
if y(i)<y( i + v) pie y(i)=0;
else
picy (i)=1; end
end
for i=1:N-v, if x(i)<x (i+v) pie x(i)=0; else
pie x(i)=1; end
end
pie y (i)=1;
end end
for i=1:N-v, if x(i)<x (i+v) pie x(i)=0; else
pie x(i)=1; end
```

13.10 Various Other Algorithms Used for the Detection of Neurological Disorders

There are several computer-assisted algorithms that are used for detection of seizures and seizure-based neurological disorders. Each algorithm takes the EEG dataset and pre-processes it. Features are then extracted from the dataset. It is at this point that the algorithms differ from each other.

The method of extracting the features from the EEG signals and the types of features are the factors that differentiate an algorithm from another. Depending on the type of feature extracted, the machine learning classifiers are used to find the various parameters like specificity, sensitivity, and accuracy of the algorithm in detecting the disorders.

Few algorithms that detect seizures and are used for diagnosis of epilepsy are given below:

- Q-wavelet-based hybrid method: This is the method of finding the seizure and normal EEG states and hence determines the occurrence of epileptic fits. This method considers EEG signals as non-linear time series. A tuneable Q-wavelet is applied that decomposes the EEG signals in smaller fragments. At that point different factual, riotous, and power range highlight sets are extricated from these portions.
- Then again, an image processing method is utilized to separate the critical surface from the pictures of the recorded EEG signals. At that point, the dark-level co-event network is applied to the picture of EEG signals, and picture-based highlights of differentiation, connection, vitality, and homogeneity are removed. These picture features and the features removed from the sub-groups are combined to make a set of feature. This dataset of features is utilized to differentiate between the seizure and non-seizure-based EEG signals. In view of a large number of separated features, a feature reduction algorithm is expected to lessen the handling time by removing the redundant features.

Generally, the firefly algorithm is used for feature reduction [19]. The block diagram of this algorithm is given below (Fig. 13.4):

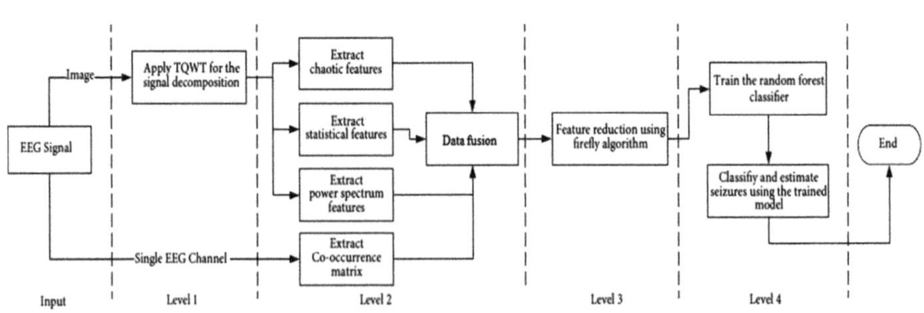

Fig. 13.4 Block diagram of a Q-wavelet-based hybrid method [19]

- Auto-regression-based method [20]: This method also extracts feature from the EEG dataset by utilizing variation mode disintegration (VMD) and auto-regression (AR) strategies.
- The crude EEG is disintegrated into decayed into a fixed number of band-limited intrinsic mode functions (BLIMFs) utilizing variational mode deterioration. At that point a logarithmic activity was forced on each BLIMF.
- When the features are extricated, they are directed to RF (random forest) model for classification purpose. This model is trained repeatedly using BLIMF, and the detection of seizure EEG states is done.
- Fourier-based Alzheimer's classification technique ([21]): This method is a time-frequency-based method which has used Fourier transform and wavelet transform for feature extraction from the EEG signal. The classification procedure is designed with the following steps:
  - Pre-processing of EEG signals.
  - Feature extraction by means of the discrete Fourier and wavelet transforms.
  - Classification with machine learning supervised methods.
- The decision tree classifier has been used, and the output of the algorithm is such that it can differentiate between the normal subjects and the subjects with Alzheimer's disease.
- Chaos theory-based method: This method was proposed by Miri and Nasrabadi [22].

This method involves noise reduction from recorded EEG dataset. Then the data is segmented, and principal component analysis (PCA) is done.

The PCA leads to the un-correlated dataset that consists all of the information that is there in the raw EEG dataset.

Finally the Poincare map is constructed, and seizure states are determined on the basis of this map.

Likewise there are many algorithms that differ on the basis of the features extracted and the classifiers used.

Few algorithms also use hybrid features, like the one proposed by Sharaf et al. [19]. Moreover, the use of machine learning-based classifiers has also improved the efficiency and performance analysis of seizure detecting algorithms.

13.11 Results and Comparisons of the Novel Algorithm with Relevant Works

The novel algorithm discussed in this chapter had yielded the range of "coupling index (ρ_π)" for the three neurological disorders that had been taken under consideration for implementing and testing this algorithm. On the basis of the value of coupling index which will be calculated from the EEG signals of the subject, one can easily find whether the subject is normal or having any of the disorder. This can be

Table 13.1 Calculated ranges of coupling index for disorders by using the proposed algorithm

Disorders	Range of coupling index (ρ_x)
Epilepsy	0.85–1
Bruxism	−15-0.40
Alzheimer's disease	0.55–0.80
Normal	0–0.14

Table 13.2 Comparison of performance on the basis of accuracy and precision in detection of epilepsy

Work	Accuracy	Precision
Sharaf et al. [19]	97%	97%
Proposed work	98.82%	99.07%

Table 13.3 Comparison of performance on the basis of accuracy in detection of seizure and non-seizure states in EEG signals

Work	Accuracy
Zhang et al. [23]	97.352%
Proposed work	98.82%

Table 13.4 Comparison of performance on the basis of accuracy in detection of Alzheimer's

Work	Accuracy
Fiscon et al. [21]	83%
Proposed work	97.64%

done by comparing the calculated value from the standard ranges that are being calculated by using the algorithm. The results are represented in the tabular form as follows (Table 13.1):

Further the results obtained from the novel algorithm have been compared with the two relevant and contemporary works that are already discussed in Sect. 10. The results are given in the tabular form as follows:

1. Comparison with the Q-wavelet-based hybrid method [19]: The comparison of the proposed algorithm based on the random forest classifier is given below in a tabular form (Table 13.2):
2. Comparison with auto-regression-based method [20]: This work has used random forest classifier, and it has only used the accuracy feature for its performance analysis. Table 13.3 is given below:
3. Comparison with Fourier-based Alzheimer's detection technique [21]: The classifier used in the work is decision tree; hence the performance of the proposed work is done using a decision tree classifier (Table 13.4).

Table 13.5 Comparison of performance on the basis of accuracy in detection of bruxism

Work	Accuracy
Heyat et al. 2019	81.25%
Proposed work	98.82%

Table 13.6 Features and advantages of the proposed algorithm

Feature used	Recurrence rate (R.R.)
Parameter used	Coupling index ($\rho\pi$)
Disorders detected	• Epilepsy • Alzheimer's disease • Bruxism
Basis of detection	Recurrences in EEG signals during seizures
Domain	Time domain
Advantages	• Simple and versatile • Single-feature-based hence feature extraction is easier • Detects disorders based on the concept of order patterns that are the matrices of zeroes and ones. Since order patterns do not deals with EEG signal voltages, the error in recording the exact values of EEG signals does not affect the detection

4. Comparison of the proposed work with bruxism detection method using EEG states [23]: Although very less work has been done in the field of algorithm development for detection of bruxism, this latest method for detection of bruxism seems to be the promising technique. Since the performance analysis has been done by the author using the decision tree classifier, the performance comparison is done in terms of the performance of decision tree only (Table 13.5).

The above comparison shows that the proposed method has been accurate and better in detection of neurological disorders. Moreover the overall features of the algorithm and its advantages have also been summarized in Table 13.6 given below:

13.12 Future Scope

This work can be further extended in the following manners:

1. Though this algorithm and its implementation have yielded good results in detecting epilepsy, Alzheimer's disease, and bruxism, still work is needed to be done in discriminating further between various types of epilepsy or different types of Alzheimer disease.
2. The phenomenon of recurrence can also be used in detecting coupling between EEG and ECG (electrocardiogram) signals or EEG and EMG (electromyogram) signals. This can help in detecting various heart ailments or muscular movement-

related disorders like muscular dystrophy. The algorithm discussed here may serve the purpose with slight changes in its coding.

3. This novel algorithm also paves the way for development of new methods for analysis of EEG signals.

References

1. UCI Machine Learning Repository: EEG Database Data Set. (2019). https://archive.ics.uci.edu/ml/datasets/eeg+database
2. CHB-MIT Scalp EEG Database v1.0.0. (2019). https://physionet.org/content/chbmit/1.0.0
3. what are neurological disorders? (2019). https://www.who.int/features/qa/55/en/
4. Khan, R. S., Ahmed, M. R., Khalid, B., Mahmood, A., & Hassan, R. (2018a). Biomarker detection of neurological disorders through spectroscopy analysis. *International Dental & Medical Journal of Advanced Research, 4*(1), 1–9.
5. Khan, A., Husain, M. S., & Khan, A. (2018b). Analysis of mental state of users using social media to predict depression! A survey. *International Journal of Advanced Research in Computer Science, 9*(2), 100–106.
6. Gourie-Devi, M. (2018). Relevance of neuroepidemiology: Burden of neurological disorders and public health issues. *Annals of Indian Academy of Neurology, 21*(4), 237–238.
7. Nadig, R., Namapally, U. S., Sarma, G. R. K., & Mathew, T. (2019). Outpatient burden of neurological disorders: A prospective evaluation of 1500 patients. *Neurology India, 67*(3), 708.
8. Kidwai, M. S., & Saeed, S. H. (2019). A novel approach for detection of neurological disorders through electrical potential developed in brain. *International Journal of Electrical & Computer Engineering, 9*, 2088–8708.
9. Shorman, O. M., & Alshorman, A. M. (2020). Frontal lobe and long-term memory retrieval analysis during pre-learning stress using EEG signals. *Bulletin of Electrical Engineering and Informatics, 9*(1), 141–145.
10. Wen, T. Y., Bani, N. A., Muhammad-Sukki, F., & Aris, S. A. M. (2020). Electroencephalogram (EEG) human stress level classification based on Theta/Beta ratio. *International Journal of Integrated Engineering, 12*(6), 174–180.
11. Raveendra Kumar, T. H., & Narayanappa, C. K. Improved feature extraction process to detect seizure using CHBMIT-dataset. *International Journal of Electrical & Computer Engineering, 11*(1), 2088–8708.
12. Kidwai, M. S., & Saeed, S. H. (2017). A novel approach to study the effects of anesthesia on respiratory signals by using the EEG signals. *International Journal of Electrical & Computer Engineering, 7*(6), 2088–8708.
13. Pikovsky, A., Kurths, J., Rosenblum, M., & Kurths, J. (2003). *Synchronization: A universal concept in nonlinear sciences* (Vol. 12). Cambridge university press.
14. Kantz, H., Kurths, J., & Mayer-Kress, G. (Eds.). (2012). *Nonlinear analysis of physiological data*. Springer Science & Business Media.
15. Heunis, T., Aldrich, C., Peters, J. M., Jeste, S. S., Sahin, M., Scheffer, C., & de Vries, P. J. (2018). Recurrence quantification analysis of resting state EEG signals in autism spectrum disorder–a systematic methodological exploration of technical and demographic confounders in the search for biomarkers. *BMC Medicine, 16*(1), 101.
16. Mihajlović, V. (2019, September). EEG spectra vs recurrence features in understanding cognitive effort. In *Proceedings of the 23rd international symposium on wearable computers* (pp. 160–165). ACM.
17. Filligoi, G., Felici, F., Vicini, M., & Rosponi, A. (2010). Recurrence quantification analysis of surface electro-myograms.

18. Boonyakitanont, P., Lek-uthai, A., Chomtho, K., & Songsiri, J. (2019). A review of feature extraction and performance evaluation in epileptic seizure detection using EEG. *arXiv preprint arXiv:1908.00492.*
19. Sharaf, A. I., El-Soud, M. A., & El-Henawy, I. M. (2018a). An automated approach for epilepsy detection based on tunable Q-wavelet and firefly feature selection algorithm. *International Journal of Biomedical Imaging, 2018.*
20. Zhang, T., Chen, W., & Li, M. (2017). AR based quadratic feature extraction in the VMD domain for the automated seizure detection of EEG using random forest classifier. *Biomedical Signal Processing and Control, 31*, 550–559.
21. Fiscon, G., Weitschek, E., Cialini, A., Felici, G., Bertolazzi, P., Salvo, D., & S.,& De Cola, M.C. (2018). Combining EEG signal processing with supervised methods for Alzheimer's patients classification. *BMC Medical Informatics and Decision Making, 18*(1), 35.
22. Miri, M. R., & Nasrabadi, A. M. A new seizure prediction method based on return map. In *Proceedings of the Iranian conference on bio-medical engineering (Tehran)* (pp. 244–248).
23. Zhang, Y., Heyat, M. B. B., Lai, D., & Khan. (2019). Sleep bruxism detection using decision tree method by the combination of C4-P4 and C4-A1 channels of scalp EEG. *IEEE Access, 7*, 102542–102553.

Chapter 14
A Prediction of Disease Using Machine Learning Approach

Surabhi Saxena, Nupur Soni, Akhilesh Kumar, and Anshul Mishra

14.1 Introduction

Driven by an expansion in computational force, stockpiling, memory, and the age of stunning volumes of information, PCs are being utilized to play out a wide scope of complex errands with noteworthy exactness. Machine learning (ML) is the name given to both scholastic control and assortment of strategies which permit PCs to attempt complex errands [1, 2]. As a scholarly order, ML involves components of arithmetic, insights, and software engineering. Machine learning is the engine that is propelling advances in the improvement of computerized reasoning. It is amazingly utilized in both scholarly community and industry to drive the improvement of "astute items" with the capacity to make exact forecasts utilizing various wellsprings of information [3]. Until now, the key recipients of the twenty-first century blast in the accessibility of large amounts of information, ML, and information science have been ventures with the ability to gather this information and recruit the important staff to change their items. The learning techniques created in and for these enterprises offer colossal potential to upgrade medical examination and

S. Saxena (✉)
Department of BCA, Koneru Lakshmaiah Education Foundation,
Guntur, Andhra Pradesh, India

N. Soni
School of Computer Applications, Babu Banarasi Das University,
Lucknow, Uttar Pradesh, India

A. Kumar
MCA Department, I.E.T, Dr. R. M. L. Avadh University, Ayodhya, India

A. Mishra
Department of IT, Baba Saheb Bhim Rao Ambedkar University,
Lucknow, Uttar Pradesh, India

M. S. Husain et al. (eds.), *Pervasive Healthcare*, EAI/Springer Innovations in Communication and Computing, https://doi.org/10.1007/978-3-030-77746-3_14

clinical care, particularly as suppliers' well-being records improve [4]. The assessment for diabetic patients, combined with the need to arrange because of the patients' keenness, causes patients to sit for long periods of time. The result of the patients' medical therapy is time-sensitive; in this way, the sooner the therapy is delivered, the better the result.

The primary point where the patient's condition is assessed happens at the beginning phase in the department. Prediction frameworks are utilized by health experts to appoint need levels to patients based on their criticality of treatment and the unpredictability of diabetic ascribes. There might be critical patients exhibiting manifestations not effortlessly perceived as indicators of criticality [5, 6].

If not distinguished in exact time, these patients need to move perception, which increases the risk of bleakness. Consequently, the requirement for a proficient forecast framework to help the health professionals in making a convenient and right choice is of critical importance.

14.2 Background

In spite of numerous long periods of examination into machine-based learning models, the order of imbalanced information is still the cause of concern [7]. For instance, the data from the UK population brings forth the fact that 4.6% of the total population has diabetes, while the rest are free of it. An expectation model that predicts the majority class accurately and the minority inaccurately will give absurd results, which may have serious consequences. Ordering anomalies comes out as the main point of contention in machine learning [8]. This issue happens in light of the fact that information tests once in a while follow a reasonable example. Specifically, some information tests may share divergent attributes with others having a place with a similar class and in this way have been removed from the majority of information of that classification.

14.3 Diabetes

Diabetes mellitus is a chronic illness caused by an increase in glucose concentration in the blood. This happens due to the pancreas and its various components failing to function properly. It may have ill effects on the heart, kidneys, eyes, etc. [9] It may occur to people of all age groups. The endocrine assistants for absorption and an exocrine secretion in the pancreas keep up the sugar level in the course framework. The pancreas is identified with various inadequacies and impacts from various organs of the body. When the glucose, or sugar level, is high in the circulatory structure, beta cells of the pancreas deliver insulin to the course system to ingest the exorbitant sugar substance from the blood into the liver, where it is later converted into a packaging criticality. Similarly, when the glucose level is low, the production of insulin is included, and the making of glucagon by the alpha cells of the pancreas will be started to maintain the glucose level in the blood. The presence of sugar in the body likewise anticipates a fundamental role in diabetes. A diabetic individual should manage his or her vision through a couple of tests and medications at the start of the disease [10].

14.4 Methodology

In diabetic infection, there were distinctive explorations finished [11]. Beforehand, numerous analysts did various explorations in medical service environments. From those analysts' funds, some of them also spent on diabetes treatment because it was a problem in the old matured examination that was done exclusively on the well-being habitats and not in the mechanized like machine learning approach [12]. The information that we utilized must be astutely formed, joined/coordinated, and prepared for examination. The dataset utilized in this investigation was obtained from the public UCI archive, which is accessible on the web. We will utilize this online accessible dataset for the examination and forecast of diabetes-related illnesses. In this investigation, this diabetes dataset comprises 768 records and 8 credits with 1 objective class (age) and is used for examination, characterization, and forecasting. And furthermore, an ensemble tree structure model with a base student for expectation is incorporated.

14.4.1 Model Development

The proposed work predicts diabetes by investigating the abovementioned instances and does execution examination as shown in Fig. 14.2. The goal of this examination is to accurately predict whether or not the patient will become infected. The data of the patient's health is taken as input for the framework that predicts diabetes. Figure 14.1 depicts the entire process.

- *Data Abstract*: It refers to taking out meaningful data and processing it for use as input to various machine learning models that are used for disease prediction.
- *Algorithm Evolvement*: Machine learning does not provide one solution or one approach for all the problems. There are several factors to be considered for choosing the right algorithm for the problem. Some problems are specific and require a unique approach, whereas others are open and need a trial-and-error approach. Getting accurate solution is not always necessary. There are problems that need only an approximate solution. It is based on the problem.*Prediction and Observation*: Prediction can possibly gain from past perceptions with the end goal that the final model can be brought in practice for determining various diseases and disorders.

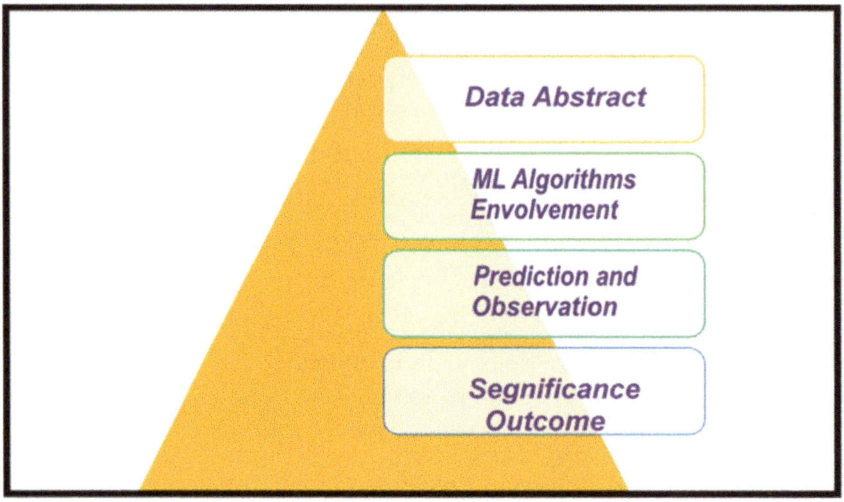

Fig. 14.1 Prediction approach

- *Significance Outcomes*: These steps have initiated to the various complete outcomes, which depend on the instances of diseases.

14.4.2 Model Implication

When the outcomes of prediction approach are given in this way, it is smarter to combine the consequences of those individual classifiers into one by consolidating the forecast of individual classifiers. An organization moves toward the issue or impediment of unmistakable calculations in order to build precision by consolidating into one. Figure 14.2 gives the better execution and precision than the single one, which is why this investigation was chosen for this examination. Data abstractions are techniques to retrieve data from open sources for prediction and analysis, which aid in the prediction approach. In step 2, we illustrate the various algorithms and apply them to a tree structure for disease conditions. The tree structure model will be illustrated (Fig. 14.2) at four levels. The tree has given various fragments at the level of diabetic patient. The goal of the tree is to create a prediction model that predicts the value of a specific value variable by learning simple decision rules inferred from data features (Table 14.1).

Figure 14.3 three depicts the relationship by applying the proposed technique to different datasets related to diabetes. The relationship with age to different variables is essential on the grounds that the connection size of the diabetes information take into account a far-reaching approval measure. The standard situation is tested on a comparable yet outside dataset. As anticipated, the rank outcomes (Fig. 14.4) follow a comparative example to the one obtained with diabetes occurrences. Aside from

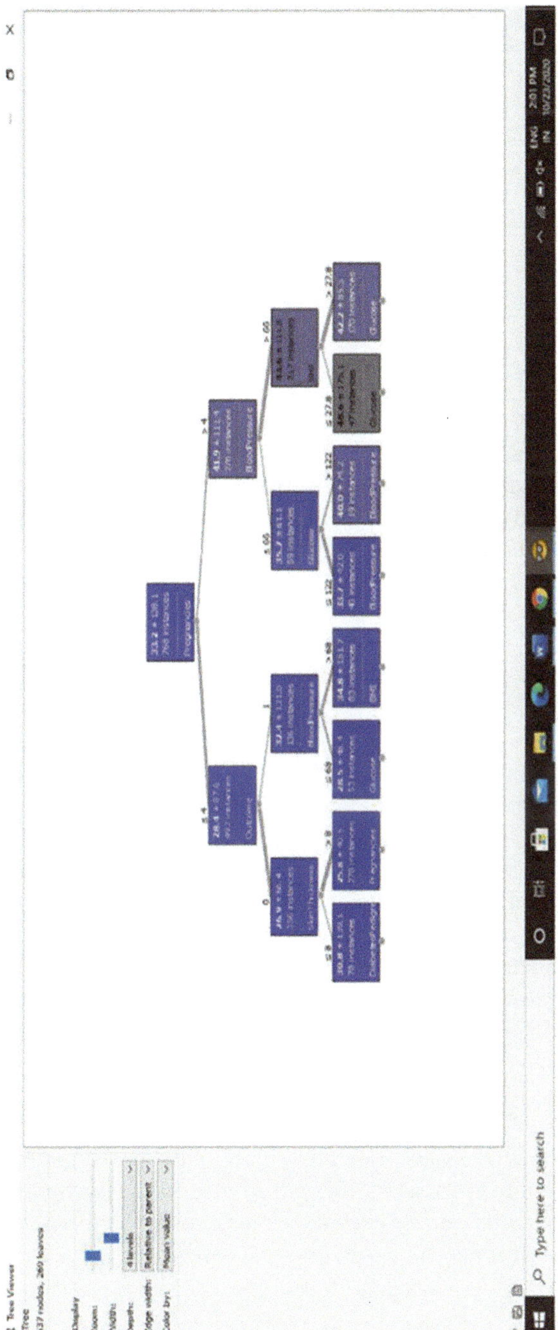

Fig. 14.2 Tree structure model

Table 14.1 Experimental data features [13]

Feature	details
1	Pregnancy instances
2	Plasma glucose fixation in a 2- h oral glucose resilience test
3	Diastolic circulatory strain (mmHg)
4	Rear arm muscle skin overlaps thickness (mm)
5	2-h serum insulin (μIU/ml)
6	Weight file (weight in kg/stature in m2)
7	Diabetes family work
8	Age
9	Class (0, 1)

exploring different avenues regarding the tree structure that created blended outcomes over the rank measurements, all the tests including information delivered the best position results within their respective gatherings. In spite of the fact that our strategy didn't generally prompt noteworthy contrast, it surely delivers some type of progress altogether. Such execution gives a foundation for additional improvement based on rank.

14.5 Conclusion

The factual models can't deal with unmitigated information with missing qualities and enormous information focuses. They don't give precise outcomes to huge dataset. That is the reason for introducing the machine learning algorithms. ML is used in many applications, from image detection to disease diagnosis. The prime objective of the ML researchers is to provide efficient learning model for better performance. The efficiency mainly focuses on the high accuracy of prediction for critical problems. It is completely data-driven and has the capability of examining the large amount of data. These algorithms are more accurate and are not prone to errors. ML algorithms are provided with priority for the development of devices that are mainly used in self-monitoring, self-diagnosis, and self-repairing. In the papers where diabetics were approved in the cases, the creators found that there was an improvement in the health experts' dynamic, prompting better ailments the executives and patients' results. Nonetheless, we found that more of the investigations fell short on this usage stage. We inferred that for these examinations, it is important to approve the effect and to characterize key execution measures so as to show the degree to which consolidation of traits can really improve care.

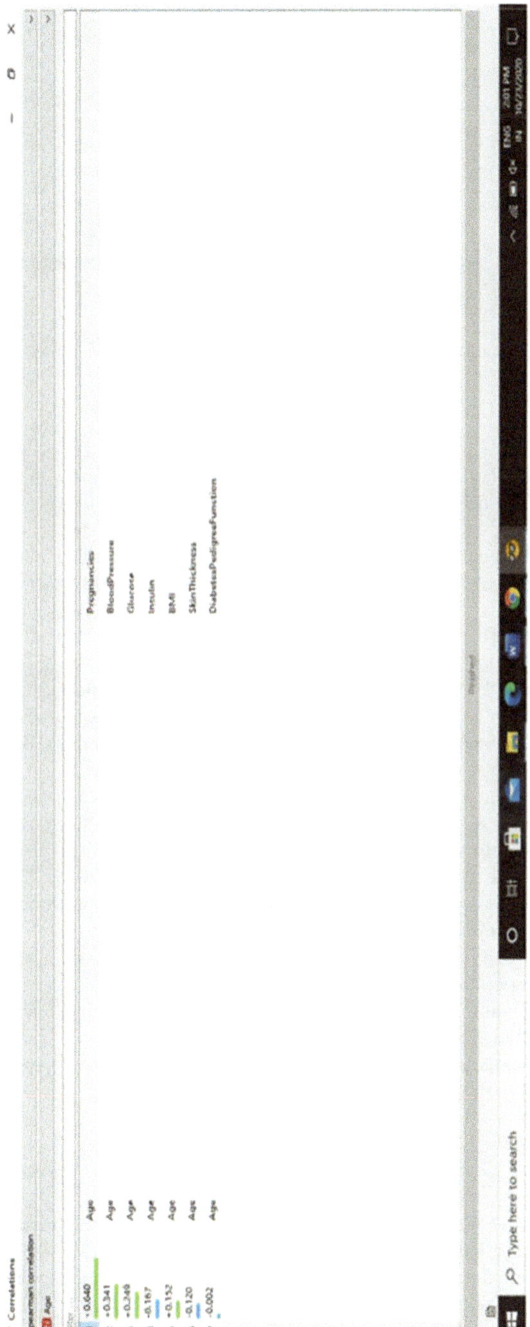

Fig. 14.3 Correlation with target class

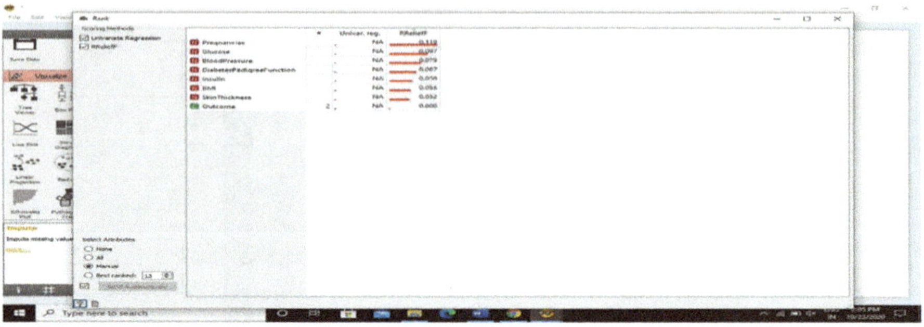

Fig. 14.4 Instance rank

References

1. Husain, M. S. (2020). Nature inspired approach for intrusion detection systems. In *Design and analysis of security protocol for communication* (pp. 171–182).
2. Adnan, M. H., Hassan, M. F., Aziz, I. A., Nurika, O., & Husain, M. S. (2020, September). Modified ISR hyper-heuristic for tuning automatic genetic clustering chromosome size. In *IOP Conference Series: Materials Science and Engineering* (Vol. 932, No. 1, p. 012065). IOP Publishing.
3. Husain, M. S. (2020). Nature inspired approach for intrusion detection systems. In *Design and analysis of security protocol for communication* (pp. 171–182).
4. Kavakiotis, G., Tzanis, I., & Vlahavas. (2014). Mining frequent patterns and association rules from biological data. In M. Elloumi & A. Y. Zomaya (Eds.), *Biological knowledge discovery handbook: Preprocessing, mining and postprocessing of biological data, Wiley book series on bioinformatics: Computational techniques and engineering*. Wiley.
5. Sharma and Singh, Sharma, N., Singh, A. (2018). Diabetes detection and prediction using machine learning/IoT: A SURVEY. In *Springer International Conference on Advanced Informatics for Computing Research* (pp. 471–479).
6. Natarajan, S., Jain, A., Krishnan, R., Rogye, A., & Sivaprasad, S. (2019). Diagnostic accuracy of community-based diabetic retinopathy screening with an offline artificial intelligence system on a smart phone. *JAMA Ophthalmology, 137*(10), 1182–1188.
7. Yi, X., Walia, E., & Babyn, P. (2019). Generative adversarial network in medical imaging: A review. *Medical Image Analysis, 58*. Art. no. 101552,
8. Zhou, L., Pan, S., Wang, J., & Vasilakos, A. V. (2017). Machine learning on big data: Opportunities and challenges. *Neurocomputing, 237*, 350–361. May.
9. Husain, M. S., & Khanum, M. A. (2017). Cloud computing in E-governance: Indian perspective. In *Securing government information and data in developing countries* (pp. 104–114). IGI Global.
10. Goodfellow, J., Pouget-Abadie, M., Mirza, B., Xu, D., Warde-Farley, S., Ozair, A., Courville, & Bengio, Y. (2014). Generative adversarial nets. In *Proc. Adv. Neural Inf. Process. Syst* (pp. 2672–2680).
11. Banerjee, Y., Ling, M., Chen, C., Hasan, S. A., Langlotz, C. P., Moradzadeh, N., Chapman, B., Amrhein, T., Mong, D., Rubin, D. L., Farri, O., & Lungren, M. P. (2019). Comparative effectiveness of convolutional neural network (CNN) and recurrent neural network (RNN) architectures for radiology text report classification. *Artificial Intelligence in Medicine, 97*, 79–88.

12. Wolterink, J. M., Leiner, T., Viergever, M. A., & Isgum, I. (2017). Generative adversarial networks for noise reduction in low-dose CT. *IEEE Transactions on Medical Imaging, 36*(12), 2536–2545.
13. Chen, M., Hao, Y., Hwang, K., Wang, L., & Wang, L. (2017). Disease prediction by machine learning over big data from healthcare communities. *IEEE Access, 5*(c), 8869–8879.

Chapter 15
Security in Digital Healthcare System

Manish Madhava Tripathi, Mohammad Haroon, Zunnun Khan, and Mohammad Shahid Husain

15.1 Introduction

In the field of healthcare system, where conventional medical investigation is being taken over by digital medical investigations, this prototype has created a number of utilization in health corporations like distance diagnosis, distance instruction, and distance surgery. But all of these applications require Internet, as information is sent from one place to another. The problem in this case is that information can be obtained from the Internet and can be modified as per interest by using different software like Photoshop editing. Since medical images can be used in legal process and money is involved through insurance of the patients, insurance companies, doctors, and patient himself can modify these medical images in their personal interest.

Our goal in this thesis is to flourish a craft that can reveal and protect these medical images and, if possible, can rescue tempered images also. Watermarking security is one of the best methods to achieve this task. It can be classified into three parts: robust, fragile, and semi-fragile. Fragile is used for authentication purposes, and upon attack, the watermark destroys. Robust is used for securing against attacks and copyright protection.

M. M. Tripathi (✉) · M. Haroon · Z. Khan
Integral University, Lucknow, India
e-mail: Mmt@iul.ac.in; Mharoon@iul.ac.in; Zunnun@iul.ac.in

M. S. Husain
Ibri College of Applied Sciences, University of Technology and Applied Sciences, Muscat, Oman
e-mail: Mshahid.ibr@cas.edu.om

M. S. Husain et al. (eds.), *Pervasive Healthcare*, EAI/Springer Innovations in Communication and Computing, https://doi.org/10.1007/978-3-030-77746-3_15

15.1.1 Security Attributes

Security [1] of medical data is very important as these days may be misused for illegal benefits. Many medical images involve insurance money; therefore, patient, insurance companies, or doctors can misuse these medical data. Despite the fact that the Data Protection Act 1998 is very useful in preventing misuse of data, due to the advancement of technology, some new techniques are necessary to protect data. Protection of data must satisfy the following conditions:

15.1.2 Confidentiality

Under this property, the doctor cannot share the patient record and data without the consent of the patient. If under any condition he has to use or share the data, he should properly justify the reasons under which he will use the data, and this data must be shared with the authorized person only.

15.1.3 Reliability

Under this property, two things have to be checked. One is authenticity of data and the other is integrity of data. Authenticity is required before the use of data, whether that particular dealer belongs to the right patient or not. The second part, which is integrity, concerns with the security of data, whether data has been stolen, modified, or fully or partially destroyed.

15.1.4 Availability

Data availability is also a prime issue for the security of medical images. Availability of data must be insured when needed. The ethical, financial, and legal issues can arise in case of data loss.

Although no damage has been reported till yet in the attack on medical health record, a lot of attacks have been identified with it, and the number of attacks on health data is increasing day by day. The study shows that 42% of sites have been accessed by unauthorized users, in which 20% do not know about this. One famous case of attack was identified in 1982, when the intruder group "414" had attacked on the patient health data record of the National Cancer Institute. But no harm was detected in this attack.

15.1.5 *Privacy and Security Issues in Healthcare*

As per survey, "70–75% of patients are concerned about healthcare sites sharing information without their permission". "Possibly this is because medical data disclosure is the second highest reported break". Some of the researchers also describe security and privacy issues in the form of medical information system:

15.2 Threats to Privacy of Information

Threat can be divided into two areas as follows:

1. Organizational threats
2. Systematic threats

Organizational threat arises when some external person gets access of the patient data. This external person may be a hacker who does not have the right to access any data from the organization. Due to relation with any of the organization member, he can do this.

15.2.1 *Web-Enabled Healthcare Information Security*

Microsoft and Google have opened the web-based healthcare system and banking access. This also has created security risk to the healthcare system and patients' personal and sensitive health information.

Mobile devices have also created a new domain of risks to patient data. Nowadays, mobile phones come with very high features. Locating the position of the person using a mobile phone can harm patient data. Smartphones also include a high-resolution camera. The intruder can at least take snapshots of the patient record, which he or she can then misuse in the future.

15.2.2 *Information Security for Authorized Data Access (Disclosure)*

In the medical field, it is necessary to share patient data from within hospitals to outside industries that are specifically involved in health-related cases. When patient data is released, it can be leaked, so a very secret procedure should be adopted when releasing the medical data of the patient. This data leakage may affect the socioeconomic condition of the patient. Technological advancements have led to consolidate all medical data into a single place. Collecting data in a single place can help researchers to use this data for research purposes and improve the algorithm.

15.2.3 Information Security and Data Interoperability

Around the world, multiple organizations store medical records in different standard formats. Using such large data formats makes it difficult to share health-related patient data across various organizations as well as in health research.

In the USA at present, 33 states have developed a plan to exchange the medical information and patient data with high security. They first try to identify the person who wants to access the medical data, and based on that, they provide them access or limited access to the data.

15.2.4 Attacks and Types

In case of medical data attacks, the following can be authorized [2]:

Mistake

This attack is characterized by mistaken or unknowing access to a record. This type of attack is the most common in the medical field.

Improper Use of Access Privileges

This happens when an authorized person violates the law of medical ethics by giving access to a friend or relative.

Unauthorized Use for Profit

This category belongs to the case when a person has limited authorization to medical records but uses his effect to access the data illegally for which he is not authorized.

Unauthorized Physical Intrusion

This is the case when an unauthorized person tries to access data.

Table 15.1 Type of attacks and its effects

Type	System authorize	Data authorize	Site access	Threat	Countermeasure
1	Yes	Yes	Yes	Mistake	Organizational and simple technical mechanism
2	Yes	Yes	N/A	Improper use of access privileges	Organizational and technical mechanisms such as authentication and auditing
3	Yes	No	N/A	Unauthorized use for spite or profit	Organizational and technical mechanisms such as authentication and auditing
4	No	No	Yes	Unauthorized physical intrusion	Physical security and technical mechanisms such as authentication and access controls
5	No	No	No	Technical break-in	Technical mechanisms such as authentication, access controls, and cryptography

Technical Break-in

This attack is the most dangerous attack. This type of attack is done by a technical person or a person who was part of the system and sacked from the job Table 15.1. The below table (Table 15.1) provides a summary of different types of attack on medical data, the threat they can have and how we can deal with them.

15.2.5 Some Existing Solutions

Some existing solutions discussed by various researchers can be described as follows:

15.2.6 Role-Based Access Security and Access Control

In an organization, workers and employees perform a variety of tasks and have different capacities. Not everybody can be given the authority, privilege, or access to the medical information of a patient. This authority must be established depending on the nature of the job of the person in the organization. The persons involving in maintenance of the medical data should be authorized by the head of the institution.

15.2.7 Authentication Mechanism

Authentication means the information sent by the sender and the information received by the receiver must be exactly the same. Suppose the sender sends the information I and the receiver receives the information I'. Then, for authentication of the information I,

$$I = I'.$$

Otherwise, the message is not authenticated and should be deleted and resent. There are a number of algorithms that can be used for authentication, some of which can be pointed out as:

- Digital signature
- Password mechanisms
- Challenge-response authentication protocol

15.2.8 Encryption

It is the process of converting plain text to cipher text so that it can be only readable by the sender and the receiver of the message. Encryption can be used to secure data and also to prevent skimming and eavesdropping. To maintain a high level of security, encryption must be done at both the hardware and software levels. Watermarking of medical data can also be done for encryption at software level.

For the encryption of medical images, several encryption algorithms were used initially, but these methods were not secure on both ends. So, signature methods were adopted before encryption. Nowadays, medical image watermarking method for securing medical data has given very promising results. It is not only used for image authentication and security but also contains other information in the form of packets within the image itself. As a result, separate transmission and storage of these information is not required.

15.2.9 Digital Watermarking [3]

In the current time, the number of Internet users is increasing exponentially every day. Every 10 years, the number of Internet users increases tenfold. Naturally, the world is moving toward the digital path. Every information is now preferable to be sent via the Internet, which simplifies our lives in a big way. But every merit has a demerit, which is why cybercrime also has increased as Internet users. As a result, data security is required. A lot of methods have been proposed by different groups of researchers in the past few years, including cryptography as well as watermarking approaches. Watermarking approach is now very popular due to its efficiency and capability to absorb extra information visible or invisible as per the need. Digital watermarking is becoming very famous due to its efficiency and reversibility nature. In reversibility, original images can be obtained back when needed. Watermarking consist of two phases: embedding phase and extraction phase. In embedding phase, watermarked information will be embedded inside the image, whereas in extraction phase, the original image can be obtained back or extracted. Several techniques by which we can apply reversible watermarking include the DCT [4] and the DWT methods. Sometimes multiple types of information are to be embedded inside the image. This case is known as multiple watermarking.

15.3 Literature Review

In networking, security is the primary concern. Data should have been confidently protected while being transmitted over the network. Data may be medical data, cloud data, or any other kinds of data.

Some of the methods classified as application-based are discussed below:

15.3.1 Authentication Code Using Cryptographic Hash Function [5]

These methods were used for security purposes for medical images. These methods were useful for those cases which are not very severe. The image is used as data in the array format message. This message will be encrypted by using hash key. Before encryption, a message authentication code will be calculated by applying mathematical function. After calculation, this code will be appended to the actual message. And then, the message will be encrypted by using some public key. At the recipient end, the message will be broken into two parts: one part will contain the message, and the other part will contain the message authentication code. A new message authentication code will be recalculated, and the two codes will now be compared. If both values match, we will say that the message is authenticated; otherwise, the message has been tampered with.

15.3.2 Digital Signature Method for Authentication [6]

With the previous method, the problem is that the message is not secure at both ends, the sender and the receiver. Both ends will be secure by using signatures or some biometric information, like a thumb impression or iris information. The rest of the procedure is the same as in the previous method (Fig. 15.1).

15.3.3 Authentication Using Content [1, 2]

This is the example of multiple watermarking. Based on the content type, the watermark will be decided. For example, if the watermark is a text, a technique such as lab embedding will be applied. But if an image or sound watermark is to be inserted, then first it has to be converted into binary embeddable formats before being embedded into the image.

15.3.4 Embedding Using Mean [3, 7]

This method is useful when using the DCT method. In the DCT method, the image is divided into blocks; then, the mean value of intensity is calculated in each block. Based on the intensity of this mean value, a threshold value will be set up, and further watermark embedding will be done on the basis of comparison with this threshold value.

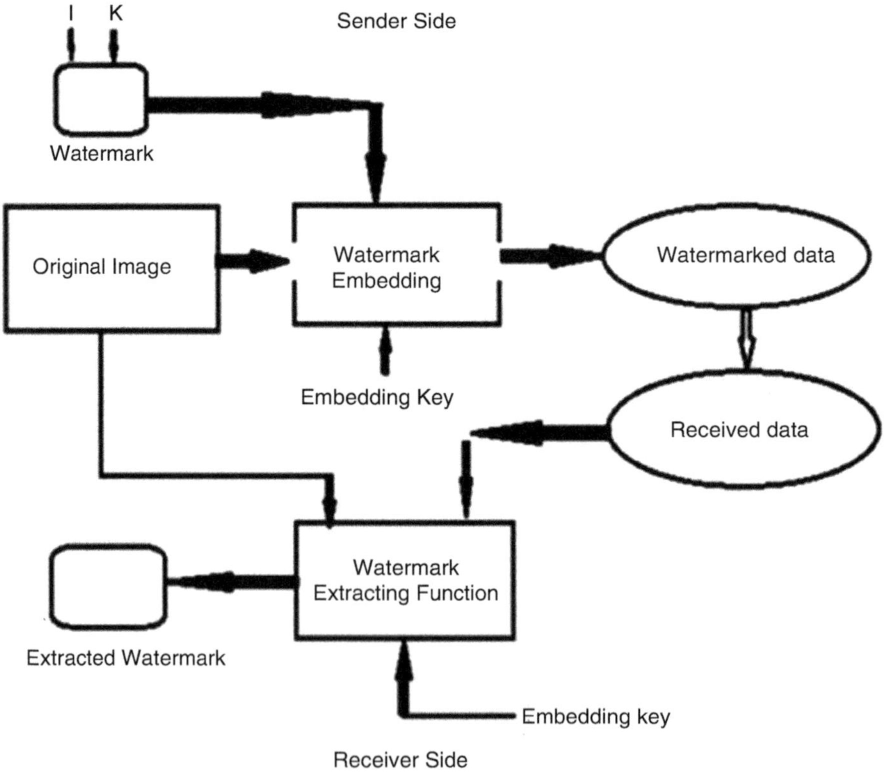

Fig. 15.1 Authentication using hash function

15.3.5 ANN-Based Approach [8, 9]

In the neural network field, we observe the working of neurons. The artificial neural network takes the idea from the human nervous system and models a computational system based on this idea. The neural network has several components like variables, vectors, activation state, hidden state, learning, neurons, etc. The neural network is very useful when large amounts of computation are involved.

In 2011, Priego et al. [15] had developed the algorithm for underwater boat security mechanism based on the neural network computational method.

Kishore et al. [16] has applied ANN computation for watermarking of medical images of MRI, CT, and X-ray types.

15.3.6 Genetic Algorithm-Based Approach [10–12]

Genetic algorithms have given very good results in the field of image processing, particularly in image classification, image segmentation, image registration, watermarking, etc. In this area, genetic algorithms are widely used and give highly optimized results.

Khanna et al., [17] have done research in the area of healthcare system by using genetic algorithm. This method also gives very good results.

15.3.7 Cosine Transform-Based Approach [3, 7, 10]

Discrete cosine transform is also used by several researchers. This method is very fast and gives non-negative values as the cosine function gives positive values in all cases. Cosine transform works in the blocks of size 8×8.

Li et al. have presented the watermarking by using a DCT approach on Haar basis.

Saad et al. have also introduced the DCT method on medical images for quality assessment of medical images.

15.3.8 Chaos-Based Approach [13]

Chaos-based encryption algorithms were also used by several researchers. These methods are smart and give very promising and good results.

Wang and Wang have applied the chaos-based approach. They used the concept of S-boxes as in the case of DES algorithm. This method has proven its capability against plaintext attack and brute force attack. As the S-box concept is very difficult to break, this method is not possible for intruders to break in any case.

Bhandari et al. [13] have developed the chaos-based method by using 256 bit of keys. The method was good despite its complexity.

15.3.9 SVD-Based Approach [11]

This approach is good for both robust and fragile watermarking methods. SVD is a very good and attractive approach as it depends on the orthonormalization of matrices. The matrix will be decomposed, analyzed, and then compiled to each other in this approach.

Hai-mei et al. [11] have disused an approach based on SVD. This method was very helpful in removing Gaussian noises. Similarly for satellite images, cuckoo optimization algorithm was used by Hai-mei et al. [11] on the basis of SVD-DWT. Four bands of DWT were used for the decomposition of images into four parts. After applying this, low-band images are obtained. Lastly, inverse DWT will be applied to get the original image back in this way.

15.3.10 Steganography-Based Approach

In stenographic approach, only the sender and the receiver know about the hidden information. Even the carrier will not be able to know whether any information is hidden in it or not.

Image staganalysis was used by Fredrik for rich images.

Texture mechanism was used by Baaziz et al. [8]. The complement of the image was extracted along with the rotational variable. By using these variables in the right way, the original image can be obtained.

15.3.11 Visual Cryptography-Based Approach [6]

For multimedia messages, this method is the most secure method.

Takore et al. [6] has applied the visual cryptographic algorithm without expansion of pixels. They have given the concept of random pixel interchange. Barni et al. [1] have also used a similar approach, but they do not use the expansion of pixels for halftone images.

15.4 Some Important Algorithms

Some methods are given as follows:

Yusuk Lim (2002): Fraser et al. [3] have developed the algorithm using fragile watermarking for image authentication. The number of Internet users was increasing day by day that time. They have used the idea of extra information insertion inside the image.

Wakatani (2002): In the previous algorithm given by Yusuk Lim, the problem was that the intruder can crop the watermark information from the image as watermarking was done only on the initial part of the image. Takore et al. [6] has given his idea that some signature should be added while watermarking so that during watermark embedding and watermark extraction process, the image can be secured. Further, if the intruder crops the image, he has to apply the signature of the sender, which an intruder cannot use. In this way, the method will become very secure. Wakatani has applied the Haar basis using the DCT method for embedding the information inside the image.

Z M Jain Algorithm (2004): Tripathi [14] has applied her algorithm on the ultrasound images. She has taken the ultrasound image and divided it into ROI and RONI parts. Then, watermark embedding is done by using the MOD function so that the watermark can be equally disputed all over his medical image. Thus, the medical image will be protected from intruders cropping the medical image. Again, before the insertion of the watermark, hash values are calculated, and by using the message digest algorithm, these hash values and watermarked information have been inserted in the image.

A. Giakoumaki Algorithm (2005) [14]: They divide the medical image into two parts, region of interest and region of non-interest, and then have applied fragile watermarking technique to authenticate the medical image by inserting text messages into the portion of non-interest.

Birgit et al. (2005): Tripathi [14] has separated the image into several regions and has identified the characteristics of each region, for example, intensity or visual quality. Based on these features, the decision to insert a watermark is taken. For example, the region with less visibility may have an inverted watermark by applying more robust methods than the region with better visibility. The region with very good visibility will not be watermarked as it contains more detailed information about the body part. In this way, this method contains both fragile and robust methods for inserting extra information in the form of watermarking.

Wang.and Rao Algorithm (2005) [14]: This fragile method algorithm was useful as this method was developed for real-time diagnosis. During diagnosis, the medical information can be leaked at embedding end. So while watermarking the information, the same chaotic sequence of the watermark information will automatically be generated and watermarked after the use of the particular image. In this way, this fragile method will be able to behave similarly to a robust one.

Sunita V. Dhavale (2013) [14]: The DCT method and hospital logo have been used as a watermark for fragile watermarking authentication purposes.

Malay.Kumar Kundu (2010) [14]: They worked for fragile watermarking in spatial domain. They used the gray-scale property for this. To measure the output of MSE, PSNR values were calculated.

Taha Jassim (2013) [14]: First-time efforts for watermarking for mobile phones were developed. In this algorithm, limited bandwidth and limited storage were considered for watermarking.

Jingbing.Li (2011): Tripathi [14] has worked a lot in the area of three-dimensional watermarking. He has applied 3D DFT and DWT for three dimensions. He took three-dimensional volume data, divided them into slices, and then applied DWT and DFT. Finally, all slices are collected together to reconstruct the medical image.

In another algorithm by Jingbing Li in 2013, he has applied the chaotic Hermite function along with DFT and DWT for three-dimensional volume data.

Mohammad Arabzadeh et al. (2011) [14]: They developed the fragile watermarking algorithm for detecting distortion regions in the image while extracting watermarks. They used the hamming distance algorithm for this purpose.

M. Kamran.Scheme (2012) [14]: Mohammad Kamran has done a lot of work in the field of medical image watermarking. In his paper published in 2012, he has used the robust method of watermarking by dividing the image into region of interest and region of non-interest.

Lingling.An (2012): Tripathi [14] has used pixel masking method by using the histogram shifting method for embedding watermarking information. Watermark information was embedded only in the portion where the histogram curve has low values, and no information were added between the maximum peaks of the histogram as it was supposed that dense information is given in that portion. This method was robust against compression attack.

Duc.M. Duong (2013): Tripathi [14] has tried counterfeit transform for robust watermarking. He has shown the results in which method was robust against geometrical and other kinds of simple attacks.

Recently, Tripathi has started working by using histogram shifting methods [14] of watermarking. In his two research papers published in 2015, he has tried to predict the watermarking capacity and error rate while histogram shifting methods were applied.

Dalel Bouslimi et al. (2012) [14]: They have applied the combined algorithm of encryption with RC4 and watermarking algorithm. The methods were tested against ultrasound images. They found that the distortion was minimized and thus the method was suited for DICOM standards.

Recently in 2015, they have applied quantization index modulation for embedding purposes with watermarking. In another paper published in 2016, they use the quantum noise modulation technique.

Lingling and.Gao (2012) [14]: They have published two research papers in 2012 for watermarking in medical images. On the first paper, they used fractional Fourier transform for watermark embedding, which makes the image rotationally invariant and thus resistant to rotational attacks.

In the second paper, they have used integer DCT method, which makes the reversible watermarking fast, but the blocks of images were overlapped. So after that, expansion methods were applied to rectify this problem.

Umaamaheshvari (2012) [14]: For her fragile watermarking for authentication, she used DWT for embedding watermark and IDWT for extracting data.

Mona.M. Soliman1 (2012) [14]: The swarm optimization technique was used along with DCT and DWT transform.

Gouenou.Coatrieux (2013): Coatrieux is a big name in the field of watermarking. He has been working in this field for a long time, and no area of watermarking is untouched by him.

In 2013, the image moment signature method was used by him for medical image watermarking. This method was robust [14].

In 2016, he published papers using watermarking with quantum noise modulation method and homomorphically encrypted image [14].

Recently (2017), he used the fractional Krawtchouk method for watermarking, which is based on eigenvalue decomposition. This method gives better robustness against attacks [14].

P. Viswanathan et al. (2014): For security enhancement and authentication purposes, they used the idea of fingerprint insertion as a watermark [14].

Syifak Izhar Hisham et al. (2015): They used a fragile watermarking method for colored medical images based on Hilbert approach. Watermarked information is checked by parity bit checker [14].

Smita Agrawal et al. (2016): They have used integer-to-integer wavelet transform idea for watermarking medical images [14].

Balamurugan G. et al. (2016): They have developed an iris-based watermarking method [14].

Ali AI-Haj et al. (2016): They have used the idea of cryptographic watermarking by fusing the concept of both cryptography and watermarking. This method is for fragile watermarking of medical images [14].

Hitesh S. Nemade et al. (2016): They have used the idea of histogram shifting for embedding watermarked information into medical images.

15.5 Conclusion and Future Scope

Based on the different approaches discussed above, we can conclude that security in the healthcare system by using classical techniques were not sufficient. Further, the healthcare system has a variety of data used for different purposes; they all should not be dealt with by a single algorithm. So, new security methods like watermarking techniques can be used by encapsulating different cryptographic approaches based on the type of healthcare data. For the simple text data, we can use simple fragile watermarking techniques, whereas for medical reports where patients' sensitive information were given, one should prefer robust watermarking techniques.

Due to excessive use of mobile phones nowadays, the healthcare system also has the scope to use it and benefit the society. There is the scope of research in this field to facilitate the patient in terms of his medical information and report. He can see and discuss his report when needed due to mobile phones. But dealing medical technology with mobile phones has some issues, like its limited storage capacity, processing power, Internet bandwidth, etc. The positive aspect is that now 4G technology is running in India, and very soon 5G is going to be launched, so bandwidth limitation problem is no longer an issue. Storage capacity and memory is also increasing day by day in mobile phones. So, research to develop security of medical images through mobile phones is a very good area.

One more area of research may be to enhance the efficiency of the watermark algorithms. Running time for fragile watermarking is good enough, but running time for robust watermark algorithms still needs some improvement.

As all variety of medical images are now coming in colored form, one can make an algorithm for colored images. But as every pixel in colored images is 24 bits, which is threefold of the size of gray images, complexity issues will arise in this case.

Research in the case of three-dimensional images can also be done. Images in the volume data can be sliced and converted into two-dimensional form. Then, two-dimensional watermarking algorithms can be applied for each slice. Finally, every slice can be combined to reconstruct the medical volume.

References

1. Barni, M., Bartolini, F., Cappellini, B., & Piva, A. (1998). DCT domain system for robust image watermarking. *Signal Processing, 66*, 357–372.
2. Madhu, B., Holi, G., & Srikanta Murthy, K. (2016). An overview of image security techniques. *International Journal of Computer Applications, 154*(6), 37–46.
3. Fraser, S. I., Allen, A. R.. (2012). A high capacity reversible watermarking techniques based on difference expansion. In: *Proceedings of signal and image processing SIP-2008*, Kailua-Kona, HI, USA.
4. Khanna, A. K., Roy, N. R., & Verma, B. (2016). Digital image watermarking and its optimization using genetic algorithm. In *International conference on computing, communication and automation (ICCCA)*. IEEE.
5. Rao, R. S. P., & Kumar, P. R. (2016). An efficient genetic algorithm based gray scale digital image watermarking for improving the robustness and imperceptibility. In *International conference on electrical, electronics, and optimization techniques (ICEEOT)*. IEEE.
6. Takore, T. T., Rajesh Kumar, P., & Lavanya Devi, G. (2016). Efficient gray image watermarking algorithm based on DWT-SVD using genetic algorithm. In *International conference on information communication and embedded systems (ICICES)*. IEEE.
7. Giakoumaki, S., & Pavlopulos, D. K. (2011). Multiple image watermarking applied to health information management. *IEEE Transactions on Information Technology in Bio-Medicine, 10*, 4.
8. Baaziz, N., Zheng, D., & Wang, D. (2011). Image quality assessment based on multiple watermarking approach. In *IEEE 13th international workshop on multimedia signal processing (MMSP)* (pp. 1–5). IEEE.
9. Usman, A. K. (2010). BCH coding and intelligent watermark embedding: Employing both frequency and strength selection. *Applied Soft Computing, 10*(1), 332–343.
10. Karras, D. A. (2005). A second order spread spectrum modulation scheme for wavelet based low error probability digital image watermarking. *ICGST International Journal on Graphics, Vision and Image Processing, 3*, 5.
11. Hai-mei, S., Tian-can, M., & Qian-ging, Q. (2004). Spread spectrum watermark based on wavelet transform for still digital image. *Wuhan University Journal of Natural Sciences, 9*(2), 203–208.

12. Enayatifar, R., & Abdullah, A. H. (2014). Chaos-based image encryption using a hybrid genetic algorithm and a DNA sequence. *Optics and Lasers in Engineering, 56*, 83–93.
13. Bhandari, K., Mitra, S. K., & Jadhav, A. (2005). A hybrid approach to digital image watermarking using singular value decomposition and spread spectrum. In *International conference on pattern recognition and machine intelligence, PReMI-05* (pp. 447–452). IEEE.
14. Tripathi, M. M. (2018). Designing a model to improve medical image watermarking. PhD Thesis, TMU Moradabad.
15. Priego, B., Souto, D., Peña, F. L., & Duro, R. J. (2011). An ANN based hyperspectral waterway control and security system. In *IEEE international conference on computational intelligence for measurement systems and applications (CIMSA) proceedings*. IEEE.
16. Kishore, P. V. V., Sai Prajwal, K., Kamal Mohan, M., Koteswarao, S. (2015) Medical image watermarking with ANN in wavelet domain. *IEEE International Conference on Electronics,Computing and Communication Technologies (CONECCT).*
17. Khanna, A. K., Roy, N. R., Verma, B. (2016) Digital image watermarking and its optimization using genetic algorithm. *International Conference on Computing, Communication and Automation (ICCCA).*

Chapter 16
Classification Algorithms for Predicting Diabetes Mellitus: A Comparative Analysis

Ravinder Ahuja, Prashant Dixit, Alisha Banga, and S. C. Sharma

Abbreviations

API	Application programming interface
ANN	Artificial neural network
BMI	Body mass index
BP	Blood pressure
DT	Decision tree
DTDN	Distributed time delay networks
ET	Extra tree
GPC	Gaussian process classifier
GNB	Gaussian Naive Bayes
QDA	Quadratic discriminant analysis
GB	Gradient boosting
ML	Machine learning
MLP	Multilayer perceptron
MICE	Multivariate imputation by chained equations
LR	Logistic regression
LDA	Linear discriminant analysis
RF	Random forest
PCA	Principal component analysis
SVM	Support vector machine
KNN	K-nearest neighbor

R. Ahuja (✉)
School of Computing Science and Engineering, Galgotias University, Noida, India

P. Dixit
Computer Science and Engineering Department, Jaypee Institute of Information Technology, Noida, India

A. Banga · S. C. Sharma
Indian Institute of Technology Roorkee, Saharanpur, India

M. S. Husain et al. (eds.), *Pervasive Healthcare*, EAI/Springer Innovations in Communication and Computing, https://doi.org/10.1007/978-3-030-77746-3_16

VT Variance threshold

16.1 Introduction

In diabetes, the sugar level of the blood rises dramatically [1]. It has become the fifth-ranked disease for disease-related deaths [2]. Due to diabetes, other problems may arise, such as an increased risk of heart attack and stroke [3]. Unfortunately, these diseases cannot be cured; the only way to treat them is to manage the glucose level in the blood. Around 8.8% of adults had diabetes mellitus in 2017 all around the world, and the projected value is 9.9% in 2045 [4]. Diabetes mellitus is classified into three categories: (a) type I, (b) type II, and (c) type III. Majority of people with diabetes are of type II [5]. The Pima are one of the most studied populations for diabetes mellitus analysis in the world [6]. Most of the Pima population has type II diabetes mellitus. Diabetes mellitus classification is a challenging issue due to the nonlinear and complex data. Due to the presence of null entries and outliers in the Pima dataset, the performance of the classifier may become low. Nowadays, machine learning algorithms are used in various applications like medicine, finance, marketing, business, etc. There are three types of machine learning algorithms, namely, unsupervised, supervised, and semi-supervised. In the supervised learning technique, the machine learns from a portion of data that has been labelled, and this learning is used to predict the label of unseen data. Data is not labelled in unsupervised algorithms, and the machine finds common properties among data points and combines data points with similar properties into one class. In the semi-supervised learning, the unsupervised and supervised techniques are combined. As we have considered a labelled dataset, we have applied supervised learning algorithms. There may be an impact on the performance of classification algorithms due to missing values and outliers [7–10]. In machine learning, data preprocessing is an important step. In data preprocessing, the missing values are replaced with the median, and outliers are identified through a box plot and replaced with median values. In the next phase five feature selection algorithms along with fifteen classification algorithms are applied.

The following contributions are made in this article:

1. Applied 5 feature selection techniques along with 15 classification techniques with k-fold cross-validation method for optimization of results.
2. No one in the literature has performed such extensive analysis and comparison of algorithms on the diabetes mellitus dataset.

The paper is divided into the following parts: Sect. 16.2 contains related work, Sect. 16.3 describes the methods and materials, Sect. 16.4 contains the methodology used and evaluation measure, Sect. 16.5 contains the results and discussion, and Sect. 16.6 contains the conclusion.

16.2 Literature Survey

Karthikeyani et al. [11] have applied ten classification algorithms, namely, CS-CRT, PLS-LDA, PNN, K-NN, MLR, SVM, BLR, C4.5, PLS-DA, and CRT to predict diabetes mellitus. They found that SVM algorithm performed better among all the algorithms, giving an accuracy value of 78.4% and an error rate of 0.29. Karthikeyani et al. [12] have applied PLS-LDA technique to classify data. PLS is used for feature extraction and LDA for classification, achieving an accuracy value of 74.40%. In their paper [13], Kumari et al. have removed the missing values from the dataset, and the remaining entries after removal become 460. Out of 460 entries, 260 were used for training and 200 for testing. They reported an accuracy value of 75.50%. In the paper [14], the LDA feature selection was applied, and two features were selected out of eight, and SVM and a feedforward neural network were applied for classification, yielding a 75.65% accuracy. Bozkurt et al. [15] have applied eight classification algorithms (six algorithms were different variants of ANN, and the other two were a decision tree and an artificial immune system). The highest accuracy of 76% was achieved by the DTNN model. Iyer et al. [16] have selected features, replaced missing values with the mean, and normalized the data. After preprocessing the data, they have applied J48 and naive Bayes classification algorithm. They found that J48 algorithm has given the highest accuracy value of 74.86%. In the paper [17], they have applied four classification algorithms, namely, C4.5, MLP, Bayes network, and random forest. They have selected features based on their rank and found the highest accuracy in blood pressure and BMI features only. Sivanesan et al. [18] have applied J48 classification algorithm with tenfold cross-validation and 65:35 ratio training and test dataset. They found that J48 classification algorithm with tenfold cross-validation performed better with an accuracy of 73.82%. Nabi et al. [19] have applied naive Bayes, random forest, logistic regression, and decision tree classification. They have evaluated these models using RRSE, CC, MAE, IC, RMSE, and RAE. They found that logistic regression is performing better, with an accuracy value of 80.43%. In the paper [20], the authors have applied four classification algorithms, namely, quadratic discriminant analysis, GPC classifier with three kernels, linear discriminant analysis, and naive Bayes with k-fold cross-validation technique ($K = 2, 3, 4, 5, 10$). They found that the GPC classifier with radial kernel is performing better among all other models. In the paper [7], the authors have proposed an ensemble model named HM-BagMoov, considering bagging and multilayer classification. They have applied the proposed algorithm with seven other classification algorithms, namely, RF, LDA, NB, KNN, ANN, LR, and SVM, on datasets of different diseases including diabetes mellitus. They found the proposed model performed better, with an accuracy value of 77.21%. In the paper [21], the authors have applied three classification algorithms, namely, naïve Bayes, support vector machine, and decision tree. They observed naïve Bayes performed better among all, with an accuracy value of 76.30%. In the paper [22], the authors have applied a combination of SVM and PCA algorithm to classify diabetes patients. PCA is used to reduce the dimension of the dataset, and SVM is used for classification. Md. Maniruzzaman et al. [23] have applied six feature selection techniques along with ten classification algorithms and two cross-validation techniques, namely, k-fold cross-validation (with $k = 2, 4, 5, 10$) and JK cross-validation. They focused on the preprocessing of data so that performance can be increased. They replaced the missing values (represented by zeros) with the median and outliers also with the median value. They found random forest classifier with random forest feature selection algorithm performed better. In [24], different techniques of classification and clustering have been applied in the medical field (on images and on numeric data), which shows the role and significance of machine learning algorithms in disease detection or prediction. In the paper [25], the authors have applied machine learning algorithms to identify fatty liver disease, and they were able to predict it quite efficiently by giving a sensitivity of 98.06%. In the paper [26], the authors have applied a modified cuckoo search with an artificial neural network to classify and detect dengue fever. They have also proposed a modified bag of feature methods to identify the most important genes in the classification. In the paper [27], the authors have applied factor analysis to reduce the dimension of the data and applied the neuro-fuzzy model and neural network fuzzy classifier to classify Crohn's disease. In the paper [28], the authors have applied linear discriminant analysis techniques for feature extraction, and five classification algorithms are applied to classify diabetes mellitus. They found that multilayer perceptron model is the best performer out of the five applied, with an accuracy of 78.70%. In the literature, various classification and feature selection algorithms have been applied to diabetes dataset. The work that thoroughly explores the predictive power of feature selection algorithms and classification algorithms in classifying diabetes disease is not presented yet. This chapter presents an exploratory analysis of diabetes mellitus, considering 5 feature selection techniques and 15 classification algorithms.

16.3 Materials and Methods

16.3.1 Dataset

The dataset has been taken from the UCI Machine Learning Repository [29]. There are a total of 768 records in the dataset. The dataset has eight attributes as shown in Table 16.1. The ninth attribute, outcome, has two values: 0 and 1. Out of 768 records, 268 records have a value of 1, indicating that they have diabetes mellitus, while 500 records have a value of 0, indicating that they do not have diabetes mellitus. The dataset has missing values in the form of zero entries, which are replaced with the median of the corresponding attribute. The outliers in the dataset are detected through box plot and replaced with the median values.

Table 16.1 Details of the attributes of the Pima Indian Diabetes Dataset

Attribute name	Type of attribute	Range	Mean ± SD
Pregnancies	Int	0–17	3.78 ± 3.27
BP (blood pressure)	Int	0–122	72.39 ± 12.09
Insulin	Int	0–846	140.56 ± 88.70
Skin thickness	Int	0–99	27.24 ± 8.86
BMI	Real	0–67.1	32.08 ± 6.29
Diabetes pedigree function	Real	0.078–2.42	0.41 ± 0.22
Age	Int	21–81	32 + 10.1
Glucose	Int	0–199	121.66 ± 30.44

16.3.2 Feature Selection Techniques

The feature selection techniques used in our study are as follows:

Linear Discriminant Analysis

It is a linear method of dimensionality reduction in which high-dimensional data is projected to low-dimensional data [30]. The data points are projected on straight lines, so data points belonging to the same class are as close as possible and data points from different classes are as far as possible.

Principal Component Analysis

PCA is an unsupervised technique for dimensionality reduction, which is used in experimental data when there is a need to analyze the variance-covariance interrelation of a group of variables by using linear relationships. In order to remove redundancy in the provided health data, PCA has been a popular choice during the development of major disease diagnosis models [31].

Random Forest

It is a widely used method for feature ranking as they are easy to apply and do not need a lot of feature engineering. With the help of the tree-based approach, random forest ranks the features according to the degree of improvement on the purity of the node. In this study, we have used mean decrease impurity method for feature selection [32].

Extra Trees

Also known as "extremely randomized trees," they are related to the random forest algorithm as they are built by choosing a random subset of *K* features for every node to determine the split. Instead of choosing the best cut-point based on the local sample as done in the random forest method, in this technique, each tree is built from the complete learning sample, and, most importantly, for every feature, a discretization threshold (cut-point) is chosen at random to determine a split [33].

Variance Threshold

Variance threshold is a simple approach to feature selection, which works on the idea that when variance within a feature is low, it has a low predictive power. The features whose variance lies below a certain cutoff are removed in this technique [34].

16.3.3 Classification Algorithms

Linear Discriminant Analysis

The basic idea of this approach is to find a linear combination of predictors which can separate the target effectively. It creates a new axis by following two conditions: (1) the distance between the means should be maximized, and (2) the variation within each target should be minimized. It is a classification technique based on the covariance matrix [35].

Quadratic Discriminant Analysis

Quadratic discriminant analysis (QDA) uses a quadric surface. In QDA, the observations in each class are assumed to be drawn from a multivariate Gaussian distribution with a class-specific mean data and covariance matrix. Contrary to LDA, the covariance matrix is not common to all the K classes [10]. QDA can perform better than LDA, but covariance matrix needs to be computed for each class.

Gaussian Naive Bayes

It uses Bayes's theorem and works on Bayesian classification techniques. In this, it is assumed that a simple Gaussian distribution is used to obtain data from each target. It has been of significant use in medical science as well as machine learning.

This classifier presumes that all the features are not related to each other by predicting the probabilities for every class [36].

Gaussian Process Classifier

Developed in the 1970s in the geostatistics field, the Gaussian process classifier is a Bayesian methodology based nonparametric classifier. Gaussian process classifier has proved to be a very effective tool, which is used in regression problems as well as in classification problems. This classifier is capable of learning from noisy data [37]. We have used the RBF kernel in our study.

Support Vector Machine Classifier

This algorithm can be used for both regression and classification [38]. In this algorithm, each data point is plotted in n-dimensional space, where n is the number of features in the dataset. The objective is to find a hyperplane in n-dimensional space with maximum margin that separates the two classes. We have used RBF kernel in our study.

MLP Classifier

MLP is also known as feedforward ANN, which consists of at least three layers, namely, input layer, hidden layer, and output layer [39]. Back propagation algorithm is used for training. The hyperparameters used in our study are learning rate of 0.01, hidden layer nodes of 100, and ReLU activation function.

AdaBoost Classifier

Boosting is the process of combining multiple weak classifiers to form a strong classifier. AdaBoost is also known as adaptive boosting. In this, each training data is given equal weight. Each classifier also gives weight on the basis of the accuracy achieved. The weak classifiers are used in successive steps to increase the performance of the model [40]. In our study, we have used n_estimators = 50 and learning rate = 1.0.

Logistic Regression

This method can be used only for classification [41]. It utilizes maximum likelihood for estimation. Suppose there are n numbers of features $A1, A2...$An and x represents the probability of occurring event. The model is represented using Eq. (16.1):

$$\log\left(x/(1-x)\right) = \text{logit}(x) = \beta 0 + \beta 1A1 +, \ldots + \beta nAn \tag{16.1}$$

where beta is the regression coefficient.

Decision Tree

This classifier forms a tree structure in which internal nodes represent a feature, the branches represent a decision mechanism, and the leaves represent the final outcome. It is easier to interpret as it mimics the human thinking process. The internal decision-making process of this classifier is known for its tree structure. This can easily process multidimensional data and takes very less time in training [42].

Random Forest (RF)

Random forest is the combination of a number of decision tree algorithms. The dataset is randomly selected, and the decision tree is formed from the randomly selected data [43]. The weight is assigned to each decision tree created, and the final output will be the weighted sum of different decision trees. The performance of a single decision tree may be affected by noise, but combining multiple decision trees, called random forest, is not affected by noisy data. In our experiment, we have used 100 decision trees and Gini for impurity index.

Bagging

Also known as bootstrap aggregation, bagging is an ensembling technique. It creates individuals for its ensemble by training each classifier on a random redistribution of the training set and then aggregates their individual predictions to form a final prediction. Such a meta-estimator can typically be used as a way to reduce the variance of a decision tree, by introducing randomization into its construction procedure and then making an ensemble out of it [44].

Gradient Boosting (GB)

This is also an ensemble of the machine learning algorithm. The decision tree is evaluated on the data points having the same weight; in the second iteration, the weight of the data points, which are not classified accurately, is increased, and another decision tree is used, which is of the form Tree1+Tree2. This process will be repeated for a specific number of times. Therefore, the final prediction is the weighted sum of all the decision tree algorithms applied [45].

K-Nearest Neighbor

This is one of the simple and easy-to-implement classification algorithms. In this, we use the distance metric (Euclidean distance in our case) to compute the distance between the test case and training data. We sort the distance metric in ascending order and find the top k elements in the list. The class of the test data is assigned based on the majority of the classes in the top k elements from the list [46]. We have taken $k = 5$.

SGD Classifier

Stochastic gradient descent is one of the best optimization techniques, due to which it is widely used in machine learning as well as medical science. It is faster than the batch gradient descent as it selects parameters randomly instead of selecting all the parameters in the training set. It is an iterative technique in which the gradient loss is evaluated with each sample at a time, and the model is updated along the way with a falling learning rate [47].

Bernoulli Naïve Bayes

This technique of classification is simple and based on the Bayesian theorem (as given in Eq. (16.2)). This approach is suitable for the multidimensional data with the assumption that attributes are independent of each other. Naïve Bayes is of two types: Gaussian naïve Bayes and Bernoulli naïve Bayes (BNB). Here we have considered BNB [48]:

$$P(X/y) = \frac{P(y/X) * P(X)}{(P(y))} \tag{16.2}$$

where $P(X/y)$ is a posterior probability, $P(y/X)$ is the likelihood, $P(X)$ is the prior probability, and $P(y)$ is the marginal probability.

16.4 Methodology Used

Figure 16.1 shows the overall methodology used in our study. This study consists of two stages. In the first stage, data is preprocessed, and feature selection algorithms are applied. In the second stage, 15 classification algorithms are applied with k-fold cross-validation technique. The dataset consists of missing values in the form of zeros and is replaced with median values, and outliers are identified using box plot and replaced with median values. Further, five feature selection techniques (RF,

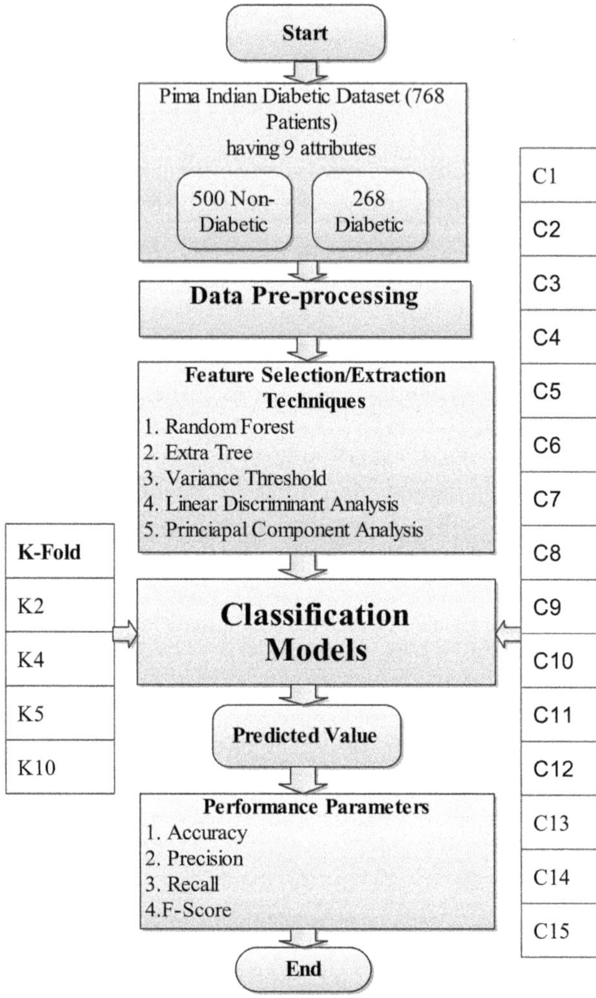

Fig. 16.1 Structure of the model designed for classification

LDA, ET, PCA, and VT) have been applied to extract features from the processed data. In the next stage, 15 classification algorithms (LDA, QDA, RF, LR, BNB, GNB, SGD, KNN, DT, GB, bagging, AdaBoost, MLP, SVC, and GPC) have been applied to predict diabetes patients with k-fold cross-validation. All the models applied are evaluated using four performance parameters, which are as follows:

Accuracy This performance parameter measures how correctly our model is performing. The formula for accuracy is given in Eq. (16.3):

$$\text{Accuracy} = \frac{(\text{TruePositiue} + \text{TrueNegatiue})}{(\text{TruePositiue} + \text{FalseNegatiue} + \text{FalsePositiue} + \text{TrueNegatiue})} \tag{16.3}$$

Precision The precision of a model is the fraction of relevant occurrences among the retrieved occurrences. It is also referred to as a positive predictive value. It is calculated by taking a ratio of true positives by the total positives in a model as given in Eq. (16.4):

$$\text{Precision} = \frac{(\text{TruePositiue})}{(\text{TruePositiue} + \text{FalsePositiue})} \tag{16.4}$$

Recall This metric of classifiers specifies the capability of the model to identify how much actual positives are identified correctly. It is the ratio of true positive by true positive+false positive as given in Eq. (16.5):

$$\text{Recall} = \frac{(\text{TruePositiue})}{(\text{TruePositiue} + \text{FalseNegatiue})} \tag{16.5}$$

F-score This parameter is a harmonic mean of precision and recall. In f1 score, both precision and recall are equally weighted as given in Eq. (16.6):

$$\text{F\_Score} = \mathbf{2}_* \frac{(\text{Precision} * \text{Recall})}{(\text{Precision} + \text{Recall})} \tag{16.6}$$

In cross-validation, the complete dataset is divided into k equal parts. We have taken the value of $k = 2, 4, 5$, and 10. In this technique, one part is used for testing, and the remaining parts are used for training. Performance is calculated in each iteration, and the final performance is the average of all the performances recorded in each iteration.

- C1: Linear discriminant analysis
- C2: Quadratic discriminant analysis
- C3: Gaussian naive Bayes
- C4: Gaussian process classifier
- C5: Support vector classifier
- C6: MLP (multilayer perceptron) classifier
- C7: AdaBoost classifier
- C8: Logistic regression
- C9: Decision tree
- C10: Random forest
- C11: Bagging
- C12: Gradient boosting
- C13: K-nearest neighbor
- C14: SGD classifier
- C15: Multinomial naive Bayes

16.5 Results and Discussion

Firstly, five feature selection methods are applied, and further 15 various machine learning algorithms for classification are evaluated over 4 parameters, i.e., accuracy, precision, recall, and f1-score. Table 16.2 shows the accuracy parameter of various feature selection algorithms along with various classification algorithms considering k-fold cross-validation with a value of $k = 2, 4, 5$, and 10. It is observed that the highest accuracy is 78.70% at a value of k=4 using a multilayer perceptron classifier with a linear discriminant feature selection technique. The recall of classification algorithms with different values of k-fold cross-validation ($k = 2, 4, 5, 10$) and five feature extraction methods is presented in Table 16.3. It is observed that the highest recall is 71.26% at a value of $k = 4$ using a multilayer perceptron classifier with variance threshold feature selection technique.

The precision of classification algorithms with different values of k-fold cross-validation ($k = 2, 4, 5$, and 10) and five feature extraction methods is presented in Table 16.4. It is observed that the highest precision is 74.45% at a value of $k = 4$ using a multilayer perceptron classifier with variance threshold feature selection technique.

The f1-score of classification algorithms with different values of k-fold cross-validation ($k = 2, 4, 5, 10$) and five feature extraction methods is presented in Table 16.5. It is observed that the highest f1-score is 72.82% at a value of $k = 4$ using a multilayer perceptron classifier with linear discriminant feature selection technique. The comparison of 15 classifiers over 5 different feature selection techniques based on the accuracy parameter is shown in Fig. 16.2. The highest accuracy of each classifier corresponding to every feature selection is considered. It is observed that the highest accuracy of 78.7% is achieved by a multilayer perceptron with a variance threshold feature selection technique.

The comparison of 15 classifiers over 5 different feature selection techniques using precision parameters is shown in Fig. 16.3. The highest precision of each classifier corresponding to every feature selection is considered. It is observed that the highest precision of 74.45% is achieved by a multilayer perceptron with a linear discriminant feature selection technique. The comparison of 15 classifiers over 5 different feature selection techniques based on the recall parameter is shown in Fig. 16.4. The highest recall of each classifier corresponding to every feature selection is considered. It is observed that the highest recall of 71.26% is achieved by a multilayer perceptron with a linear discriminant feature selection technique. The comparison of 15 classifiers over 5 different feature selection techniques based on the f1-score parameter is shown in Fig. 16.5. The highest f1-score of each classifier corresponding to every feature selection is considered. It is observed that the highest f1-score of 72.82% is achieved by a multilayer perceptron with a linear discriminant feature selection technique. Overall, it is observed that a multilayer perceptron classifier, along with a linear discriminant analysis feature selection algorithm, outperforms all other classifiers at the value of $k = 4$.

Table 16.2 Accuracy over different feature selection techniques with different classification algorithms

Linear discriminant analysis															
K-fold	C1	C2	C3	C4	C5	C6	C7	C8	C9	C10	C11	C12	C13	C14	C15
$K = 2$	77.8	77.8	77.6	77.3	77.6	77.5	73.2	77.8	69.0	69.9	70.3	77.3	72.3	77.8	75.4
$K = 4$	77.8	78	77.8	77.6	77.6	78.7	75.6	77.6	69.9	70	68.7	77.6	71.3	62.4	75.4
$K = 5$	77.8	77.8	77.8	77.8	77.5	78	76.3	77.6	71.5	72.9	73.7	77.8	75	60.9	75.4
$K = 10$	77.6	77.8	77.8	77.5	77.5	77.6	75.2	77.6	69.5	70	70	77.5	74.7	72.1	75.4
Principal component analysis															
$K = 2$	76.7	72.4	74.4	76.5	76.0	76.2	74.1	77.0	70.6	76.0	73.6	76.5	69.7	75.9	74.3
$K = 4$	77.5	74.5	75.2	76.7	75.7	77.5	76.0	77.3	67.9	72.3	72.9	76.7	69.0	69.5	74.1
$K = 5$	76.7	74.1	75.2	77.2	75.9	77.8	74.1	77.2	70.0	73.9	72.8	77.1	70.0	68.2	72.9
$K = 10$	77.0	74.9	75.0	77.0	77.2	77.2	74.6	77.5	71.4	71.6	72.6	77.0	70.6	72.3	73.4
Random forest feature selection technique															
$K = 2$	78.0	76.8	77.3	77.2	77.0	77.9	73.1	76.7	68.2	72.4	74.1	77.2	74.1	75.7	65.1
$K = 4$	77.4	76.0	76.7	77.8	77.6	77.6	75.4	77.3	70.2	73.1	75.0	77.8	73.9	66.9	65.1
$K = 5$	77.5	76.2	76.5	77.3	77.2	77.3	76.5	76.8	67.5	74.4	73.4	77.3	73.3	73.6	65.1
$K = 10$	77.5	76.3	76.5	77.3	77.0	77.2	75.8	76.8	67.9	74.6	74.0	77.3	72.6	71.6	65.1
Extra tree feature selection technique															
$K = 2$	78.0	76.8	77.4	77.2	77.0	77.2	73.1	76.7	68.9	74.2	74.1	77.2	74.1	77.4	65.1
$K = 4$	77.4	76.0	76.7	77.8	77.6	77.3	75.4	77.4	68.7	74.8	74.9	77.8	73.9	68.2	65.1
$K = 5$	77.5	76.2	76.5	77.3	77.2	77.2	76.5	76.9	66.6	75.2	73.9	77.4	73.3	69.8	65.1
$K = 10$	77.5	76.47	76.5	77.3	77.0	77.3	75.8	76.8	67.5	73.1	72.6	77.4	72.6	73.1	65.1
Variance threshold feature selection technique															
$K = 2$	77.7	74.6	75.9	77.0	76.5	77.6	72.3	76.2	71.5	75.0	73.7	77.0	70.5	69.5	65.1
$K = 4$	77.3	76.0	76.2	77.4	76.0	78.7	74.9	76.4	72.0	74.3	74.4	77.4	70.8	68.9	65.1
$K = 5$	76.8	74.7	76.5	76.7	76.2	77.8	74.7	76.2	70.0	74.4	74.8	76.7	71.9	74.1	65.1
$K = 10$	77.2	74.8	76.2	77.2	77.0	77.8	73.3	76.7	71.2	73.7	73.8	77.2	72.0	66.9	65.1

16.6 Discussions

- In this paper, 15 classification and ensemble algorithms with 5 feature selection algorithms have been explored to find a best combination that predicts the diabetes mellitus efficiently. It was found that multilayer perceptron classifier with linear discriminant feature selection algorithm has given the highest performance in terms of accuracy of 78.70%, precision of 74.45%, recall of 71.26%, and f-score of 72.82%.
- The results show that machine learning algorithms, along with feature selection techniques, can give better results on medical data.

Table 16.3 Comparison of classifiers using recall over different feature selection techniques with different k-fold values

K-fold	C1	C2	C3	C4	C5	C6	C7	C8	C9	C10	C11	C12	C13	C14	C15
Linear discriminant analysis															
$K = 2$	58.21	57.28	57.28	59.63	57.75	69.15	51.67	58.21	59.14	60.08	56.8	59.63	61.97	53.49	59.79
$K = 4$	57.72	57.17	57.17	59.79	57.60	71.26	57.45	57.70	59.15	56.81	58.86	59.79	58.99	59.60	59.86
$K = 5$	56.85	55.86	55.86	59.64	55.86	65.36	60.03	56.86	58.50	57.68	58.19	59.64	62.30	51.56	49.56
$K = 10$	57.25	56.58	56.58	59.11	57.45	66.92	59.34	57.25	56.42	56.37	55.73	59.11	60.27	45.03	59.65
Principal component analysis															
$K = 2$	56.33	54.47	53.98	51.65	44.60	58.68	59.15	52.11	52.54	47.42	45.99	51.64	51.17	46.86	49.76
$K = 4$	57.70	58.31	55.22	52.70	46.41	61.83	61.43	53.36	48.99	52.53	53.82	52.70	50.67	56.66	50.67
$K = 5$	56.97	55.97	54.42	53.62	48.07	61.24	56.16	54.04	59.79	48.13	52.33	53.62	52.12	53.00	46.56
$K = 10$	55.88	58.65	54.92	52.11	50.43	58.08	58.04	54.61	61.42	43.48	52.57	52.11	52.91	58.51	48.36
Random forest feature selection technique															
$K = 2$	58.68	56.32	59.61	52.11	53.99	55.85	60.09	50.69	54.45	49.29	55.38	52.11	63.85	61.05	65.38
$K = 4$	57.60	54.81	57.68	55.89	56.22	56.94	60.36	52.92	59.39	56.23	58.15	55.89	59.93	62.23	60.15
$K = 5$	57.31	55.15	57.57	54.19	54.61	56.85	61.29	51.23	52.24	54.12	56.02	54.19	56.33	58.21	59.02
$K = 10$	57.88	55.28	56.77	55.51	55.45	57.35	59.86	52.14	50.87	53.75	49.85	55.51	55.45	32.14	69.85
Extra tree feature selection technique															
$K = 2$	58.68	56.32	59.61	52.11	53.99	57.26	60.09	50.69	55.85	52.58	56.81	52.10	63.85	48.06	60.09
$K = 4$	57.60	54.81	57.68	55.89	56.22	58.09	60.36	52.92	62.11	53.17	53.15	55.89	59.93	46.36	62.36
$K = 5$	57.31	55.15	57.57	54.19	54.61	57.43	61.29	51.23	52.83	54.87	51.97	54.19	56.33	65.98	61.29
$K = 10$	57.88	55.28	56.77	55.51	55.45	57.43	59.86	52.15	53.11	52.36	53.43	55.51	55.45	60.97	69.86
Variance threshold feature selection technique															
$K = 2$	58.21	55.87	63.37	52.11	46.01	56.33	57.74	48.83	56.78	47.42	51.14	52.11	52.12	48.58	59.10
$K = 4$	57.77	59.28	63.72	55.36	47.37	59.22	58.68	50.73	61.63	51.12	53.33	55.36	54.18	82.91	61.25
$K = 5$	56.97	56.62	63.09	53.73	48.64	59.51	58.56	50.49	55.32	48.19	51.31	53.73	53.39	65.37	62.45
$K = 10$	57.4	56.92	62.74	53.61	49.61	58.54	54.82	51.76	58.11	47.79	54.93	54.26	55.83	57.35	64.76

Table 16.4 Comparison of classifiers using precision over different feature selection techniques with different k-fold values

K-fold	C1	C2	C3	C4	C5	C6	C7	C8	C9	C10	C11	C12	C13	C14	C15
Linear discriminant analysis															
$K = 2$	72.51	73.06	72.61	70.57	72.43	70.33	64.64	72.53	55.14	55.72	57.11	70.57	59.92	73.37	61.12
$K = 4$	72.56	73.34	72.82	70.92	72.11	74.45	67.37	72.12	56.05	59.02	57.77	70.92	58.87	71.96	61.75
$K = 5$	71.94	72.28	72.28	70.26	71.35	72.27	67.36	71.52	58.92	61.33	59.75	70.26	64.81	43.97	60.73
$K = 10$	73.01	73.30	72.30	71.31	72.48	71.10	64.66	73.02	56.39	57.51	60.02	71.31	64.28	54.99	61.45
Principal component analysis															
$K = 2$	70.59	61.7	66.21	72.84	72.83	69.09	63.63	74.01	55.41	64.69	66.29	72.84	57.16	64.12	67.59
$K = 4$	71.80	64.62	66.72	72.18	71.66	71.27	66.62	73.74	50.92	66.43	65.89	72.18	55.64	66.95	67.19
$K = 5$	69.05	63.58	67.03	71.67	71.48	69.95	64.14	71.41	56.01	64.99	63.51	71.67	58.99	72.11	65.45
$K = 10$	72.49	66.08	67.28	72.80	71.07	71.76	65.22	73.01	59.15	61.34	63.92	72.81	60.73	62.86	67.29
Random forest feature selection technique															
$K = 2$	70.67	71.01	70.55	71.51	70.80	71.48	61.74	71.98	53.76	68.85	62.35	72.51	62.58	65.44	70.44
$K = 4$	71.17	69.44	69.70	72.64	71.88	71.74	65.84	72.95	55.50	63.99	64.04	73.64	63.02	61.98	70.98
$K = 5$	70.51	68.69	68.49	72.03	71.19	69.76	66.46	72.12	50.74	63.49	62.52	72.03	62.33	54.11	71.11
$K = 10$	71.57	70.90	69.37	71.22	71.23	71.18	66.03	72.79	53.45	65.65	61.74	72.22	61.38	54.19	70.19
Extra tree feature selection technique															
$K = 2$	72.67	71.01	70.55	72.51	71.08	72.41	61.74	71.08	53.28	64.85	62.67	72.51	62.58	67.19	70.98
$K = 4$	71.17	69.44	69.70	72.64	72.88	71.85	65.84	72.95	54.94	63.18	65.81	73.64	63.02	69.55	69.95
$K = 5$	70.51	68.69	68.49	72.03	71.19	71.15	66.46	72.19	52.37	65.41	63.98	72.03	62.33	47.87	72.19
$K = 10$	71.57	70.90	69.87	72.22	71.23	70.99	66.02	72.78	54.01	64.40	63.68	72.22	61.38	59.65	67.78
Variance threshold feature selection technique															
$K = 2$	72.13	65.84	65.84	73.27	71.28	71.94	60.61	72.74	58.02	69.45	68.15	71.50	58.53	72.81	70.81
$K = 4$	71.41	67.28	66.19	72.84	71.70	71.95	65.15	72.71	60.12	69.34	64.83	72.84	58.23	64.22	64.22
$K = 5$	69.41	64.68	66.28	70.48	72.38	70.72	63.81	71.28	59.63	64.18	65.71	70.48	60.19	52.01	62.01
$K = 10$	72.08	65.33	66.32	72.22	71.31	73.22	62.25	72.03	59.21	70.87	66.27	71.22	60.57	60.70	70.45

Table 16.5 Comparison of classifiers using f1-score over different feature selection techniques with different k-fold values

K-fold	C1	C2	C3	C4	C5	C6	C7	C8	C9	C10	C11	C12	C13	C14	C15
Linear discriminant analysis															
$K = 2$	64.58	64.21	64.04	64.62	64.20	65.15	57.06	64.59	57.02	55.47	55.10	64.62	60.90	62.83	60.27
$K = 4$	64.27	64.25	64.04	64.85	64.02	72.82	61.75	64.09	57.51	59.76	57.94	64.86	58.71	54.63	59.13
$K = 5$	63.43	62.95	62.95	64.36	62.60	63.94	63.10	63.24	58.54	58.91	58.84	64.36	63.27	61.53	58.78
$K = 10$	63.52	63.29	63.29	63.94	63.09	65.58	61.42	63.52	55.91	56.18	55.95	63.94	61.99	48.64	58.89
Principal component analysis															
$K = 2$	62.66	57.86	59.43	60.43	56.41	63.45	61.31	61.15	55.41	51.25	55.74	60.43	53.99	65.79	57.35
$K = 4$	63.97	61.28	60.36	60.89	56.92	65.05	63.79	61.90	50.76	53.59	54.98	60.89	52.94	58.73	57.57
$K = 5$	62.39	59.51	60.02	61.31	57.44	63.54	59.79	61.48	55.43	49.96	61.68	61.31	55.16	50.17	54.27
$K = 10$	62.25	61.37	59.93	59.92	59.54	64.44	61.03	61.80	58.45	53.62	58.55	59.92	55.63	56.13	55.65
Random forest feature selection technique															
$K = 2$	64.93	62.78	64.58	61.31	61.99	63.33	60.84	60.14	54.95	58.79	57.78	61.31	63.12	58.16	63.58
$K = 4$	63.63	61.25	63.11	63.48	63.42	63.22	62.86	61.65	57.29	61.34	60.77	63.48	61.29	54.39	63.11
$K = 5$	63.13	61.06	62.45	61.73	61.77	62.94	63.71	59.80	52.74	60.64	58.14	61.73	58.95	57.62	62.45
$K = 10$	63.31	61.24	62.13	62.16	61.89	62.66	62.28	60.16	53.45	58.17	57.67	62.16	57.94	57.91	62.13
Extra tree feature selection technique															
$K = 2$	64.93	62.78	64.58	61.31	61.99	63.71	60.84	60.14	57.43	60.84	58.31	61.31	63.13	54.62	63.14
$K = 4$	63.63	61.25	63.11	63.48	63.42	63.66	62.86	61.65	58.72	60.98	58.71	63.48	61.29	55.43	61.65
$K = 5$	63.16	61.06	62.45	61.73	61.77	63.68	63.71	59.80	51.79	58.14	57.62	61.74	58.95	59.42	59.85
$K = 10$	63.31	61.24	62.13	62.16	61.89	62.50	62.28	60.16	51.84	58.38	54.67	62.16	57.94	52.99	64.16
Variance threshold feature selection technique															
$K = 2$	64.46	60.44	64.58	61.15	57.66	62.02	59.13	58.75	60.53	59.79	64.50	61.15	55.13	62.04	56.17
$K = 4$	63.82	62.98	64.86	62.90	57.74	65.00	61.69	59.72	58.52	61.84	60.00	62.90	56.07	61.34	57.93
$K = 5$	62.55	60.23	64.54	60.93	58.12	64.28	60.97	59.07	54.63	54.48	58.05	60.93	56.58	56.74	57.16
$K = 10$	63.14	60.35	64.21	61.27	59.05	63.50	57.78	59.46	58.75	56.03	61.11	61.27	56.91	51.62	58.69

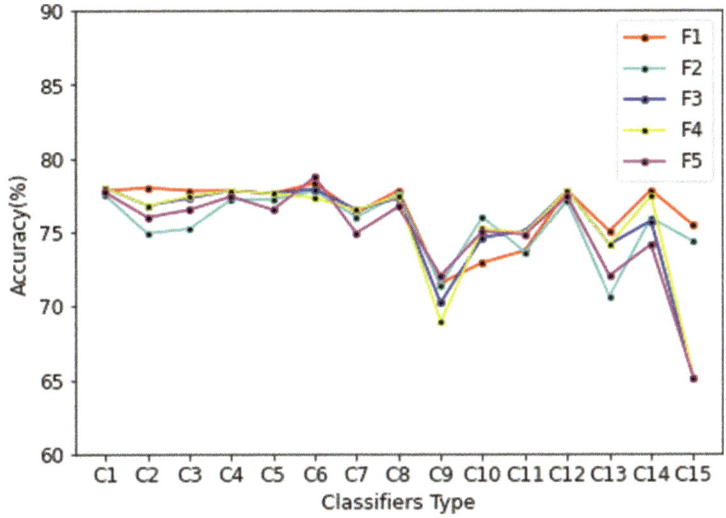

Fig. 16.2 Comparison of accuracy over different feature selection techniques

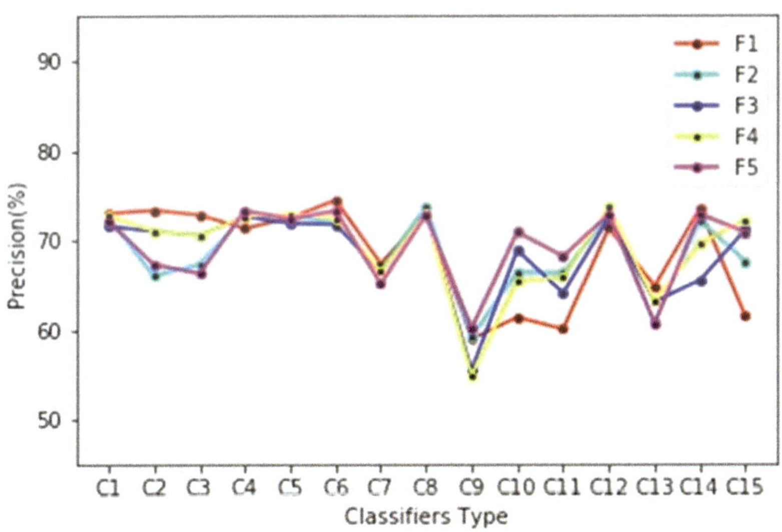

Fig. 16.3 Comparison of precision over different feature selection techniques

- The dataset (780 instances) considered is very small, which is why we have implemented classification algorithms with k-fold cross-validation considering the values of $k = 2, 4, 5$, and 10. In the future, large dataset can be collected and processed using deep learning approaches.

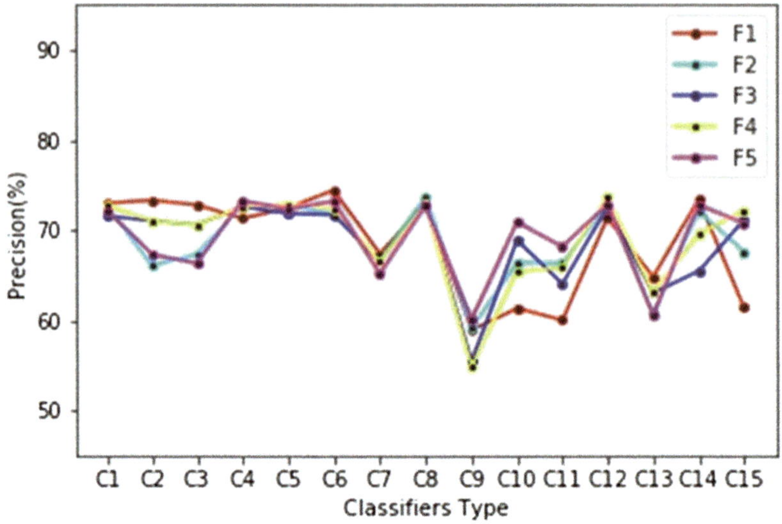

Fig. 16.4 Comparison of recall over different feature selection techniques

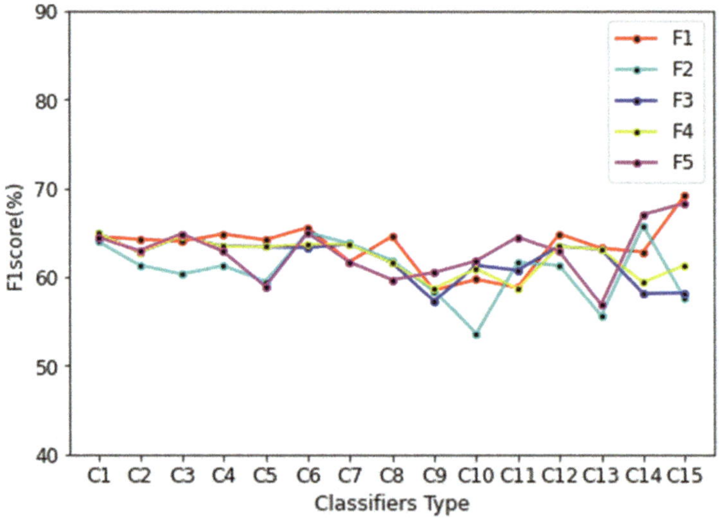

Fig. 16.5 Comparison of f1-score over different feature selection techniques

16.6.1 Limitations of the Study

- This study has considered the mean data imputation technique only. The other imputation techniques, like KNN, MICE, and deep learning techniques, are not explored, which may give better result. Similarly, outliers are handled by taking the logarithm; however, other outlier handling techniques such as Minkowski error, univariate method, and multivariate methods can be explored.

16.7 Conclusion and Future Work

We have considered the PIMA Indian Diabetes Dataset in this study, which has been taken from the UCI Machine Learning Repository. The dataset is preprocessed by replacing the missing values and outliers with the median. Further, five feature selection techniques (LDA, PCA, RF, variance threshold, and extra tree) are applied to get the best features. On the optimal features selected, 15 classification algorithms (LDA, QDA, GNB, GPC, SVM, RF, DT, MLP, AdaBoost, gradient boosting, KNN, bagging, LR, BNB, SGD) with k-fold cross-validation considering k = 2, 4, 5, 10 are applied. In this way, exploratory data analysis was performed to know optimal results. The highest accuracy of 78.70% is achieved with a multilayer perceptron with linear discriminant feature selection at the value of $k = 4$ in k-fold cross-validation. The other observation is that almost similar results are found for the different values of k in all the performance parameters. In the future, other classification algorithms, including deep learning and feature selection techniques, can be applied for further analysis.

References

1. Muntner, P., Colantonio, L. D., Cushman, M., Goff, D. C., Howard, G., Howard, V. J., Kissela, B., Levitan, E. B., Lloyd-Jones, D. M., & Safford, M. M. (2014). Validation of the atherosclerotic cardiovascular disease pooled cohort risk equations. *JAMA, 311*(14), 1406–1415.
2. Kager, V. A., & Holden, E. W. (1992). Preliminary investigation of the direct and moderating effects of family and individual variables on the adjustment of children and adolescents with diabetes. *Journal of Pediatric Psychology, 17*(4), 491–502.
3. American Diabetes Association. (2014). Diagnosis and classification of diabetes mellitus. *Diabetes Care, 37*(1), S81–S90.
4. Fitzmaurice, C., Allen, C., Barber, R. M., Barregard, L., Bhutta, Z. A., Brenner, H., Dicker, D. J., Chimed-Orchir, O., Dandona, R., & Dandona, L. (2017). Global, regional, and national cancer incidence, mortality, years of life lost, years lived with disability, and disability-adjusted life-years for 32 cancer groups, 1990 to 2015: A systematic analysis for the global burden of disease study. *JAMA Oncology, 3*(4), 524–548.
5. Shi, Y., & Hu, F. B. (2014). The global implications of diabetes and cancer. *Lancet (London, England), 383*(9933), 1947.
6. Knowler, W. C., Pettitt, D. J., Saad, M. F., & Bennett, P. H. (1990). Diabetes mellitus in the pima Indians: Incidence, risk factors and pathogenesis. *Diabetes/Metabolism Reviews, 6*(1), 1–27.
7. Bashir, S., Qamar, U., & Khan, F. H. (2016). Intellihealth: A medical decision support application using a novel weighted multi-layer classifier ensemble framework. *Journal of Biomedical Informatics, 59*, 185–200.
8. Kaiser, J. (2014). Dealing with missing values in data. *Journal of Systems Integration, 5*(1), 42–51.
9. Leys, C., Ley, C., Klein, O., Bernard, P., & Licata, L. (2013). Detecting outliers: Do not use standard deviation around the mean, use absolute deviation around the median. *Journal of Experimental Social Psychology, 49*(4), 764–766.
10. Webb, G. I., Boughton, J. R., & Wang, Z. (2005). Not so naive bayes: Aggregating one-dependence estimators. *Machine Learning, 58*(1), 5–24.

11. Karthikeyani, V., Begum, I. P., Tajudin, K., & Begam, I. S. (2012). Comparative of data mining classification algorithm (cdmca) in diabetes disease prediction. *International Journal of Computer Applications, 60*, 12.
12. Karthikeyani, V., & Begum, I. P. (2013). Comparison a performance of data mining algorithms (cpdma) in prediction of diabetes disease. *International Journal on Computer Science and Engineering, 5*(3), 205.
13. Kumari, V. A., & Chitra, R. (2013). Classification of diabetes disease using support vector machine. *International Journal of Engineering Research and Applications, 3*(2), 1797–1801.
14. Parashar, A., Burse, K., & Rawat, K. (2014). A comparative approach for Pima Indians diabetes diagnosis using LDA-support vector machine and feed forward neural network. *International Journal of Advanced Research in Computer Science and Software Engineering, 4*(11), 378–383.
15. Bozkurt, M. R., Yurtay, N., Yilmaz, Z., & Sertkaya, C. (2014). Comparison of different methods for determining diabetes. *Turkish Journal of Electrical Engineering and Computer Sciences, 22*(4), 1044–1055.
16. Iyer, A., Jeyalatha, S., & Sumbaly, R. (2015). Diagnosis of diabetes using classification mining techniques. *arXiv preprint arXiv:1502.03774.*
17. Dewangan, A. K., & Agrawal, P. (2015). Classification of diabetes mellitus using machine learning techniques. *International Journal of Engineering and Applied Sciences, 2*(5), 145.
18. Sivanesan, R., Devika, K., & Dhivya, R. (2017). A review on diabetes mellitus diagnoses using classification on pima Indian diabetes data set. *International Journal of Advance Research in Computer Science and Management Studies, 5*, 1.
19. Nabi, M., Wahid, A., & Kumar, P. (2017). Performance analysis of classification algorithms in predicting diabetes. *International Journal of Advanced Research in Computer Science, 8*, 3.
20. Maniruzzaman, M., Kumar, N., Abedin, M., Islam, M. S., Suri, H. S., El-Baz, A. S., & Suri, J. S. (2017). Comparative approaches for classification of diabetes mellitus data: Machine learning paradigm. *Computer Methods and Programs in Biomedicine, 152*, 23–34.
21. Sisodia, D., & Sisodia, D. S. (2018). Prediction of diabetes using classification algorithms. *Procedia Computer Science, 132*, 1578–1585.
22. Aishwarya, R., & Gayathri, P. (2013). *A method for classification using machine learning technique for diabetes*. ACM.
23. Maniruzzaman, M., Rahman, M. J., Al-MehediHasan, M., Suri, H. S., Abedin, M. M., El-Baz, A., & Suri, J. S. (2018). Accurate diabetes risk stratification using machine learning: Role of missing value and outliers. *Journal of Medical Systems, 42*(5), 92.
24. Dey, N., & Ashour, A. (2016). *Classification and clustering in biomedical signal processing*. IGI Global Hershey.
25. Saba, L., Dey, N., Ashour, A. S., Samanta, S., Nath, S. S., Chakraborty, S., Sanches, J., Kumar, D., Marinho, R. T., & Suri, J. S. (2016). Automated stratification of liver disease in ultrasound: An online accurate feature classification paradigm. *Computer Methods and Programs in Biomedicine, 130*, 118–134.
26. Chatterjee, S., Dey, N., Shi, F., Ashour, A. S., Fong, S. J., & Sen, S. (2018). Clinical application of modified bag-of-features coupled with hybrid neural- based classifier in dengue fever classification using gene expression data. *Medical & Biological Engineering & Computing, 56*(4), 709–720.
27. Ahmed, S., Dey, N., Ashour, A. S., Sifaki-Pistolla, D., Bălas-Timar, D., Balas, V. E., & Tavares, J. M. R. S. (2017). Effect of fuzzy partitioning in Crohn's disease classification: A neuro-fuzzy-based approach. *Medical & Biological Engineering & Computing, 55*(1), 101–115.
28. Ahuja, R., Sharma, S. C., & Ali, M. (2019). A diabetic disease prediction model based on classification algorithms. In *Annals of emerging technologies in computing (AETiC)* (p. 2516). AETiC.
29. Frank, A. (2010). *Uci machine learning repository*. Retrieved from http://archive.ics.uci.edu/ml

30. Song, F., Mei, D., & Li, H. (2010). Feature selection based on linear discriminant analysis. In *2010 international conference on intelligent system design and engineering application* (Vol. 1, pp. 746–749). IEEE.
31. Shrivastava, V. K., Londhe, N. D., Sonawane, R. S., & Suri, J. S. (2016). Computer-aided diagnosis of psoriasis skin images with hos, texture and color features: A first comparative study of its kind. *Computer Methods and Programs in Biomedicine, 126*, 98–109.
32. Hasan, M. A. M., Nasser, M., & Pal, B. (2013). On the kdd'99 dataset: Support vector machine based intrusion detection system (ids) with different kernels. *International Journal of Computer and Communication Engineering, 4*(4), 1164–1170.
33. Geurts, P., & Louppe, G. (2011). Learning to rank with extremely randomized trees. *Proceedings of Machine Learning Research, 14*, 49–61.
34. Mwadulo, M. W. (2016). A review on feature selection methods for classification tasks.
35. Sapatinas, T. (2005). Discriminant analysis and statistical pattern recognition. *Journal of the Royal Statistical Society: Series A (Statistics in Society), 168*(3), 635–636.
36. Renuka Devi, M. (2016). Analysis of various data mining techniques to predict diabetes mellitus.
37. Nickisch, H., & Rasmussen, C. E. (2008). Approximations for binary Gaussian process classification. *Journal of Machine Learning Research, 9*, 2035–2078.
38. Akay, M. F. (2009). Support vector machines combined with feature selection for breast cancer diagnosis. *Expert Systems with Applications, 36*(2), 3240–3247.
39. Reinhardt, A., & Hubbard, T. (1998). Using neural networks for prediction of the subcellular location of proteins. *Nucleic Acids Research, 26*(9), 2230–2236.
40. Kégl, B. (2013). The return of AdaBoost. mh: Multi-class hamming trees. *arXiv preprint arXiv:1312.6086*.
41. Tabaei, B. P., & Herman, W. H. (2002). A multivariate logistic regression equation to screen for diabetes: Development and validation. *Diabetes Care, 25*(11), 1999–2003.
42. Acharya, U. R., Molinari, F., Sree, S. V., Chattopadhyay, S., Ng, K.-H., & Suri, J. S. (2012). Automated diagnosis of epileptic EEG using entropies. *Biomedical Signal Processing and Control, 7*(4), 401–408.
43. Breiman, L. (2001). Random forests. *Machine Learning, 45*(1), 5–32.
44. Dhakate, P., Rajeswari, K., & Abin, D. (2015). Analysis of different classifiers for medical dataset using various measures. *International Journal of Computer Applications, 111*(5), 20–25.
45. Schapire, R. E. (2003). The boosting approach to machine learning: An overview. In *Nonlinear estimation and classification* (pp. 149–171). Springer.
46. Cunningham, P., & Delany, S. J. (2020). k-nearest neighbour classifiers. arXiv preprint arXiv:2004.04523.
47. Srivastava, S. K., Singh, S. K., & Suri, J. S. (2020). A healthcare text classification system and its performance evaluation: A source of better intelligence by characterizing healthcare text. In *Cognitive informatics, computer modelling, and cognitive science* (pp. 319–369). Elsevier.
48. McCallum, A., & Nigam, K. (1998). A comparison of event models for naive Bayes text classification. In *AAAI-98 workshop on learning for text categorization* (Vol. 752, pp. 41–48). Citeseer.

Chapter 17
Blockchain Technology for Healthcare Record Management

Mohammad Faisal, Halima Sadia, Tasneem Ahmed, and Nashra Javed

17.1 Introduction

In 2019, the world healthcare market size was estimated at around 281.8 billion US dollars and is expected to increase from 2021 to 2030 at a compound annual growth rate (CAGR) of 7.9%. The demand for value-based healthcare as per patient's preferences has seen a visible rise with the growing population across the globe. By 2050, the number of older individuals is expected to double to 1.5 billion. More patient-centered healthcare services are needed by the ageing population, which is further increasing the demand for healthcare human resource and agencies, which is going to actually drive the business growth [1–5]. A representation of previous years' healthcare expenditure across the world is shown below in Fig. 17.1:

The creation of the healthcare industry was motivated by increased spending on chronic pathologies, including cancer, diabetes, and hypertension, in both general and specialty medicine. These now account for 75% of the world's diagnosed illnesses.

Healthcare covers all of the programs, goods, equipment, and facilities used in disease prevention, treatment, and management for protecting mental and physical well-being. Various industries cover the entire market, such as the alternative medicine market, the organization of health facilities and medical equipment, the supply

M. Faisal (✉) · T. Ahmed · N. Javed
Advanced Computing and Research Laboratory, Department of Computer Application, Integral University, Lucknow, Uttar Pradesh, India
e-mail: mdfaisal@iul.ac.in; tasneemfca@iul.ac.in; nashra@iul.ac.in

H. Sadia
Department of Computer Science and Engineering, Integral University, Lucknow, Uttar Pradesh, India
e-mail: halima@iul.ac.in

M. S. Husain et al. (eds.), *Pervasive Healthcare*, EAI/Springer Innovations in Communication and Computing, https://doi.org/10.1007/978-3-030-77746-3_17

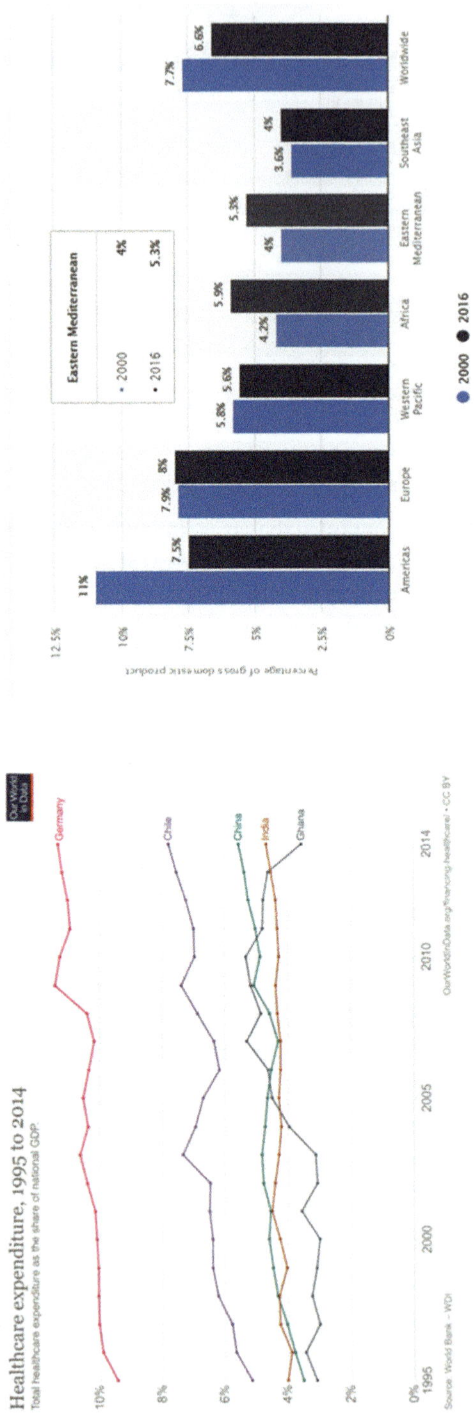

Fig. 17.1 Previous years' analysis of healthcare expenditure [2]

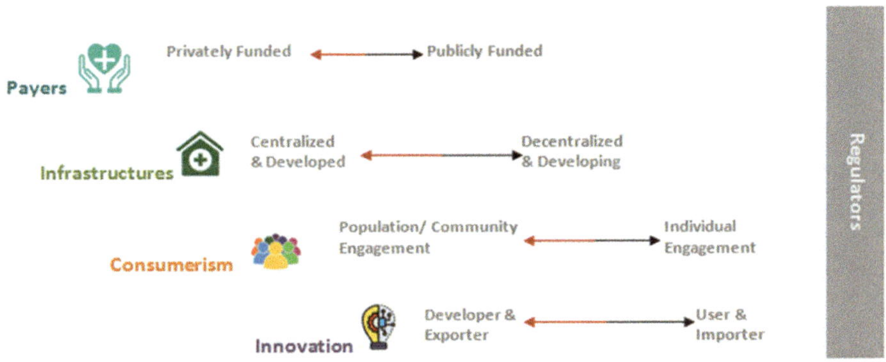

Fig. 17.2 Different components of a healthcare system

of organs, and, more indirectly, veterinary services. The e-healthcare industry is also gaining traction, thanks to broadband and telecommunication technologies.

Health insurance, prescription drugs, medical devices, biologics, and veterinary healthcare are segmented by type in the healthcare industry. The largest segment of the healthcare sector was healthcare facilities, accounting for 79.4% of the total in 2018. Pharmaceutical products, medical devices, and then the other segments followed. There are common components to health systems, even though the levels of growth and speed of change vary across countries. The various components of a healthcare system include funding from different payers, a decentralized infrastructure, dedicated service to an individual, and effective innovative solutions (Fig. 17.2).

17.1.1 Major Challenges in the Healthcare Industry

All over the world, health services are having problems that lead to increased costs [6] or lower results for health (mortality and morbidity) [7]. The healthcare area is diverse and comprises doctors from more than 120 health specialties and subspecialties [8], containing other professionals, scientists, and patients who face a range of challenges associated with increased patient data fragmentation. This is further exacerbated by diverse data systems and workflows. Data protection concerns created by the law of data sharing and the risk of financial consequences associated with data sharing have impeded the exchange of health information among other things [9]. The main challenge that persists is the capacity to share a patient's health information among numerous healthcare continuum [10].

The varied features listed in Fig. 17.3 were found to be of high importance across customer segments.

Challenge #1: How Can We Reduce Healthcare Costs?

The life spans of humans have increased compared to the past, and this indicates how we have progressed in the medical advancements. But the challenge is the

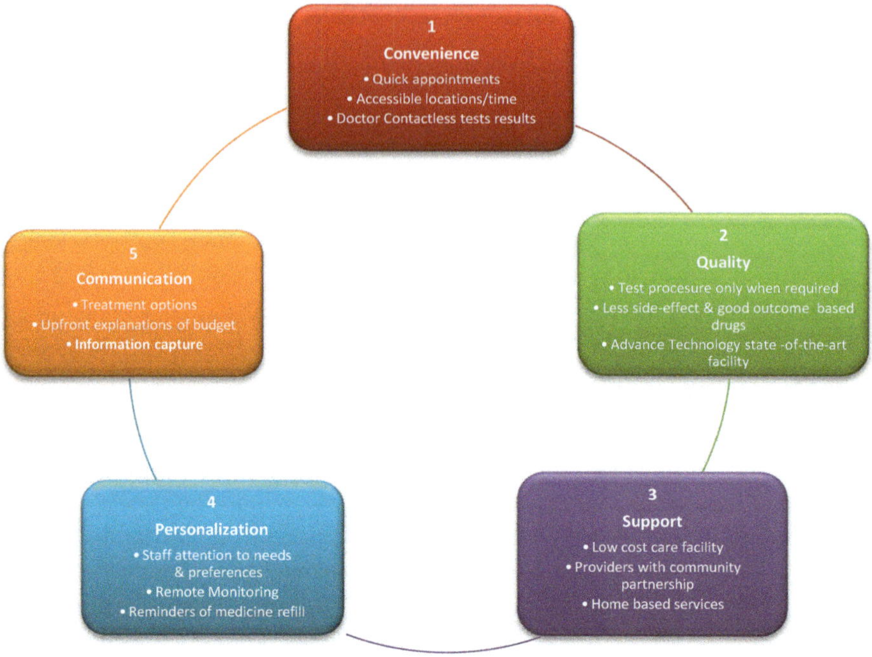

Fig. 17.3 Five pillars of customer healthcare services for patients

longer the people live, more healthcare resources must be manufactured in order to provide good health and better lifestyles. This rise in demand has escalated the cost of medical facilities for living beings. As per the Centers for Medicare and Medicaid Services (CMS) in the United States, health spending is about to increase by an average rate of 5.5% from the year 2017 to 2026, by which point it will account for approximately 20% of the US economy. Overall, by 2026, US health spending is projected to exceed at least $5.7 trillion, led largely by higher drug costs. Prevention as a solution will serve as an essential step in solving the issue of increasingly rising healthcare costs. Efforts should be taken to avoid a chronic illness that, in the short term, is more cost-effective than the cure of the disease. Although a multipronged response plan would follow the path to avoiding any epidemic in order to be successful, technical innovations are likely to play a crucial role.

Wearable devices or sensors offer real-time tracking of anything from the level of movement to heartbeat, blood pressure, and blood glucose levels—a benefit of on-the-go health monitoring. By infusing the pervasive adoption of this technology with data analytics, the future of contactless patient health monitoring is promising, and it will directly intervene to reduce the cost incurred from chronic diseases.

Challenge #2: How Can We Minimize the Inadequacies in Healthcare Services?

Healthcare is an odd industry, as in some countries, it uses both extremely high-tech solutions, such as genome sequencing and augmented reality, and extremely low-tech processes, such as paper records, which later need to be digitized.

This is not only counterproductive but is also uneconomical. Moreover, administrative expenses play a major role in the increase of healthcare costs. It is a proven fact that half of the money spent yearly on healthcare management is mostly wasted in some countries. The action taken for reducing these inefficiencies will work as a solution to address broad-ranging concerns afflicting healthcare. One of such processes that needs an immediate automation is patient record sharing.

Each time a patient changes doctor or hospital, the records are usually physically copied or delivered as paper copies or faxed to a new healthcare provider, which takes time and often results in incomplete records. This would have a disastrous result on patients who are undergoing some complex treatments, and for them, complete records are a must to avoid any type of risks.

Numerous tools and technologies have been explored to address these concerns. One potential solution may be the use of blockchain for storing and sharing patient records. It would lead to the preservation of accurate and precise records with efficient protection in the transmission of medical records such that patient privacy is protected along with data integrity.

Challenge #3: How Can We Improve Accessibility of Healthcare Facilities?

To benefit from the recent advancements in medical industry, the foremost thing is that every individual must have proper accessibility. But this is not the case, and access to healthcare is not uniformly spread both in socioeconomic and geographical terms.

As per the Office of Disease Prevention and Health Promotion (ODPHP), accessibility to healthcare is categorized into three distinct problems:

1. Insurance coverage: To check if a patient can afford the cost of treatment for both acute and chronic illness
2. Geographic availability: To ensure what geographic proximity does a patient have for accessing healthcare services and facilities
3. Timeliness of care: To track whether a patient treats a medical problem adequately in a timely way or whether it is a life-threatening accident or a recurrent illness that progresses slowly

The problems of timeliness of care and geographic availability have already been reported via modern technology, with support from devices like laptops, tablets, and smartphones that can simplify an online appointment without physically visiting the doctor. The rapid rise in the prevalence of telemedicine and e-visits enables patients to virtually interact with their caregivers—an ultimate aid to those who are living in hard-to-reach locations and remote areas. Technological advancements addressed the healthcare services for maximum possible access to the healthcare workers.

Challenge #4: How Can We Enhance the Quality of Care?

As we discuss about healthcare, most of the time, we spent inquiring queries about improving or enhancing the "quality of care." As we discuss healthcare, most of the time is spent querying about how to improve or enhance the "quality of care". These questions try to address: 'how do we confirm that a patient receives the needed support and treatment in order to receive a fruitful result?'

The question is quite common, but the solution is not that easy to list out, as it often needs a multifaceted methodology. Healthcare providers can significantly enhance the quality of care by always maintaining their patient-focused thinking, and acknowledged challenges, especially for an excessively burdened and chronically understaffed healthcare system. There is no threshold deciding the number of patients that can be treated by a single physician or a team of nurses, that ensures the standard of treatment does not deteriorate.

Although solving the shortage of physicians and nurses should be a top priority, it is likely that technology will act as a backbone and buffer against mistakes that could have significant adverse effects on patient outcomes before this is sorted out.

The inclusion of telemedicine or virtual visit can facilitate specialist consultations when a physician is not available. Also, modern technologies such as machine learning (ML), artificial intelligence (AI), and big data analytics are contributing to the identification of patients with postoperative infections, higher risk of hospital-borne illness, or other issues, helping their caregivers to avoid any complications.

Challenge #5: How Can We Make Patient-Specific Medicines?

The advent of medications which could be used to cure vast quantities of the population at once was a game-changer for the field of medicine. Broad-spectrum antibiotics and mass-produced pharmaceuticals have ushered in the era of industrialized medicine that we now live in.

Unfortunately, these therapies have often had a range of severe effects. For example, overuse and overdependence on broad-spectrum antibiotics have contributed to an increase in antibiotic-resistant diseases, while our overreliance on universal pharmacology has often led to catastrophic and unintended consequences for some patients.

It is for this reason that the future of medicine and pharmacology is likely to be patient-specific care, medication, and therapies. For instance, doctors are progressively conducting tests to determine the particular antibiotic that would be most effective in treating a disease as a substitute of using a broad-spectrum antibiotic to treat any infection. Doctors are gradually developing medications to be patient-specific to confirm efficacy, especially essential in diseases like cancer, instead of predicting that a patient will respond well to a certain medication.

This treatment is primarily driven by the emerging field of nanomedicine, which facilitates the development and implementation of patient-specific drugs and molecules for more efficient treatment. Tools such as sensors and wearable trackers that enable healthcare professionals to track the results of their cures and the use of artificial intelligence that can analyze vast quantities of data to decide which treatments are ideally suited to a specific condition or patient are also significant.

17.1.2 Solution via ICT for Healthcare Challenges

When the Declaration of Alma-Ata was agreed four decades ago, ICT (information and communications technologies) freshly emerged. The implementation of these innovations in health services at that time was limited, expensive, and complicated. There were no ubiquitous innovations such as laptops, notebook, and smartphones of today. These technologies have demonstrated remarkable significance in the health sector as they have become more extensive and more integrated in all areas and progressive in the community.

Through ICT, the quality of care that patients receive can be given in their comfort zone and home environments, with access to the needful resources to assist in times of crisis. A blended environment is delivered to reduce the immediate requirement of hospital facilities, and the need to visit will be limited to only severe emergencies. If that's the case, all emergency services would be fully linked by necessity to address urgent or immediate concern. To successfully provide greater service efficiency and self-care, home care facilities and hospitals should be combined. A remarkable trend in national healthcare technology policies (over 120 countries by 2015) ensures a valuable adherence to just using digital technologies to meet production goals, facilitate universal health insurance, and influence healthcare services. ICT advances are increasingly transforming and modernizing the functionality of the healthcare sector as well as how people can communicate to the sources of healthcare. As well as different geographical populations, medical researchers require access to comprehensive clinical trials which provide unique perspective in genes, illnesses, and consequences of treatment. Healthcare workers may link patient records with several different patients, predict the risk, and incorporate the modern technology to recommend proactive treatment. ICT has given medical tourism a massive boost, enabling patients to interact for advice and additional opinions with experts in virtually every part of the world, no matter where they are situated by themselves. Via virtual contact like videoconferences/video calls, patients will then fly to several other countries to undergo specialist care or clinically superior treatment. The new technologies have also taken a significant and beneficial move forward in the medical industry. Patients are now exposed to some of the latest medical procedures, new and cutting-edge treatments, and even some slightly invasive operations, leading to decreased pain and quicker recovery.

Better clinical results or an overall superior healthcare service has resulted in remote specialist consultations, customized therapies, and the availability of interactive mobile applications. Increase of quality in patient's health with the advancement of emerging treatments leads to better outcomes. Various classes with healthcare facilities through ICT applications are shown in Fig. 17.4.

Some of the major factors are explained below, which defined how the healthcare industry has been changed with the inclusion of the information and communications technology. The factors are defined as:

1. Switching to digital health records: Slow, dusty, and heavy paperwork allows access to secured simplified digital documents remotely accessible to patients

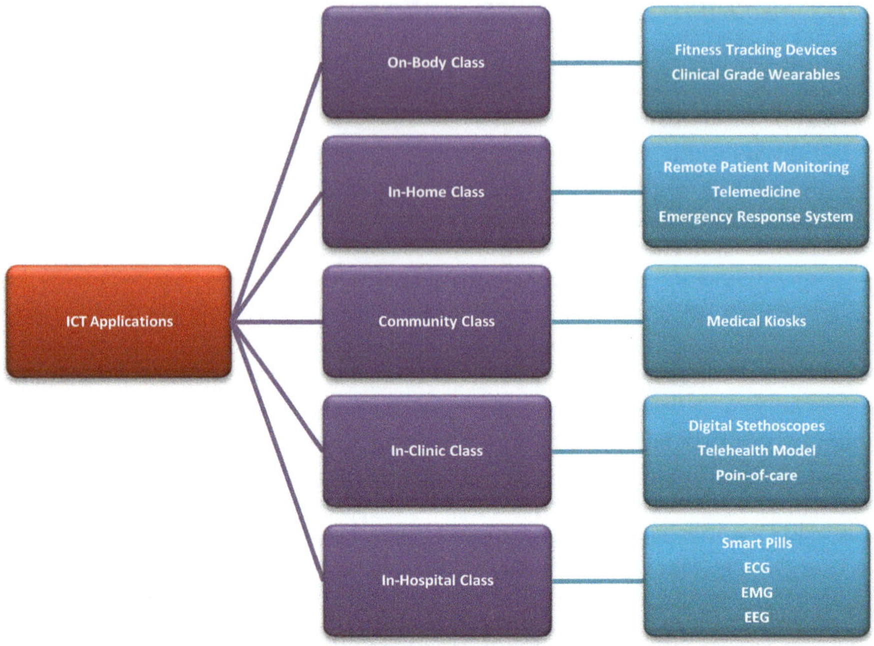

Fig. 17.4 Different classes with healthcare facilities through ICT applications

and healthcare providers. It simplifies and speeds up the storage, management, and transmission of data. Guidance to professionals and patients is delivered for professional decisions, making it easier and safer for more informed medical decisions. Health record digitization also promotes quality and accessibility to remote or inaccessible areas. This modernization is capable of streamlining operations, enhancing patient quality, and reducing costs.

2. Use of wearable devices and smartphone applications in healthcare: Patients not only have access through their mobile devices to fast and reliable medical records but can also use the applications to make appointments and receive medication reminders. Health and fitness apps help people become healthier by tracking food consumption and activity levels. They also offer customized solutions and diet plans for an individual to track daily calories.

   By minimizing the time spent on registrations, updating records, and other repetitive steps, software can help doctors in high-stress jobs. Mobile applications offer accessibility to medication knowledge to prevent side effects and interactions, solve complications, and boost diagnostics. Specialists can communicate directly with their patients, record their vital signs correctly, keep track of visits and appointments, and achieve higher procedural efficacy.

   A smartwatch software that is used on a regular basis by patients to monitor their moods and thoughts can also track major depressive disorder (MDD). Wearable technology has definite potential to do more than count steps; in this case, it could be used in real time to measure the effects of depression. A depression app may give patients and healthcare providers more insight into the situation, like other IoT healthcare applications.

Many apps will help you manage depression and anxiety, such as Moodpath, TalkLife, Daylio, Youper, etc. Apple has recently released an anti-depression app that is compatible with an Apple smartwatch. It studies patients' moods and offers knowledge that lets doctors deliver the treatment they need for patients.

3. Preferring electronic medical records (EMR) and electronic health records (EHR): These are defined as automated accounts of patient medical histories, in which diagnosis, laboratory findings, information about hospital admissions, surgical procedures, and medicines can be included. They provide a description of the patient's condition, which allows for more detailed diagnosis and treatment of the patient. Without time and money investment on paper delivery, these electronic documents promote the simple exchange of knowledge and cooperation between laboratories and specialists. EHRs provide knowledge, particularly relevant if the patient is ignorant, about patient allergies and intolerances and anything else that could be appropriate to healthcare practitioners. EHR guidelines could also enhance compliance and decrease malpractice when adequately managed and implemented. It is easier to design and operate electronic archives and takes less time to create and maintain them. For medical accountants, they make things simple and reduce the risk of making errors.
4. Managing big data on cloud: Big data is a fast-growing and promising field, especially in healthcare for identifying high-risk and high-cost patients. That is why it is currently able to make and gather huge amounts of data from a wide range of various sources in the field of healthcare. This information is then used for analytics, preventing casualties and ultimately anticipating possible pandemics. Cloud data storage, while minimizing data storage waste, encourages efficiency and accessibility to be improved. It further aids in the understanding and advancement of better medical and pharmaceutical preventive drug procedures. In fact, cloud systems can be useful for medical science, offer vast volumes of health data for research and analytics, and promote the efficient exchange of health data. Cloud computing delivers reliable and cost-effective computing options but without the difficulty and complexity of maintaining extra server infrastructure, including backup and recovery capabilities.
5. Improving patient care: ICTs have provided the medical community with a range of powerful tools for improving patient care. Increase easy access to EHR doctors so patients can see complete medical history and make medical decisions. Possible medication errors could be quickly identified by the doctors. With applications such as barcode scanners, they can achieve this and, as a result, increase patient protection. The patients' vitals and temperature can also be received through Radio Frequency Identification Technology (RFID), which is helpful in improving patient care. This makes it easier to track location, communication, and identification in real time. 3D printing is also used to improve healthcare technology and patient care, which nowadays is used in hearing aids, prosthetics, and customized dental equipment. In older individuals and patients

with mental disabilities, augmented reality systems and software help to relieve symptoms of anxiety and stress and can also aid adults in their postoperative rehabilitation process. Virtual reality may also play an important role in healthcare, which ensures that surgeons and their teams have accurate, complex procedures. In particular, interactive and virtual reality devices for physicians can improve health and fitness performance as well. The availability of procedures such as robotic knee replacement and the use of gene therapy in the treatment of cancer, as well as the role of technology in healthcare, have been determined to expand rapidly in the near future.

6. Introducing Telemedicine or e-Health: It conveys the digital transformation of healthcare toward the next big thing: nearly everywhere in the world, empowering patients to consult with doctors. This is a healthcare system infrastructure used to resolve distance barriers and promote medical care in case of an emergency, possibly trying to save lives. Telemedicine has made it much easier for patients to access e-health equipment through different software and videotelephony to obtain home treatment and assistance. In telehealth, to allow asynchronous appointments (that would not require all patients to be available or online at the same time), the store-and-forward functionality helps to transfer biosignals, diagnostic images, or other data to an expert. This will dramatically decrease patients' waiting time and will also accelerate methods of healthcare services. Telemedicine makes online supervision of patients by medical practitioners simpler. With the help of multiple applications and devices, it will serve to efficiently and economically treat critical health illnesses. In addition, real-time digital systems make it easier for individuals to consult healthcare providers remotely. Basically, this is possible through videoconferencing, which assists in the patient's counseling, disease diagnosis, and therapy management.

17.2 Pervasive Computing and Healthcare

In the past few years, ubiquitous or pervasive computing systems have made crucial advancements in the healthcare sector. This has been used to develop sensor design and development, wearable devices, wireless and mobile networks, and smart places and houses. In this chapter, current and evolving developments in pervasive computing have been addressed first and then presented how ubiquitous computing will contribute to pervasive healthcare. The most common examples are smart emergency management assistance, mobile health-related equipment, telemedicine, lifestyle promotion, inventory management systems, and access to health information. We also identified the various healthcare requirements and suggest challenges and open disputes for research in this area.

One of the most important quotes on computers is the words of Mark Weiser: "The most profound technologies are those that disappear. They weave themselves into the fabric of everyday life until they are indistinguishable from it" [11]. It is so deeply ingrained in our lives that technologies are no longer seen as something separate, which can have a strong impression or influence on us. This phenomenon is the base of pervasive and ubiquitous computing. Ubiquitous is anything that is accessible at any moment everywhere, and anything that is permeated in the atmosphere is ubiquitous. Implanted, wearable, compact, and environmental are the four separate implementations of ubiquitous technology. On both of these, the degree of indistinguishably varies, as implantable technology may be fully transparent, wearable devices could be slightly noticeable, and handheld devices may be more prominent. Environmental technologies could also become indistinguishable, based on the degree of integration, like using televisions with smart displays.

17.2.1 Pervasive Healthcare

Increased connectivity of healthcare facilities, more productive procedures, and significantly higher level of healthcare services contribute to the implementation of telecommunication technology in the healthcare industry. However, challenges around the world including medical errors, stress on health workers, and partial coverage of services in rural areas still persist [12, 13]. It has created major challenges for government, healthcare professionals, clinics, health insurance companies, and patients, along with a rapid increase in price for medical services. There is an unprecedented rise in the number of seniors and retirees in developing countries. Improving healthcare services for a growing number of people who are using limited financial and human resources remains a huge challenge. New and evolving wireless technology will improve the overall QoS (quality of services) for patients in urban and rural areas by changing the overall quality of patient care by removing the strain and stress of healthcare workers, increasing their efficiency, and providing standard of living and quality of life. Mostly medical errors are caused by a lack of accurate and complete information about the place and time of consumption, resulting in misdiagnosis and problems with drug interactions [14]. Patients can receive the required medical information at anytime from anywhere using sophisticated equipment and widespread wireless networks. Wireless technology can be efficiently and economically exploited by connecting infrastructure services to healthcare requirements. To improve the availability of healthcare facilities, fast, flexible, and versatile wireless communications based healthcare services such as the use of smart devices, user interface, location tracking, short-range wireless communications, and the use of body sensors to monitor health are used. It provides a trustworthy communication between medical teams, patients, healthcare professionals, and vehicles for effective emergency management. Wireless infrastructure access, portability, and reuse for long-term patient surveillance and preventive treatment would minimize the total expense of health services. The implementation of wireless wellness technology and the usage of wireless sensors in seamless health surveillance applications that are minimally invasive are discussed [15]. In a maritime multilingual telemedicine infrastructure, using satellite and ground-based networks to facilitate multimedia communications is represented [16]. Using the network sensors and databases and the deployment of pervasive computing technologies at the facility's emergency room where residents are alerted when they need immediate help is implemented [12]. Further, the health-promoting helper is designed to sense pulse waves, user movements, and shapes and to capture contextual images and regular sounds. With the help of the obtained contextual information, the state of high pressure (stress) is determined by the high pulse rate [13]. The data is maintained on a website and retrieved and needs adjustment to fit on smaller portable devices. It has been reported in [17] that as long as they really promote independent living, the elderly are able to continue using wireless technologies. A summary of m-general health's problems can be found in [14]. In [15], an overview of "personal wellness programs" and associated technology and use scenarios is given. The use of current wireless and mobile technologies in healthcare includes tablets, handheld devices, pagers, and other intelligent devices to interconnect with health specialists and can acquire patient data. Wireless paging networks (a combination of terrestrial and satellite networks) and wireless LAN were used earlier for the same purpose. Surveillance systems, including smart shirts, are becoming widely available to acquire, record, and track one or more significant signals, such as blood pressure. Wired networks, such as mobile networks, are used for most modern control systems. Many ongoing tests include a medical app and a wireless connection.

Pervasive healthcare could be described as "the provision of medical care to any person and to any person, by improving both the quality and quality of medical care and the removal of land, time and other restrictions." This covers diagnosis, preservation, and supervision of healthcare; short-term surveillance (home healthcare supervision), long-term tracking (nursing home), and customized tracking of healthcare; and diagnosis and management of incidence, emergency response, and transport and care. Health promotion applications include comprehensive health surveillance, an emergency management system, health information dissemination, and telemedicine everywhere. Wireless networking solutions comprise of wireless LAN, temporary wireless networks, networks focused on mobile/GSM/3G infrastructure, and satellite-based systems as shown in Fig. 17.5.

17.2.2 Open Issues and Challenges in Pervasive Computing Implementation

There are a number of challenges and open issues in implementing the pervasive approach to healthcare. This included the lack of comprehensive wireless and wireless network coverage, the reliability of wireless networks, the overall shortcomings of available technology, the clinical need for devices and control equipment, patient learning, other system intrusion, privacy and protection, and common health problems. It is observed that in pervasive computing data, security issues are very challenging and may create several controversies. From a brief literature, it is observed that patients use a wide range of healthcare systems if the information obtained

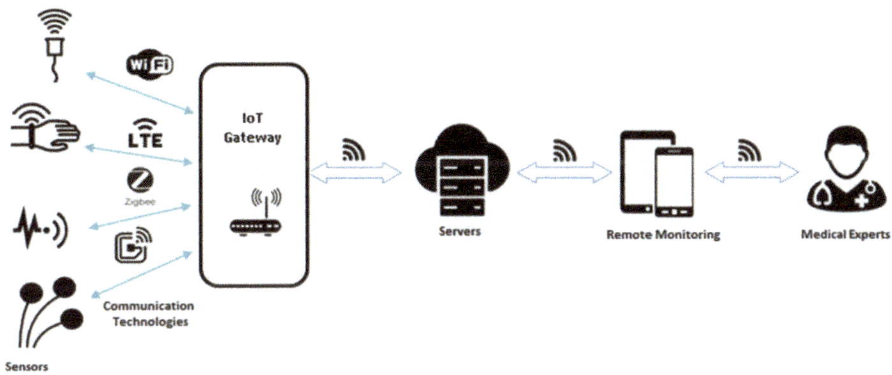

Fig. 17.5 Components of pervasive healthcare

from them can only be retrieved and used by reliable individuals, such as their family members, caregivers, and health professionals.

More investigation is required for pervasive healthcare to overcome these challenges. Technology issues related to ubiquitous healthcare include network support like site tracking, scalable architectures, reliability, access quality, routing, in what way to deliver health nursing in different environmental conditions (hospital, nursing home, assisted living, indoor, and outdoor), continuous vs. patient-based tracking, use of mobile devices for data storage, updating and broadcast of medical information, detection and transmission of vital signs via LAN, formation of ad hoc wireless networks for better patient monitoring, management of emergency medical care vehicles, and routing of network support for mobile telemedicine. The development and implementation of a robust wireless health monitoring system can overcome wireless health monitoring problems in terms of reliability.

Detailed investigation will also be required to measure the adverse effects of using long-term tracking systems on patient, and the implementation of pervasive healthcare may be affected due to these reasons. In the realization of a broad-scale application of wireless in healthcare, medical implications are very important. It is important to discuss the concerns of how healthcare is handled and how medical records should be interpreted and the interests of different patients. The most important issues are the development of appropriate health applications, the requirements of important health indicators, the variety of patients and their special requirements, the coverage of medical information in the general medical field (multimedia, solutions, processing, and care requirements), medical role protocols, healthcare improving services, and the use of wireless solutions in healthcare. This control can be used to monitor the behavior of children and how to avoid confusion and delusion for patients with dementia. A major problem is the use of uncomfortable infrastructure for people with mental illnesses caused by limited functional intelligence or memory impairment (e.g., mental retardation). Most patients are paranoid of wireless technology, particularly those that require the patient to wear a tracking device or other wearable gadgets. Any of the problems may be solved by supplying patients with training on the utility and accessibility of their treatment technology. Such type of circumstances can be ignored as a result of tracking of equipment by healthcare providers and others, as few patients must not be informed that their device is malfunctioning or not working properly.

In the future, it may be wise to self-check devices for malfunctions. Healthcare promotion management can lead to a small revolution in how wireless communication are implemented, proposed, and properly managed in the health sector. Many complex and diverse management concerns need to be addressed, including wireless healthcare protection and safety, preparing healthcare practitioners for pervasive healthcare, wireless integration management, growing wireless healthcare coverage, legal and regulatory issues, insurance incentives and costs, as well as the possible effects of the HIPAA (Health Insurance Portability and Accountability Act 1996). The main challenge is the accessibility and application of wireless-based technologies in healthcare. The systems should be configured to provide user-friendly interfaces capable of learning from individuals. Many of the population's less tech-savvy segments have been shown to be willing to learn and use mobile wireless technology to allow them to live very comfortably. As more and more of them use mobile and wireless technology, training healthcare professionals to use mobile and wireless technologies efficiently will become more challenging. Another important issue is how to reduce the cost of medical treatment for as many individuals as possible using mobile technology. Legal and regulatory concerns, such as liability issues and the risk of insurance providers not covering or paying accordingly for treatment through mobile devices, and other problems face the large-scale deployment of cellular networks in healthcare. Another big problem is privacy and potential abuse of patient care records. The HIPAA, intended to secure such records, has received some criticism in the United States and has been viewed differently by key parties, healthcare providers, insurers, and lawyers. Therefore, work is required to resolve wireless and mobile network privacy and related issues where protection is still seen as lacking. It should be found that in the short term, universal and widespread computing will contribute to the expense of healthcare, but particularly when treating chronic diseases, it can minimize the long-term cost. Many of the pervasive healthcare technologies have been reality before; further effort is required to change the financial and regulatory system to facilitate study, growth, and implementation of technical solutions for widespread healthcare.

17.3 Electronic Medical Records (EMR) and Electronic Health Records (EHR)

Systems focused on electronic medical records (EMR) have historically helped to address the digitization and exchange of health information within a health institution. In a similar way, personal health records (PHR) systems were also promoted to effectively monitor patient data in the healthcare continuum.

The essence of the continuum of healthcare, however, has changed to some extent. A dynamic multi-to-many knowledge sharing regime is required to support instruments such as machine learning and other innovations for enhanced treatment. Earlier, health organizations resolve this sharing need by trust agreements on a case-to-case basis.

A trusted third party is required to exchange information, including patient data, in the modern digital environment. Network associations for the health information exchange (HIE) have now emerged and are used to execute exchange deals between hospitals, clinical areas, regulators, insurers, and even patients [18]. They are assisting to make comprehensive health systems with the complete electronic health records (EHR) [19]. This current approach has been criticized for less transparency and for having a centralized ownership of authority, attacks, and failure [20]. Trust deficit on the protection and privacy of patient information entrusted by these intermediaries' intentional or unwitting acts is on the rise.

EMRs are digital representations of the clinical details of patients including identification, laboratory reports, diagnostic tests, prescriptions, and doctor's notes. One of the biggest healthcare challenges is the amount of sources from which the data may come and the sheer volume of data produced. Not all of this information is applicable to a specific illness or procedure, so it is also a great challenge to decide what is appropriate and what is not. EMR is an effort to bring together the most relevant data collection available for patient care. Therefore, the history of the patient, different tests and drugs, and billing details are generally included.

17.3.1 Benefits of Using EMR

As an important perspective, EMRs can be used concurrently by several users as opposed to paper-based documents, which are accessible round the clock to nearby and remote locations and are often readable [3]. The availability of EMR saves the patient, perhaps with errors of memorizing, from entering details in multiple pages of medical history and current care. EMR has shown a remarkable success in medical decision-making, although it entails substantial initial costs, which may reduce healthcare costs in the future. It has been proven that EMR also reduces the duration of stay in hospitals, decreases medication adverse effects, improves the quality of care, and decreases the practice gap [21]. Such benefits are titled as the most valuable information that is readily available in the medical records for effective decision-making, detection of possible drug reactions, and more standardized treatment of the patient. Moreover, written notes and prescriptions don't need to be interpreted and medical errors of old paper-based documentation will not exist in EMR. In Fig. 17.6, a procedure for representing the steps of EMR process is described.

The healthcare industry faces a challenge in the transitioning of EHR systems to combine paper-based records and EMRs. Different elements of clinical notes and laboratory findings have been processed using these systems [21]. Improving patient safety by avoiding errors and increasing access to information [22] has been

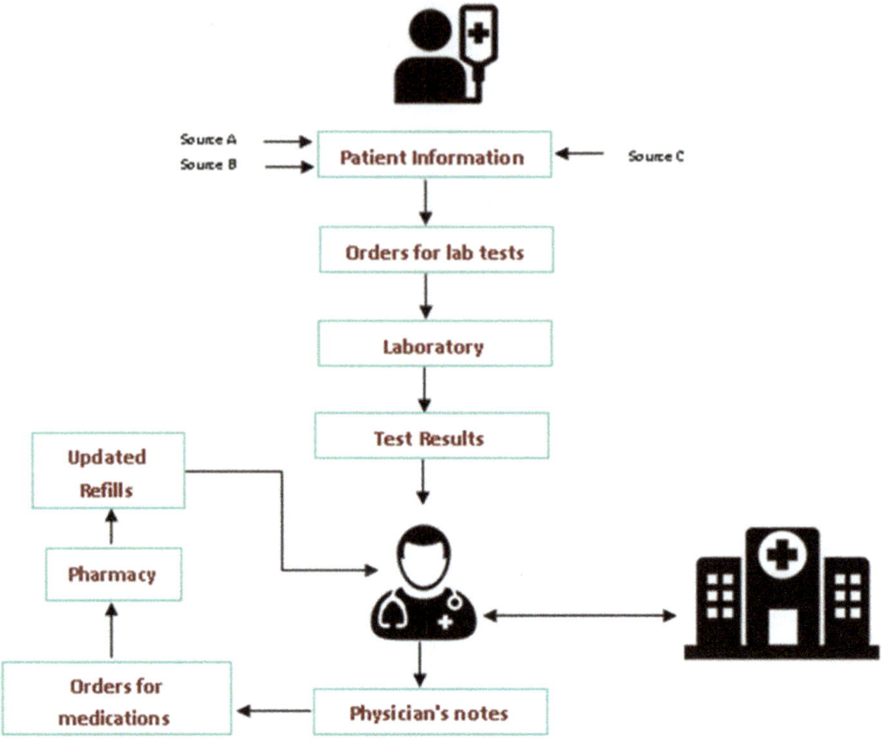

Fig. 17.6 Representation of EMR stepwise process

suggested. The premise behind the introduction of EHR programs was to address the concerns involved with the healthcare records in hardcopy and to include an effective mechanism that would enhance the healthcare industry's state of affairs [23].

Due to the advantages it offers, primarily the enhancement of protection and its cost-effectiveness, the implementation of EHR systems is done among a range of hospitals across the globe. They are considered as a critical part of the healthcare sector as it provides medical facilities with diverse functionalities [4]. Electronic medical record storage, patient appointment scheduling, billing and accounts, and laboratory testing are such functions which are easily available in most areas of the EHR scheme in the healthcare industry. The major emphasis is to provide temper-proof and safe shared medical information across several channels. Even though the motive behind the accumulation of EHR healthcare systems was to make improvement in its efficiency, these systems confronted few problems and did not meet their associated demands and standards [21]. A study in order to determine the practices of nursing/medical staff with the EHR was performed in Finland, and it concluded that these EHR systems have certain problems associated with them, like being unreliable and having a poor user-friendliness state [22].

The following are some issues faced when using the EHR method:

1. Interoperability: It's the way in which information can be exchanged between different information systems. Information should be exchangeable and available for additional purposes. A significant aspect of EHR systems is the health information exchange (HIE) or, in general, the sharing of data. Besides, the medical documents being shared should be interpreted at a technical level, and this piece of information may be used further [19].
2. Information asymmetry: Knowledge asymmetry is the biggest problem described by critics in the healthcare sector today, which means one party having more access to the information compared to the other party. While implementing EHR schemes, this issue undergoes when doctors or hospitals have to access the patient's records. Whenever a patient decides to retrieve his own medical records, very lengthy and frustrating processes have to be followed to access this information. The data is stored centrally by only a single healthcare agency, and authority to access it is only limited to very few hospitals or organizations.
3. Data breaches: In the healthcare sector, data breaches also call for the requirement of a stronger forum. A research [7] was conducted to examine data breaches in the EHR systems and revealed that approximately 173 million data entries since October 2009 have been compromised in EHR systems. One more study by Argaw et al. [8] summarizes that hospitals have turn out to be the center of attraction for cyberattackers [24–26]. In addition, many EHR systems are not configured to meet patients' needs and requirements and are faced with problems due to their inefficiency and poor adaptation [27].

The research also indicates that the use of EHRs has an adverse effect on the processing of information. EHRs were not designed to accommodate medical records that were multi-institutional and lifelong. Data is dispersed across multiple organizations as the patient's life events take them away from the data silo of one provider and into another. They lose easy access to previous data in doing so, as primary stewardship is usually held by the provider, not the patient [28, 29]. The blockchain architecture will certainly help to resolve this problem by positively developing the specifications and standards for interoperability, which addresses privacy and permits for the sharing of data securely across the systems. Adding flexibility to the framework by providing interoperability and open standards plays an important role in exchanging health data [28].

These issues make it reasonable to find a method to transform the patient-centered healthcare industry, i.e., blockchain, which would be most effective. Furthermore, a data integrity portal is secure and transparent and also provides the medical history of patients. The world should have a stable population in order to accomplish the desired improvement, and health records are estimates of a person's health over time. The world is moving toward progress. The centralized approach to the management of health records leads to data breaches.

According to the Data Breach Report of 2017 by Ponemon, the expected cost of data breach is projected to be $380 per record for healthcare organizations 27,314,647 patient records were affected, according to the 2016 Breach Barometer Survey. So, the shift toward an institution-driven record management strategy did not make any difference from the previous one. The risks of data being misused are high because the patient has no control over the data. So we need a fully decentralized, patient-centered solution that can detect data thefts, avoid data abuse, and provide the right to access control for patients.

Blockchain technology is the ultimate solution for resolving all issues and meeting healthcare requirements. As a decentralized and distributed ledger, it will also impact billing, sharing of record, medical testing, fraud identification, and financial data crimes in days to come. Implementing smart healthcare contracts will simplify things even further. It will be done using blockchain, during invocation, record creation, and validation.

17.3.2 EHR and EMR Integration with Blockchain

The exchange of key medical data with stakeholders while protecting data confidentiality and safeguarding patient privacy is one of the most critical issues faced by the healthcare industry today. It's true that the expectations for data are higher than they ever were. However, inconsistent workflows and a lack of ownership can also fall foul of EMRs. This can have a bad effect on decision-making and data veracity, which in turn, of course, affects the patient's treatment and care. At every step, there is now an increasing emphasis on organizing treatment and engaging the patient more. At each point of treatment, EMRs need to be available, and multiple stakeholders need to be able to display, edit, and exchange data while maintaining a reliable and up-to-date prescription and diagnosis record.

It makes perfect sense to use blockchain, considering that personal health data is so sensitive and subject to the challenges outlined above. It will update and secure the information stored inside an EMR and exchanged on a blockchain distributed ledger, ready to be used by anyone with permission to access it. A blockchain-based EMR solution will also decrease the time taken to access the data of the patient while improving the quality of data and interoperability.

Satoshi Nakamoto's Bitcoin white paper [30] popularized blockchain: a combination of two well-known technologies, i.e., peer-peer communication and cryptography. Initially conceptualized during the global financial crisis of 2008, the resulting Bitcoin blockchain inspired the widespread implementation of blockchain [31]. As an alternate solution to the largely centralized operating system for several sectors beyond finance, supporters of blockchain also highlighted high speed, lower costs, and security, amputation of a central point of authority, attacks, failures, less mistakes, and fault tolerance [31]. However, additional problems have arisen, which restrict its scalability [32].

Blockchain is a distributed ledger technology form of an increasingly ordered collection of documents database saved in a vast computer archive, that is, a shared ledger. This database consists of numerous interconnected devices that are not geographically restricted [32]. It does not require the network participants to trust each other because it has an integrated trust mechanism [33] that is cryptographically enabled. This network does not require mutual trust between network participants, as it contains an integrated trust mechanism enabled in cryptographic form [33]. Each entry in this ledger is referred to by cryptographic hashes as a connected and time-stamped block [34] and verified by peers in the network.

17.3.3 Components of a Blockchain

The basic components of blockchain technology are:

Block

As stated earlier, blockchain is defined as a peer-to-peer network designed by combining a number of blocks that are linked together, resulting in a decentralized application. A chain of blocks is formed where one block header has the hash of the preceding block. The data typically depends on the type of blockchain. The data is made up of coins, an electronic currency, as in the case of Bitcoin. The hash includes a cryptographic SHA-256 algorithm used to classify a block on the chain in a specific way.

The block contains the information given below:

1. Previous cryptographic hash: It is defined as the unique identifier which has been referenced from the previous (parent) block.
2. Timestamp: A timestamp value is associated with every block and denotes the approximate time of the respective block creation.
3. Merkle root hash: It is defined as the root hash of the Merkle tree. This hash value summarizes all the transactions used in a block.
4. Nonce: Abbreviated as "number used only once." It is defined as the number of cryptographic challenges that a node resolves to suggest a new block. It is a unique number assigned to a hashed block and satisfies the restrictions of the difficulty level when rehashed. This number is linked to algorithms for consensus.

Consensus Algorithm

Every block that has been added to the blockchain follows a set of rules for consensus. Blockchain technology makes use of consensus algorithms for this purpose. The most popular consensus algorithm used in the Bitcoin network is the proof of work (PoW) algorithm. The algorithm was used by Nakamoto [30]. According to this, a blockchain is a network that has a number of nodes or members, which uses mining to determine when a transaction is to be added to the network. Miners are the nodes performing these calculations [16].

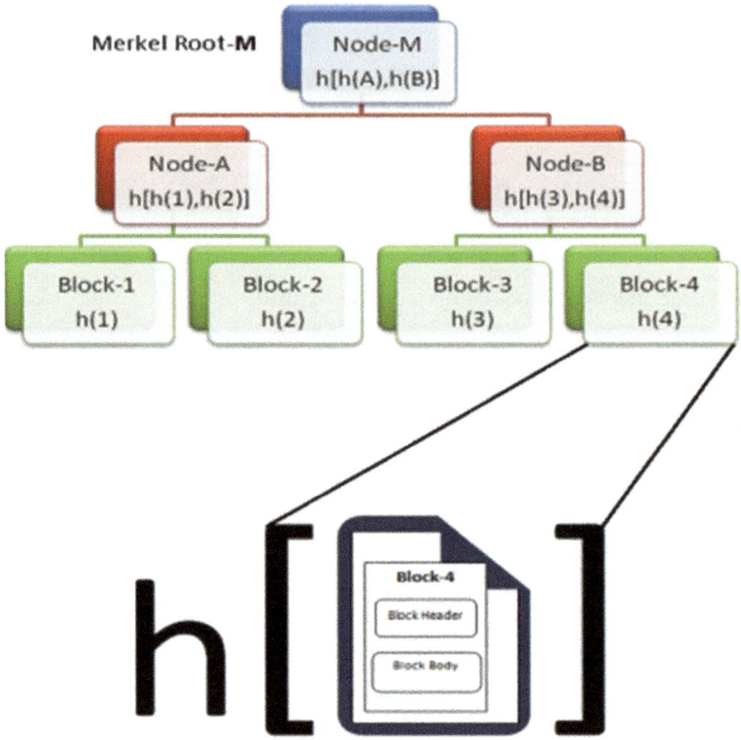

Fig. 17.7 Block in a public blockchain

Figure 17.7 shows the structure and content of a typical block used in a public blockchain network.

Bitcoin and Ethereum, the two largest public blockchain networks, make use of the binary hash structure used in the Merkel tree [10]. The hash value is the information to be registered in a block on these blockchains. A header and the message body are largely included in such details. A block edition, timestamp, Merkel root hash, nonce, parent hash, and complexity level are also included in the header. As the basic blockchain requires, the body of the block includes all the transactions that are packed altogether and represented as a list. A hash is an alphanumeric value string obtained on the data (header of the block) using a hash algorithm (e.g., SHA-2, SHA-256, etc.). The Merkel tree is a common method for confirming the integrity of a file or data against accidental malpractice or byzantine tempering in a distributed network.

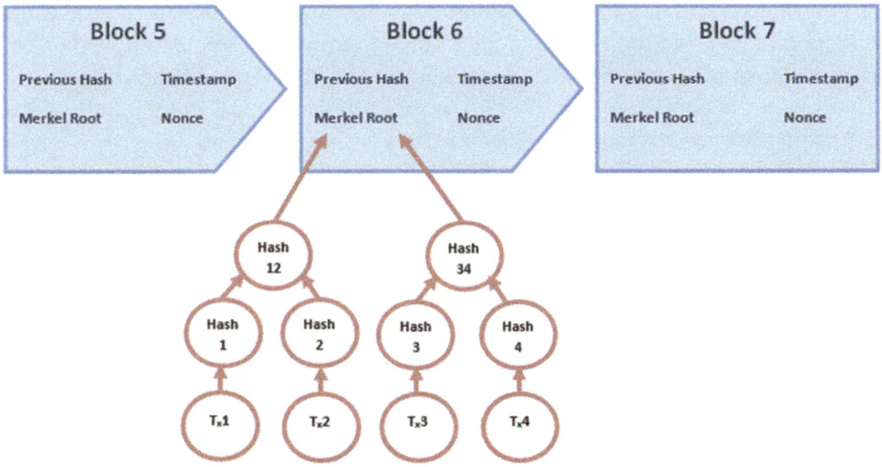

Fig. 17.8 Representation of blocks via the Merkle tree

Cryptography

Cryptography is being used in general to encrypt a message that cannot be deciphered by intermediaries or outside actors. It is a process of two-way exchange of the cipher to maintain confidentiality. The cipher can be encrypted or decrypted by each party to access the payload of the document. Cryptography is often used for the blockchain to verify data integrity. Using the message and key, the cryptographic algorithm produces a cipher text, defined as an encrypted style of the message. A key is always used for the decoding of cipher text into the original one, which can be shared with the sender and the receiver.

Merkle Tree It is used to minimize the amount of data and allow the data on the blockchain to be validated effectively. For each block, a Merkle root hash is stored. This is generated by hashing the transactions data (Fig. 17.8). There are four transactions in the following diagram (Tx). A hash of 1–4 reflects each of these transactions. Every hash pair is hashed again, i.e., hashing is applied twice (Hash 12 and Hash 34). The same is represented as the Merkle root hash in the parent block. It is used for summarizing all the transactions, hence resulting in an efficient validation. Since it produces a digital fingerprint of all the transactions that have happened, there is no need to verify the data per block. It is a binary hash tree where each transaction is hashed and the hash values per transactions are stored at the leaf nodes. The individual hashes are then paired, combined, and concatenated by hashing them together. A parent node is produced by doubly hashing the string.

The system uses a binary approach where the concatenation of siblings' hash values is contained by a parent node. The true power of the approach to the Merkel tree lies in its capability of verifying the transactions by only using the hash (Merkle path), instead of downloading the whole transactions. The timestamp is the value denoting the occurrence time associated with the respective transaction, and the nonce is a counter value used by miners for the proof of work. A value changed periodically within each blockchain network is the complexity level. Blockchain network users benefit from the freedom to perform and record transactions on the blockchain network with untrusted third parties.

The members in the blockchain network are provided with a pair of public and private keys. These pair of keys are used to send encrypted asymmetric cryptographic [32] messages using an underlying untrusted network. The encryption of a message or a transaction using a public or a private key enables the message to be read only by the holder of one of the corresponding key pair [33]. This message, called a validated message, is stored on the blockchain network and is connected using a one-way cryptography to the predecessor block and corresponding message metadata that is hashed to make sure of the immutability. With a minor change to the code, the "hash" value (fixed length text representing the transaction file) will also change. Hence, the block integrity is maintained this way.

At present, blockchains are the most common type of DLT [35]. It is possible to break blockchain technologies into three different categories [36]:

1. Public blockchains: In this variant of blockchain, all the nodes present in a distributed network may take part in the tracking and verification of data transactions and also in the process of consensus-making.
2. Consortium blockchains: A consortium blockchain is a partially decentralized network. The nature of the data can be either transparent or private. Typically, a node having jurisdiction and business-to-business partnerships has a probability of getting selected.
3. Private blockchains: In this, the nodes are limited. The blockchain has strict data access authority policies and will not include anyone.

17.4 Blockchain Networks

A blockchain network is created by a network of nodes, where the transaction ledger is stored, maintained, and updated. A copy of the shared database transactions is maintained by each and every node in the network. All the nodes synchronize continuously with the other nodes present on the network. The aim of the network is to reach a consensus, and at the same time, it ensures that every copy of the database that is shared on the network ledger is consistent and correct. The network is also responsible for validating each new block that has been added in the database. Networks provide algorithms or protocols to reach a consensus determining how nodes connect and communicate with each other. As consensus is achieved, every node performs synchronization of its copy, according to that network's particular consensus protocol. The consensus protocol guarantees the accuracy as well as authenticity of each and every copy of distributed ledger running on the network node. Networks may be registered or illegal (Fig. 17.9).

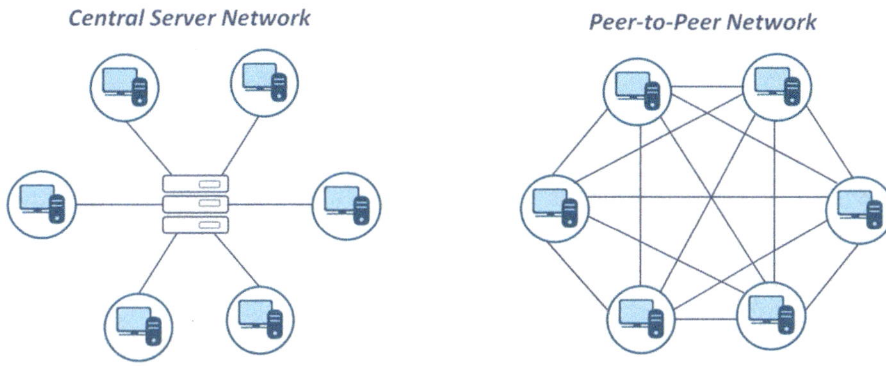

Fig. 17.9 Types of blockchain networks

The public is open to permission less network, and anyone may enter. However, the registered networks require participating parties to verify and approve them beforehand as they are private. These organizations that participate in preapproved private networks are called consortiums.

17.4.1 Peer-to-Peer Network

In DLT, "distributed" is a notion defining a peer-to-peer network (P2P). In comparison to a central server network, in P2P network, the nodes are connected with each other directly. The transactions are processed directly.

In this model, no updates to records are communicated by centralized authorities. Every node in the peer-to-peer network executes in the form of blocks. These blocks are added to the shared set of transactions, and consensus algorithms are used to trigger the updates.

17.4.2 Public Networks (Permissionless)

In this type, it is possible for everyone to join, and the participants are pseudonymous. Ethereum networks are an example of this category of blockchain networks. Trust is built in the data due to its public nature, where consensus is used by the nodes to agree. These permissionless systems are trustless in the sense that the blockchain should not be used for exchanging data. However, the validity of the records is trusted.

17.4.3 Private Networks (Permissioned)

In a private network, only trusted entities and their respective nodes participate. They are licensed network where only private entities and nodes are allowed to access blockchain network. The participation of these trusted nodes is managed by an overall authority that offers a user authentication and an identity management membership program.

Features of blockchain:

- Decentralization: In a blockchain-based system, the data is distributed over nodes on the network instead of being on a single centralized source. It also makes it possible to manage the distribution and handling of information by mutual feedback reached through consensus from the related nodes on the network. Several trustworthy organizations currently manage the knowledge that was formerly consolidated at one central stage.
- Data transparency: Data transparency is defined as a trust-based relationship among organizations. The documents should be safe and temperature-proof. Information on the blockchain is not centralized and neither operated by a single node. Instead, it is distributed over the network of connected nodes. The ownership of the data is private and is protected from third-party intruders.
- Security and privacy: A trust-based relationship among organizations is the achievement of data transparency in any technology. The information or records at stake should be secure and temperature-proof. Any information stored on the blockchain is not centralized in one location and is distributed across the network rather than run by one node. One of the strongest features is cryptographic hash that makes data extraction impossible. Blockchain, a decentralized network that is protected through cryptographic approaches, makes it a reasonable option to maintain privacy for certain applications.

17.5 Blockchain Technology Challenges

17.5.1 Scalability and Storage Capacity

Storing of data using a blockchain generates two main issues: scalability and confidentiality. The information on a blockchain is exposed to one and all existing on the chain that makes it vulnerable, an undesirable outcome for any decentralized network. Patient medical records/observations, laboratory results, MRI and X-ray reports, etc. will be included in the data stored on the blockchain. It creates ample data to be stored on the blockchain, which will have a huge impact on the blockchain's storage capacity.

17.5.2 Lack of Social Skills

Since this technology is in the evolving phase, there are very few individuals who know the way blockchain technology works. Moreover, when hospital and healthcare institutions require to entirely migrating their existing systems to blockchain, it will take time to switch from trusted EHR systems to the blockchain.

17.5.3 Lack of Globally Acknowledged Standards

Since the technology is still in the development phase, it lacks for the defined specification. Introduction of blockchain in healthcare industry would require added budget and time. It would be requiring certified standards from international authorities who set the regulation phase of any evolving technology [19]. These common regulations and standards will be very helpful to decide on the type, size, and format of the data to be stored and managed through the blockchain.

17.6 Managing Healthcare by Implementing Blockchain

By introducing new members and shifting organizational partnerships, the blockchain directory model supports the potential to evolve and change dramatically over the life of blockchain. In particular, the software is useful for tracking the steady and persistent growth of transactions. There is an upper limit on the number of reports for the EHR system, which is the number of people it serves. Development in the population is relatively slower than that of, for example, the number of money transactions in the Bitcoin network [37].

The layout of the blockchain chain also helps to preserve growing medical records by keeping an increasingly connected list of health records, in which each block consists of a timestamp and a connection to the previous block [38]. Another solution could be a blockchain containing off-chain data pointers; metadata related with the pointers may provide the details required to allow interoperability [39, 40].

Using this process, heavyweight data, including imaging analysis results, might be stored off-chain. A few studies also recommended that secure medical records be held directly on the blockchain in the case of the sharing of imaging test results; nevertheless, storing encrypted image data of all patients will result in a huge blockchain, which would be too outsized to import, archive, and verify for a node built on a mobile device and even a modern machine.

The size of the blockchain is a problem that has been seen to be a limiting factor for chains that store general transactional information, smaller than the big blocks needed to store medical imaging information [41]. If the blockchain continues to evolve, the scalability of the framework could be diminished, because only users with large storage spaces and high computing capacity will act as miners or complete nodes in the blockchain.

Usually, blockchain maintains three types of nodes, like full nodes, light nodes, and archive nodes, to solve such type of problems. The nodes are as follows:

1. Full Nodes: In this node, each block in the blockchain is stored, and each transaction is processed [41].
2. Light Nodes: Without a full network node being run, transactions can be verified. Adequate security should be provided by requiring users to request the network before obtaining the longest chain [30]. By keeping the head of the block, check the variable conditions of the light node transaction without adding large chunks of memory to the blockchain. Lighting networks can use similar information.
3. Archive Node: On the blockchain, they are responsible for storing any transaction and block. In addition, it also holds purchase receipts and the whole state tree [42].

17.6.1 Advantages of Managing Healthcare Using Blockchain

When a blockchain is adopted to handle electronic medical records, it becomes the centralized digital health data management method that has long been sought after. To access patient records, hospitals and medical providers will no longer need special software or databases. For example, the decentralized blockchain will enable physicians, nurses, managers, and other authorized individuals, instead of relying on a private network between local hospitals, to participate in an exchanging network without the need for external data exchange infrastructure across the organizations.

1. Patient data protection: The most common blockchain healthcare application at the moment is keeping our critical medical data safe and secure, which is not surprising. In the healthcare sector, security is a big concern. Between 2009 and 2017, over 176 million data breaches were reported in medical records. Credit card and banking data as well as health and genetic research documents were stolen by the perpetrators. Blockchain's potential to maintain an upright, decentralized, and transparent archive with all patient records provides it with a variety of security development technologies. However, it is well-known that blockchain is private and transparent; it can also be used for hiding any person's identity with protected and complicated codes that can secure the sensitivity of medical information. The decentralized design of technology also enables patients, physicians, and healthcare professionals to easily and safely access the same information.
2. Streamlining the medical records and preventing costly mistakes: Improper communication between health workers costs the healthcare system $11 billion a year. Inefficient method of a patients' medical data accessibility exhausts the resources of personnel and causes the delay of patient care. Blockchain-based

medical records provide these ills with a cure. The decentralized design of technology provides a single patient data ecosystem that can be referenced easily and securely by clinicians, clinics, pharmacists, and everyone else interested in care. The blockchain can thus lead to faster diagnosis and tailored care plans.

3. Medical supply chain management and drug safety: Blockchain has a huge effect on supply chain management of pharmaceutical drugs, and its decentralization basically assures complete accountability in the shipping process. The point of origin will be marked whenever a drug ledger is established. The log will also begin to log data every step of the way, including who received it and where it has been, before it reaches the user. Labor costs and waste emissions can also be monitored by the process.
4. Revolutionizing genomics: The potential of genomics to improve the future of human health, once a fantasy, is now a science and financial reality. In 2001, it costs $1 billion to process a human genome. Today, it costs around $1,000, and organizations bring DNA samples to millions of homes that unlock our health and history buttons. For this growing field, blockchain is a perfect fit, since it can store billions of genetic data points securely. It has now become a forum where people can sell their encrypted genetic records in order to create a bigger database, enabling scientists to obtain valuable data quicker than ever before.
5. Enhance the security of healthcare transactions: One of the most recent inventions simplifies the processing of claims and the management of sales periods. It allows hospitals and health facilities to control claims and remittances, maximize patient payment processing, reduce denials and underpayments, and more efficiently manage daily revenue cycles and business operations. Blockchain-based EMR may also offer the patient personalized health advice, delivered via an app or email, with wearables and smartphone apps producing additional data.

This suggests that a doctor may review the recovery of a patient from surgery or disease in real time, recognizing food, exercise, and vital signs such as heart rate opportunities or complications, without the need for face-to-face consultation.

17.7 Blockchain Use Cases in Healthcare During the COVID-19 Pandemic

Because of the technology's capacity to allow better data consistency and authentication, the biggest advantages provided by blockchain are correlated with greater confidence and privacy. Blockchain changes ownership and control of data from one centralized source to various data-contributing sources at the most simple level. The following are few examples of blockchain use in healthcare linked to COVID-19:

1. Contact tracing: Many governments have embarked on contact tracing to follow the possible transmission of the novel coronavirus, in which infected individuals are asked to identify any other persons they have come into contact with for a

certain period of time. Data decentralization helps to promote vital healthcare operations, such as contact tracking, since the mechanism relies on the use of granular, confidential data to notify public health officials who, based on their activities and connections, may be at risk of exposure. Holding the privacy of people is important in contract tracing. Nodle's blockchain network released a contact tracing app called "Coalition" earlier this year, which emphasized user privacy.

2. Patient record sharing: The collection of patient information during a crisis or catastrophe to build a "light" electronic health record system is another useful use case for blockchain when it applies to COVID-19, which can be used by disparate groups of clinicians to exchange patient records when treating new patients during pandemics or other emergencies and natural disasters. Such a platform will allow providers to collaborate with patients who are unable to reach their regular provider but who still receive the full spectrum of care and medications required. The key principle of the approach is that the electronic health records of patients accompany them wherever they go.
3. Clinical trial management: As it becomes usable, blockchain technology can assist researchers and clinicians in capturing clinical data in real time. This increases precision, facilitates data exchange, and maintains compliance with regulations. It can also monitor and keep track of who has accessed which portion of the datasets, providing an audit trail that enhances data protection and privacy.

   Civitas, an app introduced by a Canadian setup that is engaged in blockchain solutions, helps to monitor the outbreak of COVID-19 by different government officials and local authorities [43]. This app can be helpful in handling COVID-19-related clinical trials as it secretly associates the ID of each person with its corresponding blockchain records without revealing their identity. It can discover whether or not a person has left his house. This is important because it helps to minimize the spread of this virus. Moreover, it will help doctors to track their patients' progress and evaluate their symptoms for any side effects.
4. Medical supply chain: The COVID-19 emergency situation disrupted supply networks around the world. Therefore, during the COVID-19 pandemic, large numbers of blockchain arrangements were in supply chain management. By expelling third-party delegates and innate delays in managing and processing processes, blockchain accelerates the validation method. The benefits include quicker time to manage and process, lower costs, lower operating risks, and faster settlements for all parties involved. The VeChain network guarantees the credibility and durability of new KN95 masks imported from China while collaborating inseparably with production offices and facilities [44]. All activities related to the manufacture of vaccines are noted and held in assigned ledgers, from codes to packages and materials.
5. Donation tracking: The pandemic condition has offered mankind with extreme hardships. The promotion of donation activities helps to assist people who face medical or economic challenges due to the spread of the infectious diseases [45]. HyperChain is a network built on blockchain that aims to combat the outbreak of

coronavirus by specializing in uniquely monitoring donations [46]. In the donation process for contaminated people, this site assists governments and healthcare organizations. This network ensures that the process of donation remains unchanged, reliable, and traceable. It offers a straightforward forum for donors to track where their funds have been used.

6. Outbreak tracking: As information managed via such a network is secure, precise, tamper-free, and transparent, blockchain technology offers an appropriate coronavirus tracking platform. Consequently, to enhance preparation and management, governments may help update the status of the coronavirus pandemic, such as predicting the outbreak, isolating potential regions, and monitoring the spread of the infection. Acoer has created a HashLog dashboard from an ever-growing collection of public data that helps individuals to understand the extent of infection spread and trend over time. In addition, the Acoer Coronavirus HashLog helps to build data visualization models associated with clinical trial data [47] through information obtained from the CDC, WHO, and patterns from social networking websites.
7. Data aggregation: The use of a blockchain-fueled framework allows compliance management, data ownership, and auditability to provide flexible sharing through multiple levels of management. The World Health Organization (WHO) introduced MiPasa, a worldwide scale control and correspondence system controlled by blockchain innovation that helps capture, collect, and research data on the spread and containment of the virus while working with major innovation organizations and governments. MiPasa is an asset that is intended to benefit public health authorities, the science and business network, and the general public [48].
8. User privacy protection: The balance between privacy assurance and data collection must be acquired in these disturbing times. Blockchain can be used to more productively capture and analyze patient data and screen the movements of patients to ensure the required social distance criteria while also protecting their identity. There is no focal force, and in a blockchain network, customers are given control of their data. In particular, they may exchange information that is useful for coronavirus relief efforts while ensuring that their privacy and identity are protected. In addition to this, through coronavirus monitoring, governments and healthcare associations can increase data collection, while consumers can be assured that their data will not be leaked or exchanged. A blockchain-based platform for COVID-19 contact tracing using Bluetooth was devised by a group of privacy specialists across Europe. In addition, a blockchain-based arrangement has been made by German tech scale-up MYNXG that uses mobile phones, thus safeguarding client security [49].

17.8 Conclusion

By 2025, if blockchain technology is implemented, the healthcare sector can save up to $100 billion a year in counterfeit-related fraud and insurance fraud, administrative costs, IT costs, data breach-related expenses, and support feature and personnel costs, according to a BIS study survey. The report also notes that from 2018 to 2025, the use of "the global blockchain in the healthcare market is anticipated to rise at a CAGR of 63.85% and will touch $5.61 billion by 2025." Due to the usage of blockchain to solve the most prevalent interoperability and non-standardization problem in healthcare information systems that have generated data silos throughout the sector, the use of blockchain for the exchange of healthcare data would contribute to the highest market share in the forecast period, hitting a valuation of $1.89 billion by 2025.

Although blockchain technology has innovative features, more research is also required to better grasp, enhance, and test this technology easily and safely. In order to strengthen the confidence of stakeholders in using this technology and to expand its acceptance in healthcare, ongoing efforts have been made to address weaknesses in scalability, protection, and privacy.

References

1. Mcclean, S., Gillespie, J., Garg, L., Barton, M., Scotney, B., & Kullerton, K. (2014). Using phase-type models to cost stroke patient care across health, social and community services. *European Journal of Operational Research, 236*(1), 190–199.
2. World Health Statistics. (2018). *Monitoring health for the SDGs*. WHO.
3. AAMC. (2019). *Careers in medicine*. Retrieved Jan 29, 2019, from https://www.aamc.org/cim/specialty/exploreoptions/list/
4. Zhang, P., Schmidt, D. C., White, J., & Lenz, G. (2018). Blockchain technology use cases in healthcare. *Advances in Computers, 111*, 1–41.
5. Hosseini, M., & Dixon, B. E. (2016). Syntactic interoperability and the role of standards. In *Health information exchange: Navigating a network of health information systems* (p. 135). Elsevier.
6. US Institute of Medicine Report. *To err is human: Building a safer health system*. Retrieved from http://www.nap.edu/books/0309068371/html/
7. JAMA Abstract. (2001). *Estimating hospital deaths due to medical errors*. Retrieved from http://jama.ama-assn.org/issues/v286n4/rfull/joc02235.html#abstract
8. Singh, M. (2002). Treating health care. *IEEE Internet Computing, 6*(4), 4–5.
9. Parsloe, C. (2003). Worlds apart? Healthcare technologies for lifelong disease management. *IEEE Engineering in Medicine and Biology Magazine, 22*(1), 53–56.
10. *US administration on aging report on demographic changes*. Retrieved from http://www.aoa.dhhs.gov/aoa/stats/aging21/demography.html
11. Boric-Lubecke, O., & Lubecke, V. (2002). Wireless house calls: Using communications technology for health care and monitoring. *IEEE Microwave Magazine, 3*(3), 43–48.
12. Anogianakis, G., Maglavera, S., & Pomportsis, A. (1998). Relief for maritime medical emergencies through telematics. *IEEE Transactions on IT in Biomedicine, 2*(4), 254–260.

13. Pattichis, C., Kyriacou, E., Voskarides, S., Pattichis, M., Istepanian, R., & Schizas, C. (2002). Wireless telemedicine systems: An overview. *IEEE Antennas and Propagation Magazine, 44*(2), 143–153.
14. Suzuki, T., & Doi, M. (2001). LifeMinder: An evidence-based wearable healthcare assistant. In *Proc. ACM conference on human factors in computing systems* (pp. 127–128). ACM.
15. Mikkonen, M., Vayrynen, S., Ikonen, V., & Heikkila, M. (2002). User and concept studies as tools in developing mobile communication services for the elderly. *Springer-Verlag's Personal and Ubiquitous Computing, 6*, 113–124.
16. Editorial, G. (2004). M-Health: Beyond seamless mobility and global wireless healthcare connectivity. *IEEE Transactions on IT in Biomedicine, 8*(4), 405–413.
17. Stanford, V. (2002). Using pervasive computing to deliver elder care. *IEEE Pervasive Computing Magazine, 1*(1), 10–13.
18. Website for HealthVault. Retrieved from http://www.healthvault.com
19. Moller, J., & Vosegaard, H. (2008). Experiences with electronic health records. *IEEE IT Professional, 10*(2), 19–23.
20. Makeham, M., Dovey, S., County, M., & Kidd, M. (2002). An international taxonomy for errors in general practice: A pilot study. *Medical Journal of Australia, 177*, 68–72.
21. Tierney, W., & Zafar, A. (2002) *EMRs: An introductory tutorial*. Retrieved from http://healthit.ahrq.gov/portal/server.pt/gateway/PTARGS_0_251_0_0_18/EMR%20Talk.ppt
22. Website for HIPAA. Retrieved from http://www.hhs.gov/ocr/hipaa
23. Wikipedia. Retrieved from http://en.wikipedia.org/wiki/Medical_informatics
24. Website for CCHIT. Retrieved from http://www.cchit.org
25. Website for Hl7. Retrieved from http://www.HL7.org
26. Wikipedia for Regional Health Information Organizations. Retrieved from http://en.wikipedia.org/wiki/RHIO
27. Website for Office of National Coordinator for HIT. Retrieved from http://www.hhs.gov/healthit/initiatives/
28. Yue, X., Wang, H., & Jin, D. (2016). Healthcare data gateways: Found healthcare intelligence on blockchain with novel privacy risk control. *Journal of Medical Systems, 40*(10), 218.
29. Guo, R., Shi, H., & Zhao, Q. (2018). Secure attribute-based signature scheme with multiple authorities for blockchain in electronic health records systems. *IEEE Access, 776*(99), 1–12.
30. Nakamoto, S. (2008). Bitcoin: A peer-to-peer electronic cash system. *Journal for General Philosophy of Science, 39*(1), 53–67.
31. Puthal, D., Malik, N., Mohanty, S. P., Kougianos, E., & Das, G. (2018). Every-thing you wanted to know about the blockchain: Its promise, components, processes, and problems. *IEEE Consumer Electronics Magazine, 7*(4), 6–14.
32. Crosby, M., Nachiappan, P., Pattanayak, S. V., & Kalyanaraman, V. (2015). *Blockchain technology beyond bitcoin*. Blockchain Technol.
33. Burniske, C., Vaughn, E., Shelton, J., & Cahana, A. (2016). *How blockchain technology can enhance ehr operability*. Gem Ark Invest Res., Tech. Rep..
34. Schneier, B. (2006). Foundations. In *Applied cryptography: Protocols, algorithms and source code in C* (2nd ed., pp. 1–5). Wiley.
35. Ribitzky, R., Clair, J. S., & Houlding, D. I. (2018). *Pragmatic, interdisciplinary perspectives on blockchain and distributed ledger technology: Paving the future for healthcare*. Blockchain Healthc Today. https://doi.org/10.30953/bhty.v1.24
36. Ichikawa, D., Kashiyama, M., & Ueno, T. (2017). Tamper-resistant mobile health using blockchain technology. *JMIR mHealth and uHealth, 5*(7), e111.
37. Cheng, E. C., Le, Y., & Zhou, J. (2018). Healthcare services across China—on implementing an extensible universally unique patient identifier system. *International Journal of Healthcare Management, 11*(3), 210–216.
38. Patel, V. (2019). A framework for secure and decentralized sharing of medical imaging data via blockchain consensus. *Health Informatics Journal, 25*(4), 139.

39. Dubovitskaya, A., Xu, Z., & Ryu, S. (2017). Secure and trustable electronic medical records sharing using blockchain. *American Medical Informatics Association Annual Symposium Proceedings, 2017*, 650.
40. Zhang, P., White, J., & Schmidt, D. C. (2018). Fhirchain: applying blockchain to securely and scalably share clinical data. *Computational and Structural Biotechnology Journal, 16*, 267–278.
41. Cyran, M. A. (2018). Blockchain as a foundation for sharing healthcare data. *Blockchain in Healthcare Today*. https://doi.org/10.30953/bhty.v1.13
42. Yang, H., & Yang, B. (2017). A blockchain-based approach to the secure sharing of healthcare data. In: Proceedings of the Norwegian information security conference, Oslo.
43. Wright, T. (2020). Blockchain App used to track COVID-19 cases in Latin America. *Coin telegraph: The future of money*. Retrieved from https://cointelegraph.com/news/blockchain-app-used-to-track-covid-19-cases-in-latin-america.
44. Blockchain and Crypto Firm VeChain Utilized to Confirm Authenticity of Coronavirus KN95 Masks. *Blockchain Magazine*, 20 April 2020. Retrieved from https://www.blockchainmagazine.net/blockchain-and-crypto-firm-vechain-utilized-to-confirm-authenticity-of-coronavirus-kn95-masks/
45. Chang, M. C., & Park, D. (2020). How can blockchain help people in the event of pandemics such as the COVID-19? *Journal of Medical Systems, 44*(5), 102.
46. Zhang, J. (2020). Chinese startup launches blockchain platform to improve donation efficiency. *Tech in Asia*. Retrieved from https://www.techinasia.com/china-blockchain-platform-donation
47. Acoer. Providing daily tracking and visualizations of the pandemic. *Coronavirus (COVID-19) Tracker*. Retrieved from https://www.acoer.com/coronavirus
48. Singh, G., & Levi, J. (2020). MiPasa project and IBM Blockchain team on open data platform to support Covid-19 response. *IBM*. Retrieved from https://www.ibm.com/blogs/blockchain/2020/03/mipasa-project-and-ibm-blockchain-team-on-open-data-platform-to-support-covid-19-response/
49. Dragov, R., Croce, C. L., & Hefny, M. (2020). How Blockchain can help in the COVID-19 crisis and recovery. *IDC-Analyze the Future*. Retrieved from https://blog-idcuk.com/blockchain-help-in-the-covid-19-and-recovery/

Chapter 18
An Experimental Approach for Prediction of Breast Cancer Diseases Using Clustering Concepts

Amit Kumar Bhasker, Rama Nandan Tripathi, and Nawazish Naweed

18.1 Introduction

Data mining has a close relationship with large datasets [1]. Over the past two decades there have been many changes in the methodology and environment of data mining concepts. Therefore, we use the data of cancer patients. The main reason for death in women is breast cancer and its effect on the overall structure of the body. If any methods and techniques are found to predict cancer tissue at an early stage, then the death ratio will be decrease day by day. Data mining concepts open the source of prediction and provide help to the medical environment in taking decisions and improving health services and activities [2, 3]. In the era of computer science, a few methods are available for early detection and indication issues. Data mining has provided supervised learning and unsupervised learning tools to achieve the aim. From this perspective, techniques are classification, clustering, decision tree, and data virtualization, which are depicted in Fig. 18.1. We carried out a complete analysis on cancer patients at various stages. Cancer analysis is dependent on tumor size [4–6]. Tumor size indicates the actual stage of cancer. The main role of clustering algorithms is to divide data sets into one or more segments and, then the appropriate algorithm is applied for the prediction of tumor size.

A. K. Bhasker (✉) · R. N. Tripathi
Department of MCA, Dr. RML Avadh University, Ayodhya, Faizabad, India

N. Naweed
University of Technology and Applied Sciences, Ibri, Oman
e-mail: nawazish.ibr@cas.edu.om

M. S. Husain et al. (eds.), *Pervasive Healthcare*, EAI/Springer Innovations in Communication and Computing, https://doi.org/10.1007/978-3-030-77746-3_18

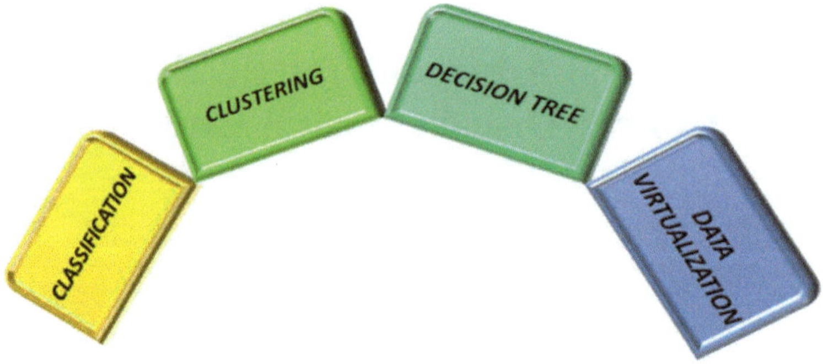

Fig. 18.1 Data mining method criteria

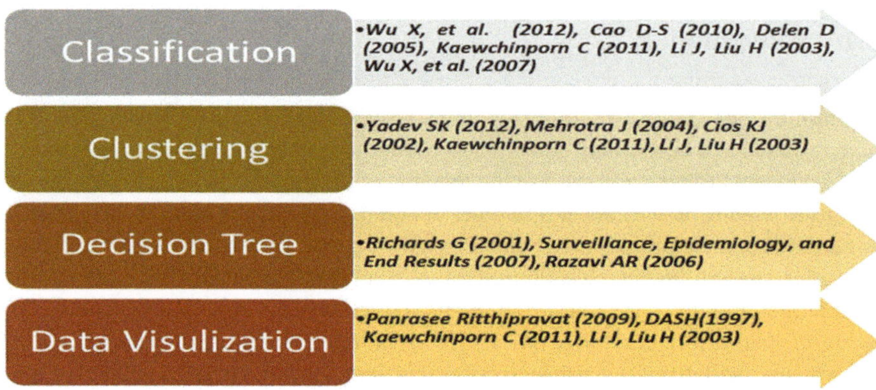

Fig. 18.2 A systematic review of approach 1

18.2 Related Work

Many of the current methodologies and techniques are based on domain clustering. Clustering techniques are most powerful and have a high level of accuracy. Various experts have indicated various algorithms, which are depicted in Fig. 18.2. Karthikeyani et al. [7] explained large-scale determinations on the basis of the clustering approach. Perspective algorithms are able to explain cancer parameter residuals, error accuracy, and variations in breast tissues. Dursun et al. [1], discussed statistical observations and a comparative study on various algorithms. This observation shows the effect on parameters with a visualization format. Tan and Gilbert [2] established the practicality of tissues in classifying data and accessing some theoretical clarifications of the performance of accuracy. As an impact, they recommend that cooperative machine learning should be measured for the task of classifying cancer patient data. Clustering can be said to be the identification of similar training of objects. By the use of clustering techniques, we can further perceive dense and sparse regions in an object area and can find out ordinary distribution

Table 18.1 Accepted approaches by experts

Experts ↓	Approaches→	Classification	Clustering	Decision table	Data visualization
Carloz Ordonez [8]	√	√	√	√	
Humar and Novruz [9]		√	√	√	
Anbarasi [10]	√	√	√	√	
Rajkumar and Reena [11]	√	√	√		
Shantakumar et al. [12]	√	√	√	√	
Sarvestan Soltani [13]	√	√		√	
Pradhan and Sahu [14]		√	√	√	
Patil and Sherekar [15]	√	√	√		
Crisóstomo et al. [16]	√	√	√	√	
Nyante et al. [17]	√		√	√	
Shu et al. [18]	√	√		√	
Sidiq [19]	√	√	√	√	

patterns and correlations among information attributes. The classification technique can also be used for powerful methods of distinguishing organizations or classes of object, but it becomes steeply priced. Clustering can be used as a preprocessing approach for characteristic subset selection and classification (Table 18.1).

18.3 Breast Cancer

Cancer is a field of innovation. As well as illness, it leads to changes in the structure of the body. The tissue growth rate is high. Tissues have damaged the cells for long periods. Cell death is called apoptosis in the medical sciences [20]. Body cells have contributed a special role in fighting diseases. Damaged tissues to burn according to the requirement of medicine. Otherwise, damaged tissue develops itself in whole body rapidly. Breast tissues destroy body function and damage other cells in the form of a tumor [21]. Breast cancer is a malicious breast tumor considered as uncontrolled cell growth in the breast. Damaged tissues is the basic cause of death. The data taken from [22] for prediction to breast cancer tissues. Clustering methods are used to find the variances at various level tissues. Source data have taken the 106 instances and 10 attributes (9 attributes and one class) for observation. Instances are divided into six segments (Carcinoma, Fibroadenoma, Mastopathy, Glandular, Connective, and Adipose). We observed six features of instances using the clustering approach. In this chapter, we quantify clustering-based data mining algorithms and five different features (I0, PA500, HFS, DA, AREA). After rigorous evaluation, we observed these algorithms to predict breast cancer or whether breast cancer will recur based on the scaling data set. And we quantify the accuracy and confusion metrics to find the most significant tissues as the predictive model of breast cancer. We have used Orange, SPSS and MATLAB to experiment with clustering algorithms. Furthermore, the accuracy of the algorithms model is depicted in the table and figures, which are completely dependent on the instances. Data visualization of clustering approach performance is shown for breast cancer datasets.

18.4 Data Interpretation Evauation

Interpretations of collected cancer patients is the process of predicting the outcome of a tissue that has been secured at an early stage of illness of the patient. This step has been established at different stages, and may be present in various steps as correlation with attributes and presentation in graph form.

Figure 18.3 explains k-means observation and correlation between attributes, and also defines the definition of process improvement activity. K-means clustering is a basic process for background checking cancer patients with regard to a new prediction.

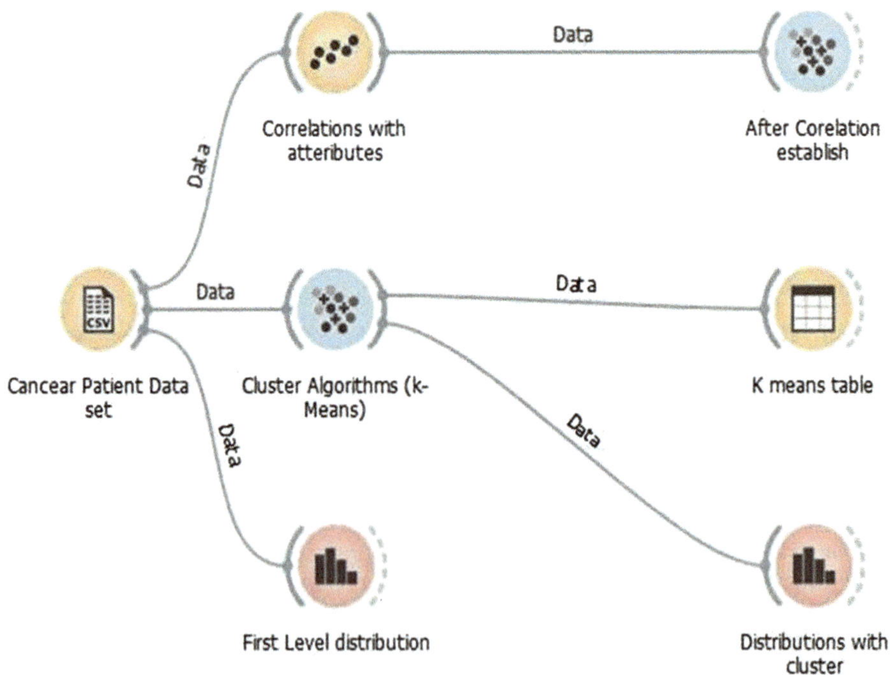

Fig. 18.3 Clustering approaches with research steps

18.5 Conclusion and Discussion

The breast cancer database consists of attributes with one class. The decisional attribute takes only 6 classfifications the values 0 or 1. As presented in Table 18.2, the clustering of all values of attributes excluding the conditional class, Carcinoma, Fibroadenoma, Mastopathy, Glandular, Connective, and Adipose are multi-valued.

Figure 18.4 shows the conditional instances impact ratio between the x axis and the y axis. Figures 18.5, 18.6, 18.7, 18.8, and 18.9 present the actual accuracy level for cancer tissues. Nevertheless, the complete cluster in Table 18.3 are shown the class label with values and two-level clusters 0 and 1. In this study, we illustrate the complete description of the clustering approach and also illustrate the impact analysis of every attribute. Table 18.4 presents the results for statistical significance of complete instances. Table 18.5 confirms the accuracy level performance of the clustering in the case of the breast cancer database.

However, inclusive k-means algorithm quantifications result that 0 cluster result and 1 clustering result is 29% and 71% in Table 18.5. In the following predictive analytics, Table 18.5 is a matrix with two rows and three columns that report the percentage accuracy and non-accuracy variances.

Table 18.2 Grouping table of patients on the basis of weight

Class label	Weight
CL^1	21.0
CL^2	15.0
CL^3	18.0
CL^4	16.0
CL^5	14.0
CL^6	22.0

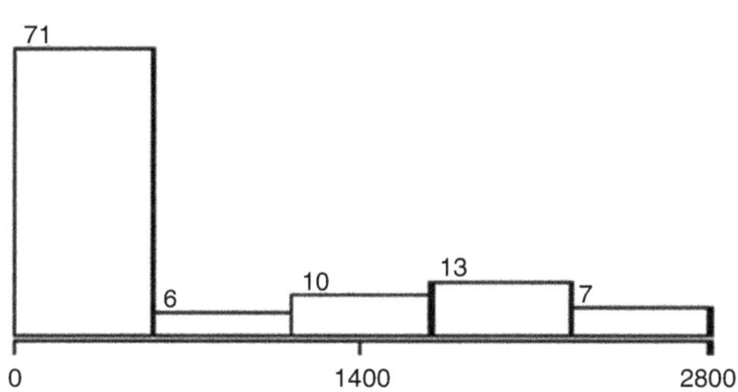

Fig. 18.4 Class level 1

Fig. 18.5 Impedivity attribute 1

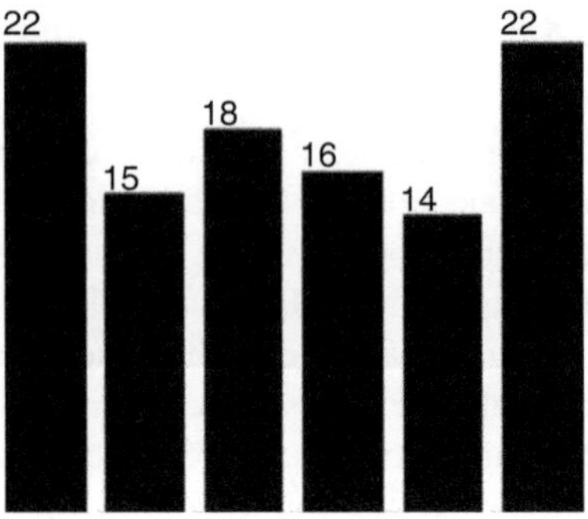

Fig. 18.6 Phase angle attribute

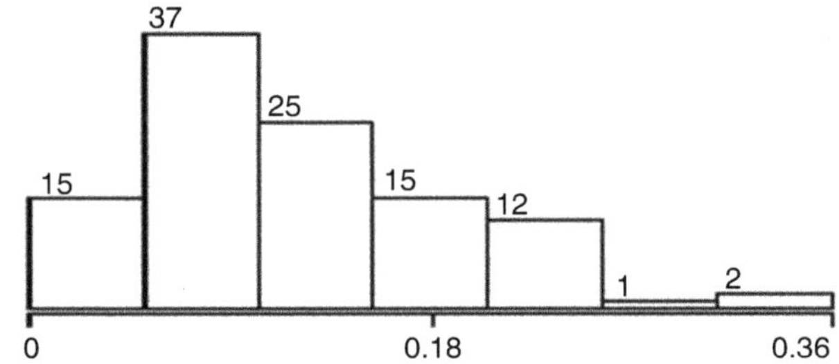

Fig. 18.7 Slope 1

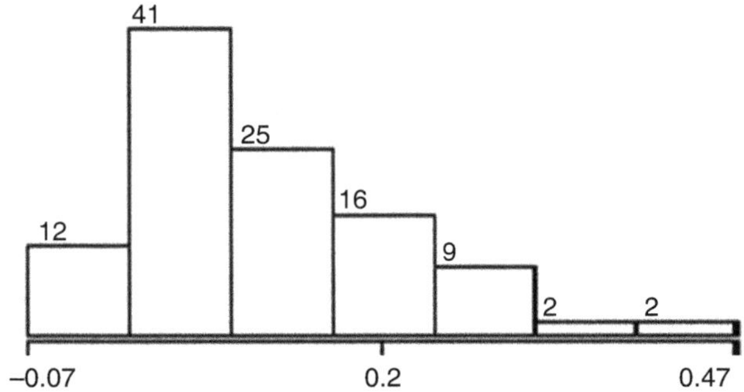

Fig. 18.8 Impedance

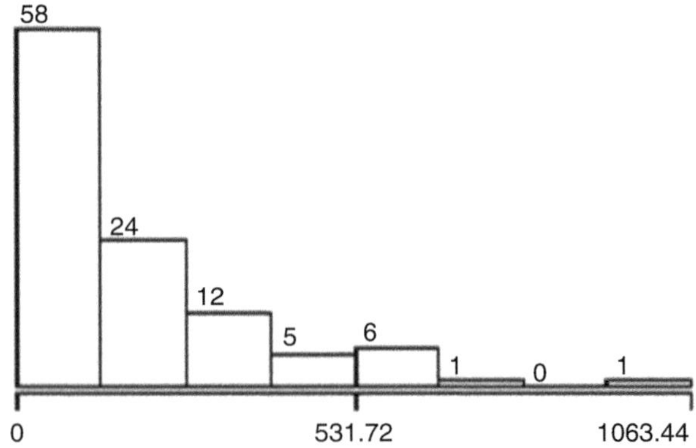

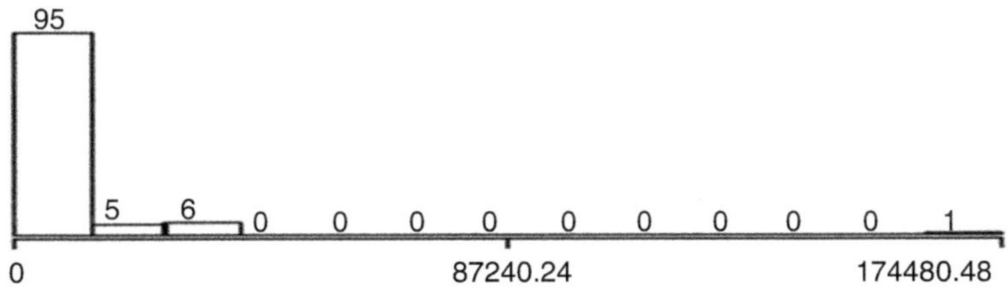

Fig. 18.9 Spectrum

Table 18.3 Clustering (K-means observation)

Class label	Instances	Cluster^0	Cluster^1
AT^1	784.2516	1879.9877	331.3474
AT^2	0.1201	0.0746	0.139
AT^3	0.1141	0.1108	0.1163
AT^4	190.5686	416.2653	97.2807
AT^5	7335.15	19,830.9045	21,702,454

Table 18.4 Statistical view of complete instances

Minimum	1
Maximum	106
Mean	53.5
Standard deviation	30.74

Table 18.5 Clustered 106 instances matrix

0	31	29%
1	75	71%

References

1. Dursun, D., Glenn, W., & Kadam, A. (2004). Predicting breast cancer survivability: A comparison of three data mining methods. *Artificial Intelligence in Medicine, 34*, 113–127.
2. Tan, A. C., & Gilbert, D. (2003). Ensemble machine learning on gene expression data for cancer classification. *Applied Bioinformatics, 2*, S75–S83.
3. Suhaib Kidwai, M., & Zunnun Khan, M. (2021) "A new perspective of detecting and classifying neurological disorders through recurrence and machine learning classifiers," 2021 International Conference on Advance Computing and Innovative Technologies in Engineering (ICACITE), pp. 200–206, https://doi.org/10.1109/ICACITE51222.2021.9404645.
4. Kaewchinporn, C. (2011). A combination of decision tree learning and clustering for data classification. In *2011 eighth international joint conference on computer science and software engineering (JCSSE)* (pp. 11–13). IEEE.
5. Delen, D., et al. (2005). Predicting breast cancer survivability: A comparison of three data mining methods. *Artificial Intelligence in Medicine, 34*, 113–127.

6. Wu, X., et al. (2007). Top 10 algorithms in data mining analysis. *Knowledge and Information Systems, 14*(1), 1–37.
7. Khan, M. Z. & Shoaib, M. (2019). Healthcare Analytics in the Modern Era: A Survey. *International Journal of Research in Advent Technology, 7*(3), 132–13.
8. Ordonez, C. (2006). Association rule discovery with train and test approach for heart disease prediction. *IEEE Transactions on Information Technology in Biomedicine, 10*(2), 334–343.
9. Humar, K., & Novruz, A. (2009). Mining classification rules for liver disorders. *International Journal of Mathematics and Computers in Simulation, 3*, 9.
10. Anbarasi, M., Anupriya, E., & Iyengar, N. C. H. S. N. (2010). Enhanced prediction of heart disease with feature subset selection using genetic algorithm. *International Journal of Engineering, Science and Technology, 2*(10), 5370–5376.
11. Rajkumar, A., & Reena, G. S. (2010). Diagnosis of heart disease using datamining algorithm. *Global Journal of Computer Science and Technology, 38*(10), 10.
12. Shantakumar, B. P., et al. (2009). Intelligent and effective heart attack prediction system using data mining and artificial neural network. *European Journal of Scientific Research, 31*(4), 642–656.
13. Sarvestan Soltani, A. (2010). Predicting breast cancer survivability using data mining techniques. *Software Technology and Engineering, 2*, 227–231.
14. Pradhan, M., & Sahu, R. K. (2011). Predict the onset of diabetes disease using artificial neural network (ANN). *The International Journal of Computer Science & Emerging Technologies, 2*(2), 303–311.
15. Patil, T. R., & Sherekar, S. S. (2013). Performance analysis of Naive Bayes and J48 classification algorithm for data classification. *International Journal of Computer Science and Applications, 6*(2), 256–261.
16. Crisóstomo, J., et al. (2016). Hyperresistinemia and metabolic dysregulation: A risky crosstalk in obese breast cancer. *Endocrine, 53*(2), 433–442.
17. Nyante, S. J., et al. (2017). The association between mammographic calcifications and breast cancer prognostic factors in a population- based registry cohort. *Cancer, 123*(2), 219–227.
18. Shu, X., et al. (2018). Associations of obesity and circulating insulin and glucose with breast cancer risk: A Mendelian randomization analysis. *International Journal of Epidemiology, 48*(3), 795–806.
19. Sidiq, U. (2018). Diagnosis of various thyroid ailments using data mining classification techniques. *International Journal of Computer Science and Information Technologies, 5*, 131–136.
20. Mehrotra, J., et al. (2004). Very high frequency of hypermethylated genes in breast cancer metastasis to the bone, brain, and lung. *Clinical Cancer Research, 10*(9), 3104–3109.
21. Richards, G., Rayward-Smith, V. J., Sonksen, P. H., Carey, S., & Weng, C. (2001). Data mining for indicators of early mortality in a database of clinical records. *Artificial Intelligence in Medicine, 22*, 215–231.
22. Khan M. Z., et.al. (2021). Hadoop based EMH framework: A Big Data approach. International Conference on Advance Computing and Innovative Technologies in Engineering (ICACITE), pp. 1068–1070, https://doi.org/10.1109/ICACITE51222.2021.9404710.

Chapter 19
Post-COVID-19 View of Indian Economy with Emphasis on Service Sector: A Regression Implementation

Alakananda Chakraborty, Muskan Jindal, and Shruti Gupta

19.1 Introduction

"Coronavirus disease" 2019 (COVID-19) is a virulent disease caused by the "SARS-CoV-2" virus, which is genetically associated with the family of viruses that was introduced by the SARS outbreak in 2003 [1–10]. This pandemic has resulted in no less than 200,000 deaths with a mortality rate of approximately 4% globally, as of April 9, 2020 [11, 12], and it has led to extensive lockdowns in major countries, mostly starting from March 10. Some of the worst-hit countries like Italy, Spain, the USA, France, India, etc. have announced lockdowns till May, and, if needed, till June, while other countries like Ireland, Norway, etc. have not [13–15]. Thus, economic shock in developed nations would soon turn to developing nations by means of exchange and venture channels, particularly those whose economy is profoundly subject to the travel industry and commodity exports, which support a great number of low-skilled workers. According to the IMF (International Monetary Fund), the global economy is going to contract by 3% in 2020 [16]. In addition, if the government of the nation neglects to give salary support and help in customer consumption, the world is probably going to confront a substantive economic recession, leaving millions of employees at a hopeless possibility of losing their jobs [17].

GDP or gross domestic product can be calculated on two bases, namely, annual basis and quarterly basis. It is being predicted by the IMF and the UN that while it

A. Chakraborty (✉) · M. Jindal · S. Gupta
Department of Computer Science and Engineering, Amity University, Noida, Uttar Pradesh, India

M. S. Husain et al. (eds.), *Pervasive Healthcare*, EAI/Springer Innovations in Communication and Computing, https://doi.org/10.1007/978-3-030-77746-3_19

Table 19.1 Categorization of subsectors

Subsector 1	Subsector 2	Subsector 3
Travel and tourism	Finance	Trade
–	Real estate	Hotels
–	Business services	Transport
–	–	Communication
–	–	Broadcasting services

was predicted earlier that the global economy will increase by 2.5% in 2020, this extensive lockdown of developed and developing countries will result in the contraction of 2020 GDP by 3% [18], which will bring a deep economic recession to the world, in other words, a black swan period. A black swan is an unpredictable event that is unusual to the normal expectation of a situation and has the potential of severe consequences [19–21].

This study explores and provides erudite insight into this problem of the major economic shock in the year 2020 and the years that follow using the concepts of machine learning and econometric models. The service sector and its respective subsectors are majorly considered for this research as the deliberated sector provides more than a quarter of the employment in India [22]. It has been divided into the following subsectors: travel and tourism, finance, real estate, business services, trade, hotels, transport, communication, and services related to broadcasting. These subsectors were classified broadly into three major subsector categories, which are shown in Table 19.1 [23].

This classification was formulated based on the fact that the proposed sectors of Indian economy are grouped into similar economic categories when taken into account for the GDP calculation of India for a particular economic year. A group of researchers and experts had collected the datasets of the last 10 years, which comprised of the overall GDP pattern of India; the three sectors, i.e., the agricultural, industrial, and, most importantly, the service sector's contribution, along with their respective subsectors' contribution to the GDP; and thereby the overall employment of the country. Table 19.2 shows the average GDP of India in the last 10 years and that of its sectoral contribution, respectively.

The entire methodology of this research consists of the application of reverse engineering technique. From the preliminary prediction of the value of GDP in 2020 provided by the IMF and UN due to the COVID-19 pandemic and the lockdowns of several countries [18], the contribution of each and every subsector of the service sector toward GDP and toward employment in 2020 would be predicted, and the change in these factors compared to the pattern of the last 10 years would be compared to predict the exact economic situation of the Indian subcontinent after the lockdown period is over. Various datasets related to the three major subsectors of the service sector selected for this research, and their overall contribution to GDP and employment of India, are analyzed, and one dataset per area is selected.

Table 19.2 Average GDP of India and contribution toward GDP by the three major groups of subsectors over the last 10 years (https://databank.worldbank.org/reports.aspx?source=2&series=NY.GDP.MKTP.KD.ZG&country=IND#;https://knoema.com/WTTC2019/world-travel-and-tourism-council-data?accesskey=ewmskkd; https://dbie.rbi.org.in/DBIE/dbie.rbi?site=publications)

Average GDP of India	7.1808
GDP contribution by travel and tourism	9.2682%
GDP contribution by subsector comprising finance, real estate, and business services	19.9064%
GDP contribution by subsector comprising trade, hotels, transport and communication, and services related to broadcasting	18.6055%

19.2 Subsector Comprising Travel and Tourism

The dataset of this subsector has four main attributes. The first attribute is the year which ranges from 2009–2010 to 2019–2020. The second is the overall GDP of India within this range of years. The remaining two attributes are the subsector's total contribution to GDP and total contribution to employment. The last two attributes determine the subsector's role in affecting the GDP of the country and how much employment is supported by it.

19.3 Subsector Comprising Finance, Real Estate, and Business Services

This subsector has five attributes. The first one is the year ranging from 2009–2010 to 2019–2020. The second is GDP within this yearly range. The third attribute comprises the subsector's contribution to GDP, and the fourth is the number of employees supported each year by this subsector. The last is the service sector's overall contribution to employment. The number of employees supported each year by this subsector describes its role in affecting the employment support of the entire service sector shown in the last attribute.

19.4 Subsector Comprising Trade, Hotels, Transport and Communication, and Services Related to Broadcasting

There are four attributes in this subsector. The year ranging from 2009–2010 to 2019–2020 is the first attribute. The second is the Indian GDP within this yearly range. The third attribute comprises the subsector's contribution to GDP, and the last is the service sector's overall contribution to employment.

19.4.1 Data Preprocessing

Before conducting any machine learning process, the data that is going to be used by the algorithm needs to be transformed and encoded in such a way that the machine learning model can easily understand and parse it. Then, each dataset was divided into a training set and test set using the order of 75% and 25%, respectively.

19.4.2 Econometric Model

An econometric is one of the tools that are used by economists to predict the afterward metamorphosis of the economy. In this research, it is applied to study the pattern of GDP over the last 10 years to contemplate on the changes in the growth and its contributing factors in different sectors.

19.4.3 Multivariate Data Analysis

To carry out the prediction using the selected machine learning models, it is important for the machine to understand what the dependent variable and the independent variables are. The multivariate data analysis technique is applied for this research. This analysis consists of a set of statistical procedures and models to explore the patterns in the multidimensional data by reviewing at once several data variables.

Travel and Tourism

After conducting the correlation analysis, it has been found out that the overall GDP growth in India are the independent variables and the total contribution to GDP and employment are the dependent variables.

Finance, Real Estate, and Business Services

It has been concluded that the GDP growth are the independent variables, while the subsector's contribution to GDP, the number of employees supported by this subsector each year, and the service sector's overall contribution to the employment are the dependent variables.

Trade, Hotels, Transport and Communication, and Services Related to Broadcasting

Following the correlation analysis, it is understood that the overall GDP growth in India are the independent variables, while the subsector's contribution to the GDP and the service sector's overall contribution to the employment are the dependent variables.

After establishing the co-dependency of the variables in each dataset, the methodology ultimately arrives at the actual prediction, which is done using two models: (1) simple linear regression and (2) simple logistic regression models. Using them, initially, each subsector's contribution to the GDP and employment is predicted from the actual GDP of India for the past 10 years, and they are compared with the actual values to calculate the total error generated in each case. Finally, using the preliminary predicted value of GDP by the IMF and the UN [18], each subsector's contribution to the GDP and employment is predicted for the economic year 2020–2021. The corresponding graphs are formed among the GDP values and the actual and predicted values of each dependent variable for each subsector of the service sector. The graphs are studied and analyzed to predict the future socioeconomic impacts due to the economic crisis caused by the lockdowns to prevent the spread of the COVID-19 infection.

19.4.4 Significance of the Proposed Methodology

Though there are multiple statistical studies which predict and comprehend the global economy along with the Indian economy in the post-COVID fiscal year, there is a paucity of research that focuses specifically on the Indian economy with predilection to service sector, its subsectors, and employability [16]. Despite the significance of this topic and its impact on the Indian economy, there are no specific studies which cater to this niche area, which was the sole motivation of this study. This study explores and provides erudite insight into this problem of the major economic shock in the year 2020 and the years that follow using the concepts of machine learning and econometric models. The service sector and its respective subsectors are majorly considered for this research as the deliberated sector provides more than a quarter of the employment of India [22].

19.5 Literature Review

To go through with this study, firstly, various articles related to the COVID-19 outbreak were scanned thoroughly. The articles of the WHO and the Scripps Research Institute provide the source and the name and family of the virus behind the COVID-19 disease [1–5], while the articles of Wetsman N., the TWC India Edit

Team, and Wikipedia webpage give information about the symptoms of the disease, the four stages of COVID-19 and at what stage India is in currently, and the first COVID-19 outbreak in China [6–13]. The Business Insider discusses the effect of pandemic on varied countries that have sealed their respective national borders, schools, colleges, offices, restaurants, movie theatres, malls, etc. and have placed extensive restrictions on their citizens from going out of their homes along with their durations [14–19]. The article released by the Press Trust of India predicts that due to extensive lockdowns, the global economy would shrink up to 1% in 2020, which would cause a great economic depression which would almost be similar to the Great Depression that took place in the year 1929–1932 [20, 21].

Accordingly, as we assayed through 30 reference studies, Zeheng Wang et al. [24] highlight the applications of traditional Chinese medicines (TCM), whether they are suitable for supplementary treatment of COVID-19 with minimum chances of side effects, and a preventive or curative vaccine which will create a substantial effect against the pandemic. Linhao Zhong et al. [25] found out that the released data related to the COVID-19 pandemic in China was unreasonable and, hence, applied simple mathematical model using Susceptible-Infected-Removed (SIR) and other fitting parameters to predict the trend of the spread of 2019-nCoV in Mainland China till the month of June. Joglas Souza et al. [26] present an innovative data science framework, known as predictive analysis framework over hybrid big data resources, and conduct cases where it can be applied in disease analytics. In this paper, the researchers assayed the climate information and online search engine data to foresee the number of patients stricken with dengue implementing a tri-kernel hybrid via a support vector machine (SVM).

Bhatnagar et al. [27] have done comprehensive work from the aspect of effect of the pandemic on India by analyzing data of patients deliberating different attributes like gender, age, and mode of communication of virus to discover substantive pattern and relationship between some of the assayed factors. Yan et al. [28] present a machine learning-based model to predict the survival rates in patients diagnosed with severe COVID-19 infection. Ronsivalle et al. [29] provide a prototype model that can be applied for georeferencing the inherent risk of contagion from COVID-19, in the nation of Italy. Each geographical unit of the country is classified into classes according to their social viscosity index (SVI), and their demographic details are taken from the following datasets [30–32] (http://opendatadpc.maps.arcgis.com/apps/opsdashboard/index.html#/b0c68bce2cce478eaac82fe38d4138b1). They apply machine learning algorithms, like k-means, k-medoids, random clustering, support vector clustering, and other deep learning methods, to predict the spread of COVID-19 in the next 10–12 days with the help of the inherent risk of contagion (IRC) mapping.

Since the infection of COVID-19 has turned out to be a global pandemic, in other words, a massive disaster, therefore, a number of research papers from known journals, which discussed the economic impacts of a disaster in a country, or in a wide region, were screened thoroughly. The prescribed reference [33] has estimated the loss in GDP due to the natural and the technological disaster-related mortality in the WHO African region. By applying the machine learning technique known as double-log econometric model and cross-sectional data on 45 out of 46 countries in the WHO African region, they concluded that capital investment, life expectancy, educational enrolment, and exports have a positive impact on GDP, while imports and disaster-related mortality are found to impact negatively. Disaster mortality of a single person could reduce GDP by US $0.018. Therefore, the policy-makers must strive to increase their investments in strengthening the national capacity to alleviate the effects of a natural disaster effectively and yield significant economic returns, which in turn would increase the GDP at a much higher rate. In the mentioned reference [34], autoregressive distributed lag (ARDL) methodology is applied to investigate the perpetual results of various categories of natural calamities on the corresponding gross domestic product in three variegated sectors for the selected Southern African countries. Having studied and analyzed all these research papers, articles, and datasets, it was evident that the main objective of this research was to predict the percentage depletion in the contribution to GDP and the associated employment from different sectors and how this depletion can be controlled. The center of this prediction would be one sector, i.e., the service sector which supports more than a quarter of the overall employment of the country [22] (Table 19.3).

19.6 Methodology

This research aims to determine the aftereffects of the COVID-19 outbreak from an economical perspective and special emphasis on the service sector of the Indi-an economy by analyzing how the potential decline in gross domestic product or GDP will affect service sectors and its various subsectors. This is done by the GDP growth prediction for the Indian economy by the International Monetary Fund or also known as IMF. According to the IMF's latest survey, GDP of the Indian economy will see a growth percentage of 1.9%, which is approximately 5.3% less than the average growth rate of the last decade. This decline will have a "domino effect" on the subsectors of the economy, while this study calibers this enervation effect on service sectors and its subsectors. This section of the research study elaborates upon the methodology used and is divided into the following sections:

- Data selection and comprehending the features dataset for each subsector
- Understanding the co-dependency of various features
- Using regression techniques to predict values
- Error calculation and results

The model development of the whole methodology is shown in Fig. 19.1, where primarily datasets are collected and conflated to get the required attributes which are then identified and assayed followed by the preprocessing of data. To get a comprehensive view of GDP pattern and their respective dependencies, econometric models are used, followed by multivariate analysis to understand the individual relationships between the selected attributes. Subsequently, to predict the subsectoral contribution to GDP and employment for service sector for the year 2020–2021,

Table 19.3 Details of research domain to identify the literature gap

Citation	Algorithm used	Dataset used	Research gaps	Conclusion
[35]	Global amalgamation of dynamic stochastic general equilibrium (DSGE) models and computable general equilibrium (CGE) models	I/O tables originated in the global trade analysis project (GTAP) database	Capital (K), labor (L), energy inputs (E), and material inputs (M) were used as input variables	This paper has described some primary estimates of the cost of the COVID-19 epidemic under seven different situations of how the disease might progress. It specifies the possible expenses that can be evaded through global accommodating asset in community health in all nations
[36]	SIR epidemiological model along with linear economy	The World Health Organization (WHO) compiled by the Johns Hopkins University Center for Systems Science and Engineering (JHU CCSE)	Total cases separated into those that have recovered and those who have died have been used. The results conclude that the population starts with 10% at the beginning of the lockdown and peaks at 60% within a month and then the curve slowly decreases to 10% again when lockdown completes	This paper investigates the optimum lockdown policy to control the mortalities of the contagion and minimalize the output expenses during lockdown. After doing the examination, it settles that the absence of testing upsurges the economic prices of the lockdown and cuts the duration of the optimal lockdown, which ends more brusquely
[37]	Review on the real-world observations of the measure adopted during the COVID-19 pandemic	Social distancing policies, fiscal policies, monetary policies, stock market policies	With the increasing lockdown days, the monetary policies and other policies greatly affect the level of economic activities and the closing, opening, and highest and lowest stock price of the major stock market indices, while,internal movement restrictions and higher fiscal policy had a negative impact on the level of economic activities	This paper answers two questions: How did a health crisis turn into an economic crisis? Why did the spread of COVID-19 disrupt the global economy?
[38]	A review on the economic impact of COVID-19	Stock market volatility, newspaper-based economic uncertainty, and subjective uncertainty in business expectation surveys	The COVID-19 pandemic has created a massive ambiguity tremor—greater than the one linked with the fiscal disaster of 2008–2009 and more alike in degree to the rise in ambiguity during the Great Depression of 1929–1933	This paper studies and symbolizes the enormous increase in the economic ambiguity in near real time using stock market unpredictability measures,newspaper-based measures of economic ambiguity, and accumulating over answers to survey questions about apparent enterprise-level ambiguity

Citation	Algorithm used	Dataset used	Research gaps	Conclusion
[39]	A review on the stock market impact of COVID-19	Automated and human readings of newspaper articles	It suggests that administration limitations on marketable activity and voluntary social isolation, functioning with influential effects in a service-oriented economy, are the main reasons the US stock market reacted so much more forcefully to COVID-19 than to the previous pandemics in 1918–1919, 1957–1958, and 1968	This paper has shown that the effects of COVID-19 expansions and strategy replies on the US stock market are without ancient instance. There were more than 1100 daily stock market changes (up or down) superior than 2.5% from 1900 to 2019
[33]	Machine learning technique called double-log econometric model	United Nations Development Programme, World Bank Data	Land, capital, labor force, human capital, and import of goods were used as input variables. Capital investment, life expectancy, educational enrolment, and exports have a positive impact on GDP, while imports and disaster-related mortality are found to impact negatively. Disaster mortality of a single person could reduce GDP by US$ 0.018	This paper has estimated the loss in GDP due to the natural and the technological disaster-related mortality in 45 out of 46 countries in the WHO African region. It has concluded that the policy-makers must strive to increase their investments in strengthening the national capacity to alleviate the effects of a natural disaster effectively and yield significant economic returns, which in turn would increase the GDP at a much higher rate
[34]	Autoregressive distributed lag approach or bound testing	The economic sectors of five selected Southern African countries	Floods, drought, epidemic, storm's effect on agriculture, manufacturing, and services were used in the analysis. It was concluded that some calamities have negative effect on GDP, while others have positive effect	This paper investigates the effect of various natural disasters on the economic performance of the five selected countries of Southern African region. It suggested that the present study for all three models has been bound together perceptually. The nations need to plan in developing flood protection systems and water storage for supply during droughts

(continued)

Table 19.3 (continued)

Citation	Algorithm used	Dataset used	Research gaps	Conclusion
[24]	Artificial neural network (ANN)	Self-created dataset consisting of name, category (hot and cold), and dosage of each medicine component in a TCM compound prescription	A BOW (bag of word) was used for this methodology, which is a dictionary of names of all TCM drug ingredients and the information of their dosage and attributes. FTS, PMSP, and SF are the harmless, which have more than 0.8 SI, whereas JHQG, LHQW, etc. are the medications that are unsafe in nature, indicating below 0.2	This paper mainly highlights the use of TCM medicines and whether they can be used as a supplementary treatment for COVID-19 without causing much side effects. Medicines like FFTS, PMSP, and SF will have minimum side effects, which means they can very well be used for treatment
[25]	Simple mathematical model using Susceptible-Infected-Removed (SIR) and fitting parameters to predict infection	(1) Wuhan Municipal Health Commission (http://wjw.wuhan.gov.cn/), (2) (http://wjw.hubei.gov.cn/), (3) (http://www.nhc.gov.cn/)	Simple analysis using the susceptibles (S), namely, the healthy population vulnerable to infection, the infectives (I), the infected population, and the removed infectives (R). Every two 2019-nCoV infectives can infect at least one person per day	This paper presents a study and a prediction on the trend of the spread of SARS-CoV-2 virus in the region of Mainland China till the month of June using simple mathematical model and susceptible-infected-removed (SIR) technique, which presents results contradicting the original released data.
[26]	Support vector machine (SVM)	(1) Environment Canada and (2) US National Centers for Environmental Information (NCEI), which is formerly known as National Climatic Data Center (NCDC) and Google trends	Total dengue cases such as CDC, NOAA Google Search Interest (GSI), and Google Trends, were the variables used. Results also show that the linear kernel with the GSI feature led to the most accurate prediction (with MAE being the smallest)	In this paper, the researchers assayed the climate information and online search engine data to foresee and forecast dengue-stricken patients and find that this hybrid framework can be used in health agencies for disease control and prevention
[27]	Data mining techniques like boxplot, Q-Q plot, normalization, chi-square, decision tree techniques, etc.	The dataset consists of the records of the patients who belong to India or have visited India. Created and maintained by the government, this dataset gets updated every 5 min	Date announced, age, gender, state, status (hospitalized, deceased, or recovered), country travelled, and transmission type were used as input variables. Age is not a significant factor in getting infected by the disease, a strong relationship is found between gender and transmission type, Maharashtra has the highest number of hospitalized patients, but the number of deaths is less in all states, young people have higher chance of recovery, and old or middle-age people especially belonging to East or North have higher chances of death	This paper presents a comprehensive work from the aspect of the effect of pandemic on India by analyzing data of patients deliberating different attributes like gender, age, and mode of communication of virus to discover substantive pattern and relationship between some of the assayed factors

Citation	Algorithm used	Dataset used	Research gaps	Conclusion
[28]	Classification concept was applied for the problem generated in this situation. XGBoost and decision tree classification were used	Blood samples of severely affected COVID-19 patients	Basic information; symptoms; blood samples; laboratory tests, including liver function, kidney function, and coagulation function; electrolytes; and inflammatory factors taken originally from severe and critical patients were used. Increase of LDH and hs-CRP and decrease in lymphocytes are the major contributing factors that can lead to the death of the patients severely infected with COVID-19	The dataset of blood sample of various patients seriously infected with COVID-19 was used to identify life-saving biomarkers of patients within a dangerous ailment variety. The concept of classification was used, in which XGBoost model and decision tree model were applied. The model predicted that LDH, hs-CRP, and lymphocytes are highly contributing factors in predicting the survival rates of patients with up to 99% accuracy
[29]	Machine learning algorithms (k-means, k-medoids, random clustering, support vector clustering, deep learning)	Census sections dataset—(https://www.istat.it/it/archivio/104317), Municipality datasets - (A)ISTAT, "Matrici di contiguità" (contiguity matrixes)—(https://www.istat.it/it/archivio/157423), (B) OpenStreetMap, maps of municipal services (2011–2019)—(https://www.openstreetmap.org), (C) ISTAT, "Confini administrative aggiornati al 1 gennaio 2019" (Administrative boundaries updated at 1 January 2019)—(https://www.istat.it/it/archivio/222527), Covid-19 case dataset—Department of Civil Protection, in the "COVID-19 Italy—situation monitoring" area, updated as of 12 March 2020: (http://opendatadpc.maps.arcgis.com/apps/opsdashboard/index.html#/b0c68bce2cce478eaac82fe38d4138b1)	Each geo-unit is defined by a vector v which contains its characteristics. These vectors were used as input variables. The real and predicted values of IRC over provinces show (1) a constant spread of contagion in the northern provinces, (2) a probable decrease in the rate of contagion in "historic" areas, and (3) the progressive potential spread of contagion in some southern provinces. The IRC values at the municipal level give an overview of the potential development of the rate of contagion in the next 10/12 days	This paper proposes a prototype model of georeferencing the COVID-19 contagion risk in Italy by classifying each geographical unit into classes according to their social viscosity index (SVI) and predicts the spread of COVID-19 in the next 10–12 days with the help of inherent risk of contagion (IRC) mapping

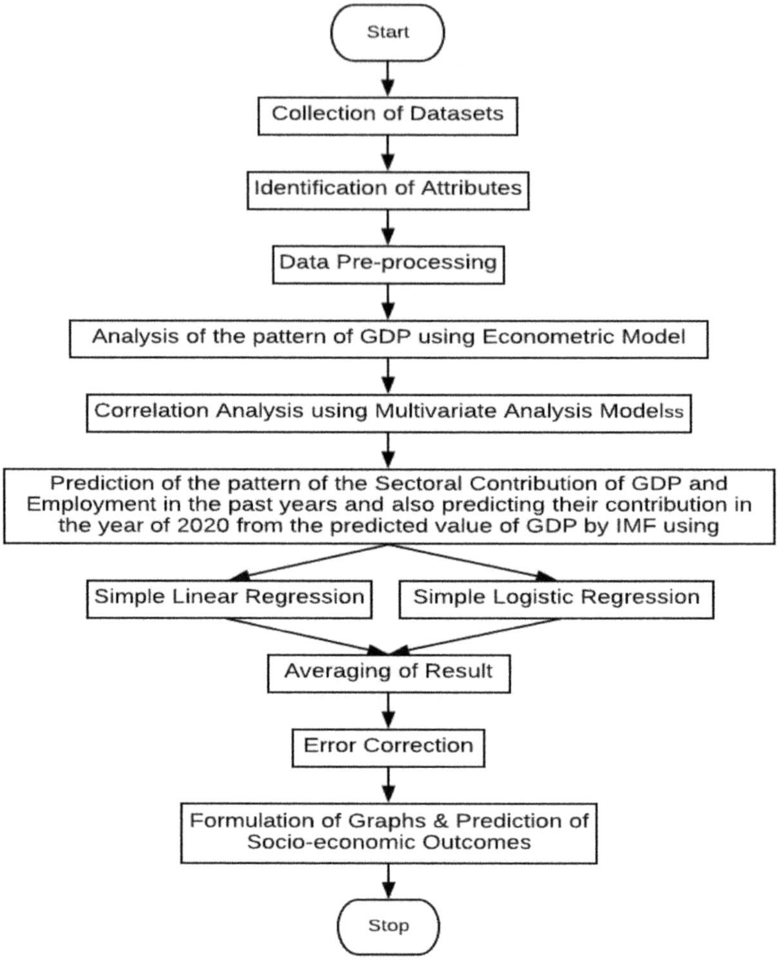

Fig. 19.1 Model development of the proposed methodology

the data from the previous decade is deliberated to understand and develop the relationship between the identified attributes using regression algorithms like simple linear regression and logistic linear regression. The mean value of outcomes is calculated, which the errors generated are deliberated using the mean absolute percentage error, and the results are visualized graphically (Table 19.4).

19.7 Subsector 1: Travel and Tourism

Figure 19.4 shows the dataset elaborating the collected data with features considering employment contribution and GDP contribution of the selected subsector 1. The specified dataset revolves on three features: GDP growth in India, also formally

Table 19.4 Dataset of subsector comprising travel and tourism (https://databank.worldbank.org/reports.aspx?source=2&series=NY.GDP.MKTP.KD.ZG&country=IND#; https://knoema.com/WTTC2019/world-travel-and-tourism-council-data?accesskey=ewmskkd; https://dbie.rbi.org.in/DBIE/dbie.rbi?site=publications)

Year	GDP growth of India	Travel and tourism's percentage share of GDP (%)	Travel and tourism's percentage share of employment (%)
2019–2020	7.9899	9.34	8.12
2018–2019	6.8114	9.24	8.08
2017–2018	7.1679	9.31	8.03
2016–2017	8.1695	9.37	7.96
2015–2016	7.9963	9.26	7.92
2014–2015	7.4102	9.19	7.93
2013–2014	6.3861	9.15	7.87
2012–2013	5.4564	9.14	7.88

known as economic growth, is defined as an increase in the production of economic goods and services, compared from one period of time to another. It can be explained as the aggregate economic growth measured in terms of gross national product (GNP) or gross domestic product (GDP). The second feature is the selected subsector's share of GDP, i.e., travel and tourism's contribution to GDP in percentage. Lastly, the third factor is the selected sector's contribution toward employment percentage provided by the Indian economy. Both GDP contribution and employment contribution are mutually exclusive in terms of de-pendency while are individually dependent on GDP growth.

For the year 2019–2020, the growth percentage of GDP was 7.98%, which is individually dependent on the given sector's share to GDP and employment contribution.

19.7.1 Subsector 2: Finance, Real Estate, and Business Services

Table 19.5 shows the dataset elaborating the collected data with features considering employment contribution and GDP contribution of the selected subsector 2. The specified dataset revolves on three features: GDP growth of India, which can be explained as the aggregate economic growth, is measured in terms of gross national product (GNP) or gross domestic product (GDP). The second feature is the selected subsector's share of GDP, i.e., finance, real estate, and business services' contribution to GDP in percentage. Lastly, the third factor is the selected sector's contribution toward employment percentage provided by the Indian economy. Both GDP contribution and employment contribution are mutually exclusive in terms of dependency while are individually dependent on GDP growth.

Table 19.5 Dataset of subsector comprising finance, real estate, and business services (https://databank.worldbank.org/reports.aspx?source=2&series=NY.GDP.MKTP.KD.ZG&country=IND#; https://knoema.com/WTTC2019/world-travel-and-tourism-council-data?accesskey=ewmskkd; https://dbie.rbi.org.in/DBIE/dbie.rbi?site=publications)

Year	GDP growth in India	Finance, insurance, real estate, and business services percentage contribution to GDP (%)	No. of employees supported each year	Contribution of service sector toward employment (%)
2009–2010	7.8619	15.98	838,769	26.27
2010–2011	8.4976	19.05	824,659	26.57
2011–2012	5.2413	18.28	926,028	27.52
2012–2013	5.4564	22.43	1,050,885	28.64
2013–2014	6.3861	25.24	1,175,149	29.04
2014–2015	7.4102	25.75	1,220,731	29.55
2015–2016	7.9963	24.55	1,253,955	30.10

For the year 2019–2020, the growth percentage of GDP was 7.98%, which is individually dependent on the given sector's share to GDP, i.e., 15.98 and employment contribution of value 26.27 with a feature of the number of employees that is redundant to contribution to employment.

19.7.2 Subsector 3: Trade, Hotels, Communication, and Broadcasting Services

Table 19.6 shows the dataset elaborating the collected data with features considering employment contribution and GDP contribution of the selected subsector 3. The specified dataset revolves on three features: GDP growth of India, which can be explained as the agglomerative economic advancement, is quantified on the grounds of gross domestic product (GDP). The second feature is the selected subsector's share of GDP, i.e., trade, hotels, communication, and broadcasting services' contribution to GDP in percentage. Lastly, the third factor is the selected sector's contribution toward employment percentage provided by the Indian economy. Both GDP contribution and employment contribution are mutually exclusive in terms of dependency while are individually dependent on GDP growth.

For the year 2019–2020, the growth percentage of GDP was 7.98%, which is individually dependent on the given sector's share to GDP, i.e., 18.30 and employment contribution of value 31.90.

Table 19.6 Dataset of subsector consisting of trade, hotels, transport, and communication and broadcasting services (https://databank.worldbank.org/reports.aspx?source=2&series=NY.GDP.MKTP.KD.ZG&country=IND#; https://dbie.rbi.org.in/DBIE/dbie.rbi?site=publications)

Year	GDP growth in India	Trade, hotels, transport, and communication and broadcasting services' percentage contribution to GDP (%)	Contribution of service sector toward employment (%)
2019–2020	7.989878	18.30	31.90
2018–2019	6.811369	20.19	31.45
2017–2018	7.167889	18.41	31.01
2016–2017	8.169527	17.53	30.59
2015–2016	7.996254	17.47	30.10
2014–2015	7.410228	20.43	29.55

19.7.3 Linear Regression and Logistic Regression

Linear regression models or procedures are applied to display or forecast the relationship between two variables or factors. In the simple regression model, a straight line resembles the relationship between the dependent variable and the independent variable. The model is represented by the following equation:

$$Y = aX + b \tag{19.1}$$

Y GDP contribution of subsector 1 toward economy, X growth of GDP for the Indian economy for the year 2020–2021, where "a" is the coefficient and "b" is the intercept with residual.

$$Y_2 = cX_2 + d \tag{19.2}$$

Y_2 employment contribution of subsector 1 toward economy, X_2 Growth of GDP for the Indian economy for the year 2020–2021, where "c" is the coefficient and "d" is the intercept with residual.

The model was firstly trained by applying the training set of each dataset and then applied on the test sets, respectively. It predicted the pattern of the contribution of each subsector of the service sector toward GDP and employment over the past 10–20 years till 2019, which was then compared with the actual values to get the error in prediction. Then, using reverse engineering technique, the model was used to predict the contribution of each subsector toward GDP and employment in 2020, given the predicted value of GDP by the IMF due to the situation around COVID-19.

Logistic regression is essentially a classification algorithm, which is only applied to situations where the dependent variable is categorical. The main aim of a logistic regression model is to identify a relationship or co-dependency between the features and the probability of a particular outcome. The logistic regression is expressed as follows:

$$\log\left(\frac{p}{p-1}\right)=y \tag{19.3}$$

where "*y*" is the dependent variable, i.e., either employment contribution or share toward GDP contribution, and "*p*" is the independent variable, i.e., GDP growth of India for the year 2020–2021 as predicted by the IMF.

The model was firstly trained by applying the training set of each dataset and then applied on the test sets, respectively. It predicted the pattern of the contribution of each subsector of the service sector toward GDP and employment over the past 10–20 years till 2019, which was then compared with the actual values to get the error in prediction. Then using reverse engineering technique, the model was used to predict the contribution of each subsector toward GDP and employment in 2020, given the predicted value of GDP by the IMF due to the situation around COVID-19.

Table 19.7 shows the averaged-out results for the regression algorithms applied; as visible, it contains eight columns or attributes, namely, years (1), GDP growth of India (2), subsector 1's contribution to GDP actual (3), subsector 1's contribution to GDP predicted (4), error calculation for GDP contribution (5), contribution toward employment actual (6), contribution toward employment predicted (7), and error calculation for contribution toward employment (8).

Attributes that are previously elaborated upon are, namely, years (1), GDP growth of India (2), subsector 1's contribution to GDP actual (3), and contribution toward employment actual (6). On the contrary, subsector 1's contribution to GDP predicted (4) and contribution toward employment predicted (7) are predicted using previously mentioned regression algorithm.

Error is calculated using the mean square error formulation that is calculated using the given formula for attributes, namely, error calculation for GDP contribution (5) and error calculation for contribution toward employment (8).

$$\frac{1}{n}\sum_{i=1}^{n}\left(Y_i-\hat{Y}_i\right)^2 \tag{19.4}$$

n number of data points, Y_i observed values, $\widehat{Y_i}$ predicted values

Moving on to subsector 2 (Table 19.8) consisting of 11 columns or attributes, namely, years (1), GDP growth in India (2), subsector 2's contribution to GDP actual (3), subsector 2's contribution to GDP predicted (4), error calculation for GDP contribution (5), number of employees actual (6), number of employees predicted (7), error calculation for the number of employees (8), contribution toward employment actual (9), contribution toward employment predicted (10), and error calculation for contribution toward employment (11).

Attributes, namely, years (1), GDP growth in India (2), subsector 2's contribution to GDP actual (3), number of employees actual (6), and contribution toward employment actual (9) are elaborated upon previously. On the other hand, subsector 2's contribution to GDP predicted (4), number of employees predicted (7), and

Table 19.7 Predicted percentage contribution toward GDP and employment by subsector comprising travel and tourism for the past 10 years and for 2020–2021

Year	GDP growth in India	Travel and tourism's percentage contribution of GDP (actual) (%)	Travel and tourism's percentage contribution of GDP (predicted) (%)	Travel and tourism's percentage contribution of GDP (error) (%)	Travel and tourism's percentage share of employment (actual) (%)	Travel and tourism's percentage share of employment (predicted) (%)	Travel and tourism's percentage share of employment (error) (%)
2020–2021	1.9		5.41485			3.1748	
2019–2020	7.9898783	9.34	9	−0.03640257	8.12	7.05	0.131773399
2018–2019	6.81136933	9.24	8.56	−0.073593074	8.08	11.36	−0.405940594
2017–2018	7.16788886	9.31	10	0.074113856	8.03	11.78	−0.466998755
2016–2017	8.16952651	9.37	10.03	0.070437567	7.96	9.08	−0.140703518

Table 19.8 Predicted percentage contribution toward GDP and employment by subsector comprising finance, real estate, and business services for the past 10 years and for 2020–2021

Year	GDP growth in India	Finance, insurance, real estate, and business services (A) (%)	Finance, insurance, real estate, and business services (P) (%)	Finance, insurance, real estate, and business services (error) (%)	No. of employees supported each year (A)	No. of employees supported each year (P)	No. of employees supported each year (error)	Contribution of service sector towardsemploy-ment (A) (%)	Contribution of service sector toward employment (P) (%)	Contribution of service sector toward employment (error) (%)
2020–2021	1.9		−13.95			113,031.5			10.53	
2019–2020	7.989878	−1.34	−3.74	−179.10	1,380,461	1,089,046	0.21109977	31.90	28.90	9.40
2018–2019	6.811369	19.71	13.71	30.44	1,349,891	1,254,891	0.070376053	31.45	29.45	6.36
2017–2018	7.167889	−26.09	−15.75	39.63	1,300,934	1,115,934	0.142205523	31.01	29.06	6.29
2016–2017	8.169527	20.55	23.98	−16.69	1,291,542	1,261,344	0.023381353	30.59	32.77	−7.13
2015–2016	7.996254	24.55	29.58	−20.49	1,253,955	2,053,657	-0.637743779	30.10	32.90	−9.30

contribution toward employment predicted (10) are predicted using mentioned regression techniques, and error evaluation is done using the MEAN or mean squared error.

Lastly, subsector 3, such as trade, hotels, transport and communication, and broadcasting services, works on similar grounds as shown in Table 19.9.

It consists of trade, hotel, communication, and broadcasting, which consist of eight columns or attributes, namely, years (1), GDP growth in India (2), subsector 3's contribution to GDP actual (3), subsector 3's contribution to GDP predicted (4), error calculation for GDP contribution (5), contribution toward employment actual (6), contribution toward employment predicted (7), and error calculation for contribution towards employment (8).

Attributes that are previously elaborated upon are, namely, years (1), GDP growth in India (2), subsector 3's contribution to GDP actual (3), and contribution toward employment actual (6). On the contrary, subsector 3's contribution to GDP predicted (4) and contribution toward employment predicted (7) are predicted using mentioned regression techniques, and error evaluation is done using the MEAN or mean squared error. Here is a concise error for the three subsectors (Table 19.10).

19.8 Results and Discussions

This research is a compendium of the aftereffects the Indian economy will face post-COVID-19 breakdown. With special emphasis on the service sector and its subsectors, below are the compiled results derived from the previously mentioned methodology and algorithms which are further categorized into four sections, namely:

19.8.1 Travel and Tourism

Figures 19.2 and 19.3 show the results predicted based upon the proposed methodology, i.e., reverse engineering applied on the GDP prediction declared by the IMF for the economic year 2020–2021, for the service sector's most prominent subsector travel and tourism. It predicts how much drop in terms of employment and GDP contribution the sector will face.

The GDP contribution by the travel and tourism subsector faces a steep drop of 20.702%, while the employment contribution of the same declines by the percentage of 59.052%. This colossal drop will adversely affect the growth and solvency of the sector and the various small trades and businesses dependent on it. Some of the tourist spots of India, such as Andaman and Nicobar Islands, Goa, Kerala, Assam, and Himachal Pradesh, to name a few, have their economy and employment majorly dependent on the lucrative tourist attention and will face major setbacks.

Table 19.9 Predicted percentage contribution toward GDP and employment by subsector comprising trade, hotels, transport, and communication and broadcasting services for the past 10 years and for 2020–2021

Year	GDP growth in India	Trade, hotels, transport, and communication and services related to broadcasting (A)	Trade, hotels, transport, and communication and services related to broadcasting (P) (%)	Trade, hotels, transport, and communication and services related to broadcasting (error)	Contribution of service sector toward employment (A)	Contribution of service sector towardsemployment (P)	Contribution of service sector toward employment (error)
2020–2021	1.9		12.24			13.33	
2019–2020	7.9898783	18.30	15.44	15.63	31.90	32.56	−2.07
2018–2019	6.81136933	20.19	24.16	−19.66	31.45	32.18	−2.32
2017–2018	7.16788886	18.41	15.63	15.10	31.01	31.99	−3.16
2016–2017	8.16952651	17.53	16.73	4.56	30.59	29.91	2.22
2015–2016	7.99625379	17.47	16.87	3.43	30.10	29.00	3.65

Table 19.10 Average error calculated for each subsector

Travel and tourism	Finance, real estate, and business services	Trade, hotels, transport, and communication and broadcasting services
0.129655013	3.860502573	0.13679675

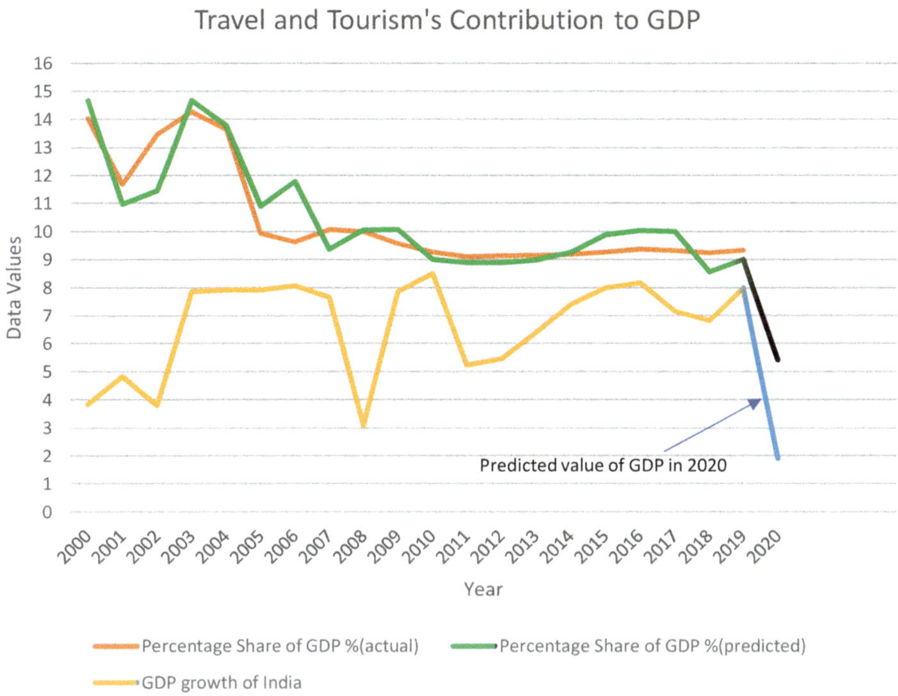

Fig. 19.2 Graph showing the predicted contribution to GDP in 2020–2021 by the subsector comprising travel and tourism

19.8.2 Finance, Real Estate, and Business Services

Finance, real estate, and business services like major banks and money lenders like SBI, ICICI, HDFC, or real estate giants like DLF, Supertech, Amrapali, or major or minor business services contribute a salient amount toward GDP alone. Figures 19.4 and 19.5 show the results cumulated by applying the proposed methodology.

The mentioned sector's contribution to GDP will see a gigantic drop of 20% in the first quarter, which will step down to 88.65% toward the last quarter of the coming economic year. On similar grounds, the sector's contribution to employment will see an enormous decline of 98.96%. The above figures are worrying enough to understand and comprehend the aftereffects of COVID-19 on the Indian economy, with special emphasis on banking, finance, and real estate subsector.

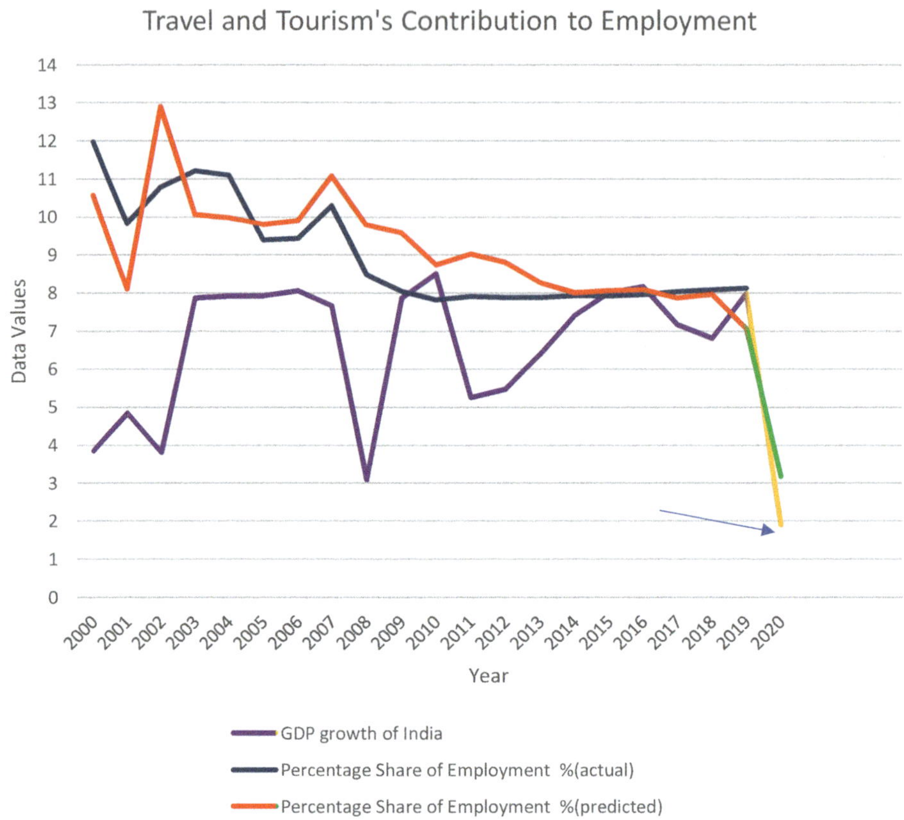

Fig. 19.3 Graph showing the predicted contribution to employment in 2020–2021 by the subsector comprising travel and tourism

19.9 Trade, Hotels, Transport, and Communication and Services Related to Broadcasting

The trade, transport, and communication industry include various minor and major industries in the field of fashion, processed agrarian industries, individual trades and businesses, etc. and major transportation and communication industries like buses, taxis, metros, trains, and airline services including entertainment industry, to name a few. Figures 19.6 and 19.7 show the predicted results based on the proposed methodology.

This sector clarifies under a vast drop of 92.007% toward its GDP contribution while a hefty decline of 63.555% toward its employment contribution. This will adversely affect businesses like Ola, Uber, the fashion industries like Biba, Nykaa, Raymond, small-scale shops, and eateries like the city-specific eating joints and processed food industries including famous restaurant chains like Mainland China,

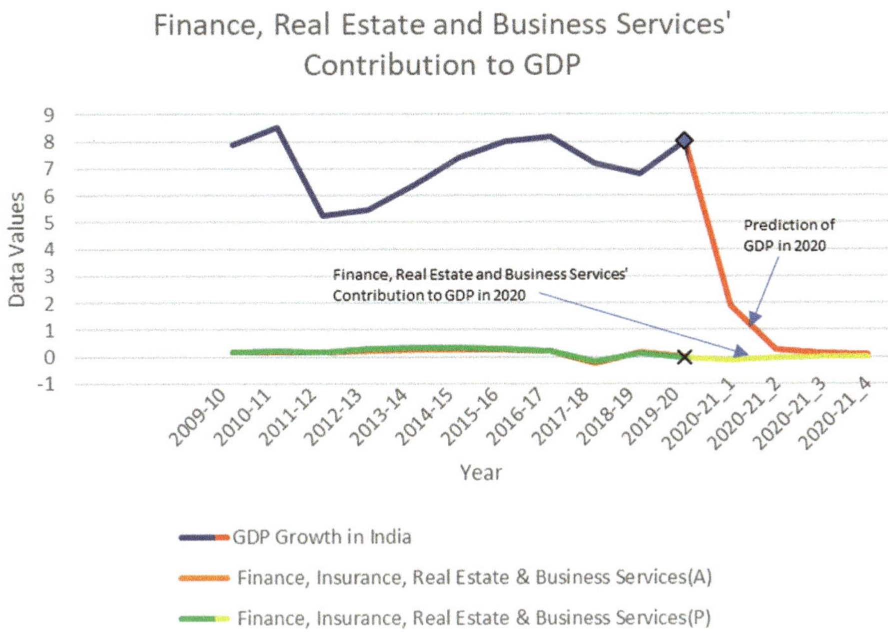

Fig. 19.4 Graph showing the predicted contribution to GDP in 2020–2021 by the subsector comprising finance, real estate, and business services

Karim's Cafe, etc. The hotels and hospitality industry will face major setbacks including brands like Taj, J W Marriott, Radisson along with millennial businesses like OYO, regional small-scale hotels, and motels. This will also adversely affect the entertainment industry like daily broadcast services like television, movies, theatres, and radio.

19.9.1 Limitations of the Study

Although this study explores and elucidates upon a niche and crucial branch of research, there are certain limitations of the study which cannot be ignored. Firstly, the approach followed in the presented study has scope of improvement as multiple attributes like developments in the equity market, policies by state and regional government authorities, and Indian trade policies among others can be considered. The pandemic, global economy, and government policies are very dynamic, in which with every passing day, multiple updates are encountered, proving the need for a dynamic data-based study. But this study deliberated the data at a static time, which can have major shortcomings. The scope of the presented study is limited to the service sector of the Indian economy. International policies, global trade, and

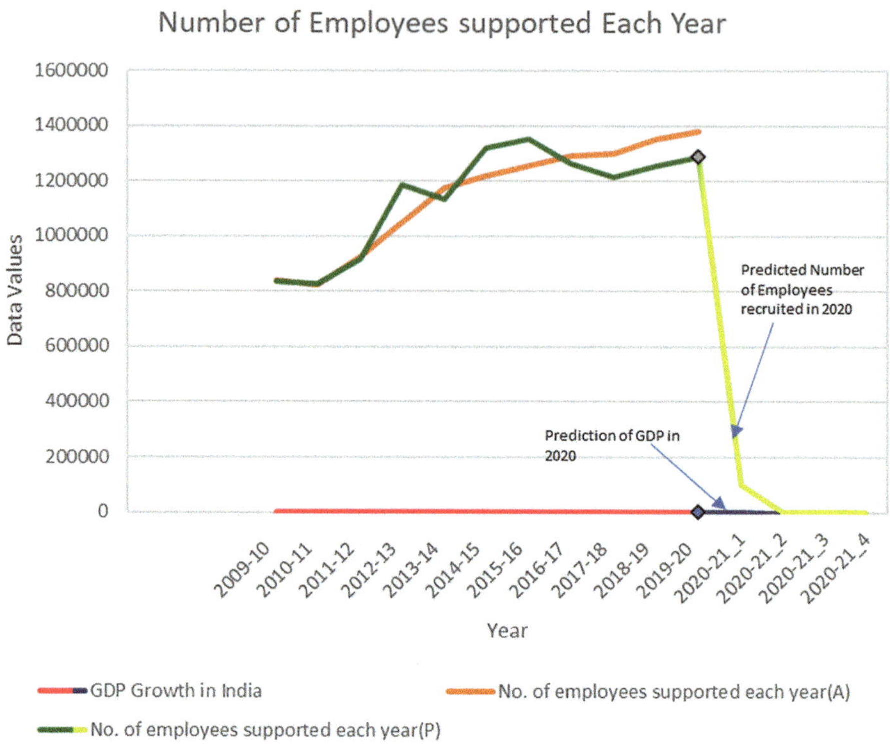

Fig. 19.5 Graph showing the predicted contribution to employment in 2020–2021 by the subsector comprising finance, real estate, and business services

international equity market have not been deliberated upon, thus limiting the scope of the study.

19.10 Implications of the Study

Conclusively, this study explicitly evaluates and elaborates the economic perspective of the aftereffects of the pandemic across each of the major subsector categories of the service sector of India for the fiscal year 2020–2021. The results discussed above conclude how each economic subsector category's trend of contribution to the GDP and employment would dwindle by the end of the year, as predicted using the regression techniques. As mentioned in the previous sections, this study successfully maps the impact of the pandemic on Indian economy, thereby paving way to identify the solutions to mitigate the same. Considering that this pattern continues, there are various socioeconomic aspects of the post-COVID-19 scenario that are likely to change with the predicted changes in the economy. Due to lack of

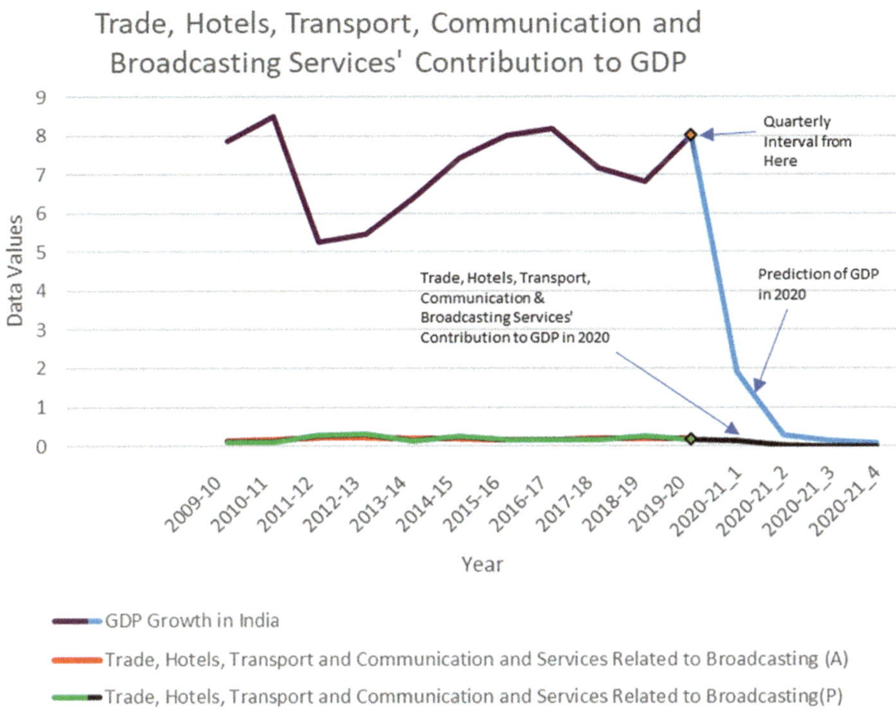

Fig. 19.6 Graph showing the predicted contribution to GDP in 2020–2021 by the subsector comprising trade, hotels, transport, and communication and broadcasting services

liquid funds and lucrative businesses, there will be a huge downfall in employment, which will create civil war situations with many occurrences of corruption and crime. Hence, criminal activities, like robbery, murder, chain snatching, cybercrimes, looting, and hacking of lucrative fund sources like banks, will become prevalent. This will adversely affect the lifestyle and physical and mental health of the citizens by increasing mental stress and depressive tendencies collaborated with increased suicides, loss of loved ones, and further scarcity of resources.

19.11 Recommended Solutions and Future Work

In future research, it is proposed to further analyze the quantized effect of the pandemic on the socioeconomic front. But below are some recommended policy solutions which can be implemented to reduce the effect to a palpable extent:

1. It is important for the government policies to be multidimensional, bold, and unbound by convention, for instance, the recent policies by RBI will have positive affect.

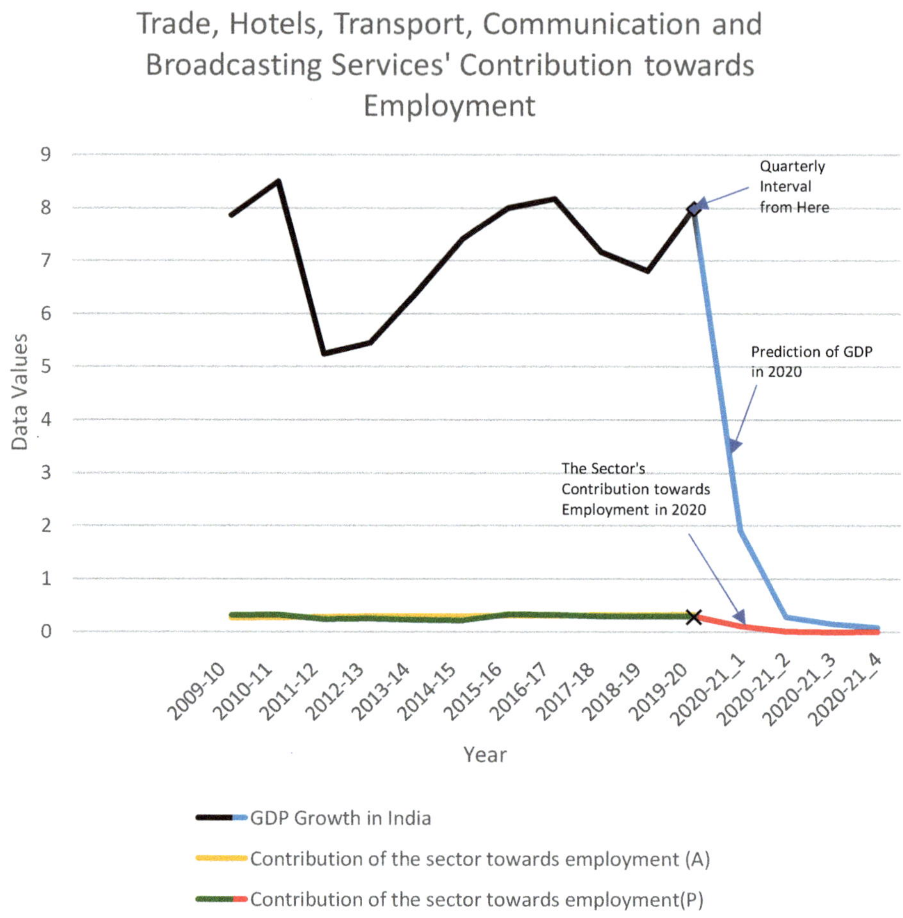

Fig. 19.7 Graph showing the predicted contribution to employment in 2020–2021 by the subsector comprising trade, hotels, transport, and communication and broadcasting services

2. Eminently, the effects of the same on healthcare will create a dense economic contraction. Thus, strict trade policies and reduced taxes will lift some of the load.
3. There can be significant policies by the government in the field research and developments toward treatment to recruitment of hospital staff and intensifying communal aid.
4. Mitigation efforts can include decrease of revenue and attenuation in spending amounts by reprioritizing daily needs.
5. India may have room for providing liquidity to solvent banks. Hence, the government must take severe measures to maintain inflow to banks. The presented solutions and socioeconomic effects can be further quantized and analyzed to

determine by how much and to what extent the proposed techniques mitigate the pandemic's effect on both social and economic fronts.

Acknowledgments Accomplishing a successful task is not an individual effort. It requires team work and cooperation to make it possible. This research study is not an exception as well; it was a task which was done by the unison and combined efforts by me and my fellow authors. Therefore, I would like to express my gratitude toward my mentor, Dr. Shruti Gupta, who guided me in the process and helped me overcome the obstacles in it. This acknowledgment would be incomplete without mentioning my coauthor Muskan Jindal, who envisioned the concept and provided enlightenment on the procedure. My mentor and my coauthor have provided immense support and were the driving force which led to the completion of this study. Without their inspiration, assistance, and astute guidance, this study would have been incomplete.

References

1. World Health Organization. (n.d.). *Naming the coronavirus disease (COVID-19) and the virus that causes it*. Retrieved April 16, 2020, from https://www.who.int/emergencies/diseases/novel-coronavirus-2019/technical-guidance/naming-the-coronavirus-disease-(covid-2019)-and-the-virus-that-causes-it
2. Alipio, M. M. (2020). 2019-nCOV scare: Situation report, role of healthcare professionals and clinical findings.
3. Dr. Sophie Vergnaud, MBBS. (2020, March 17). *GoodRx - error*. Retrieved May 12, 2020, from http://blocked.goodrx.com/blog/what-does-covid-19-mean-who-named-it/
4. Rogers, A. (2020, March 26). Coronavirus has a name: The deadly disease is Covid-19. Retrieved May 12, 2020, from https://www.wired.com/story/coronavirus-has-a-name-the-deadly-disease-is-covid-19/
5. Scripps Research Institute. (2020, March 17). *COVID-19 coronavirus epidemic has a natural origin*. Retrieved April 16, 2020, from https://www.sciencedaily.com/releases/2020/03/200317175442.htm
6. Wetsman, N. (2020, April 1). *Coronavirus outbreak: everything you need to know*. Retrieved April 21, 2020, from https://www.theverge.com/2020/1/23/21078457/coronavirus-outbreak-china-wuhan-quarantine-who-sars-cdc-symptoms-risk
7. Reguera, J., Mudgal, G., Santiago, C., & Casasnovas, J. M. (2014). A structural view of coronavirus–receptor interactions. *Virus Research, 194*, 3–15.
8. WHO–China Joint Mission. (2020). *Report of the WHO-China Joint Mission on coronavirus disease 2019 (COVID-19)*. World Health Organization.
9. Stewart, K., Connelly, Dawn, & Robinson, Julia. (2020, May 11). *Everything you should know about the coronavirus outbreak*. Retrieved May 12, 2020, from https://www.pharmaceutical-journal.com/news-and-analysis/features/everything-you-should-know-about-the-coronavirus-outbreak/20207629.article?firstPass=false
10. Nania, B. R. (2020, May 11). *Latest updates on coronavirus: Older Americans urged to continue 'distancing.'* Retrieved May 12, 2020, from https://www.aarp.org/health/conditions-treatments/info-2020/coronavirus-facts.html
11. OWID; ECDC. (2020). *China: Novel coronavirus case death rate trend 2020 [Dataset]*. Retrieved from https://www.statista.com/statistics/1108866/china-novel-coronavirus-covid19-case-fatality-rate-development/
12. Coronavirus Cases: Statistics and Charts - Worldometer. (2020). [Dataset]. Retrieved from https://www.worldometers.info/coronavirus/coronavirus-cases/
13. Business Insider India. (2020, April 17). *A third of the global population is on coronavirus lockdown — here's our constantly updated list of countries and restrictions*. Retrieved

April 23, 2020, from https://www.businessinsider.in/international/news/a-third-of-the-global-population-is-on-coronavirus-lockdown-x2014-hereaposs-our-constantly-updated-list-of-countries-and-restrictions/slidelist/75208623.cms#slideid=75209210
14. Salcedo, A. (2020, May 8). *Coronavirus travel restrictions and bans globally: Updating list*. Retrieved May 12, 2020, from https://www.nytimes.com/article/coronavirus-travel-restrictions.html
15. Richardson, P. (2020, May 8). *Weekly update: Global coronavirus impact and implications*. Retrieved May 12, 2020, from https://www.counterpointresearch.com/coronavirus-weekly-update/
16. PTI. (2020, April 2). *Global economy could shrink by almost 1% in 2020 due to COVID-19 pandemic: United Nations*. Retrieved April 24, 2020, from https://economictimes.indiatimes.com/news/international/business/global-economy-could-shrink-by-almost-1-in-2020-due-to-covid-19-pandemic-united-nations/articleshow/74943235.cms
17. Associated Press. (2020, April 2). *Coronavirus pandemic could shrink global economy almost 1% in 2020: UN Report*. Retrieved May 12, 2020, from https://www.hindustantimes.com/world-news/coronavirus-pandemic-could-shrink-global-economy-almost-1-in-2020-un-report/story-hVDxf03ST6emhZT7MQrXMJ.html
18. Singh, Y. (2020, April 2). *Global economy could shrink by almost 1% in 2020 due to COVID-19 pandemic: UN*. Retrieved May 12, 2020, from https://theprint.in/economy/global-economy-could-shrink-by-almost-1-in-2020-due-to-covid-19-pandemic-un/393605/
19. World Economic Survey 1932–33. League of Nations: 43.
20. History.com Editors. (2020, February 14). *Great depression history*. Retrieved May 12, 2020, from https://www.history.com/topics/great-depression/great-depression-history
21. Pells, R. H., & Romer, C. D. (n.d.). *Great depression|definition, history, causes, effects, & facts*. Retrieved May 12, 2020, from https://www.britannica.com/event/Great-Depression.
22. World Bank. (2020). *India - Distribution of the workforce across economic sectors 2019* [Dataset]. Retrieved from https://www.statista.com/statistics/271320/distribution-of-the-workforce-across-economic-sectors-in-india/
23. Jain, D., Nair, K., & Jain, V. (2015). Factors affecting GDP (manufacturing, services, industry): An Indian perspective. *Annual Research Journal of SCMS Pune, 3*, 38–56.
24. Wang, Z., Li, L., Yan, J., & Yao, Y. (2020). Evaluating the traditional Chinese medicine (TCM) officially recommended in China for COVID-19 using ontology-based side-effect prediction framework (OSPF) and deep learning.
25. Zhong, L., Mu, L., Li, J., Wang, J., Yin, Z., & Liu, D. (2020). Early prediction of the 2019 novel coronavirus outbreak in the mainland China based on simple mathematical model. *IEEE Access, 8*, 51761–51769.
26. Souza, J., Leung, C. K., & Cuzzocrea, A. (2020). An innovative big data predictive analytics framework over hybrid big data sources with an application for disease analytics. In *International conference on advanced information networking and applications* (pp. 669–680). Springer.
27. Bhatnagar, V., Poonia, R. C., Nagar, P., Kumar, S., Singh, V., Raja, L., & Dass, P. (2020). Descriptive analysis of COVID-19 patients in the context of India. *Journal of Interdisciplinary Mathematics*, 1–16.
28. Yan, L., Zhang, H. T., Goncalves, J., Xiao, Y., Wang, M., Guo, Y., & Huang, X. (2020). A machine learning-based model for survival prediction in patients with severe COVID-19 infection. medRxiv.
29. Ronsivalle, G. B., Foresti, L., & Poledda, G. A prototype model of georeferencing the inherent risk of contagion from COVID-19.
30. Basiterritoriali e variabilicensuarie. (2020). [Dataset]. Retrieved from https://www.istat.it/it/archivio/104317
31. Matrici di contiguità, distanza e pendolarismo. (2019). [Dataset]. Retrieved from https://www.istat.it/it/archivio/157423

32. Confini delleunitàamministrative a finistatistici al 1° gennaio 2020. (2020). [Dataset]. Retrieved from https://www.istat.it/it/archivio/222527
33. Kirigia, J. M., Sambo, L. G., Aldis, W., & Mwabu, G. M. (2002). The burden of natural and technological disaster-related mortality on gross domestic product (GDP) in the WHO Africa Region. *African Journal of Health Sciences, 9*(2), 169–180.
34. Abdelhak, S., Sulaiman, J., & Mohd, S. (2011). A bound testing to cointegration: An examination of natural disasters and GDP relationship in Southern Africa region. *International Journal of Applied Economics, Finance, 5*, 213–225.
35. McKibbin, W. J., & Fernando, R. (2020). The global macroeconomic impacts of COVID-19: Seven scenarios.
36. Alvarez, F. E., Argente, D., & Lippi, F. (2020). *A simple planning problem for covid-19 lockdown (No. w26981)*. National Bureau of Economic Research.
37. Ozili, P. K., & Arun, T. (2020). Spillover of COVID-19: impact on the global economy. Available at SSRN 3562570.
38. Baker, S. R., Bloom, N., Davis, S. J., & Terry, S. J. (2020). *Covid-induced economic uncertainty (No. w26983)*. National Bureau of Economic Research.
39. Baker, S. R., Bloom, N., Davis, S. J., Kost, K. J., Sammon, M. C., & Viratyosin, T. (2020). *The unprecedented stock market impact of COVID-19 (No. w26945)*. National Bureau of Economic Research.

Chapter 20
Diabetes Management System in Mauritius: Current Perspectives and Potentials of Pervasive Healthcare Technologies

Geshwaree Huzooree, Kavi Khedo, and Noorjehan Joonas

20.1 Introduction

Pervasive healthcare is a new discipline involving the use of ubiquitous computing technology to provide emergency and preventive healthcare services. Pervasive healthcare is an emerging area with the widespread plethora of health sensors, communication protocols, and intelligent context-aware applications [1, 2]. Pervasive healthcare systems (PHSs) aim at proactive detection of significant vitals of patients, ensuring preventive care and continuous monitoring solutions, thereby improving both system reliability and efficiency [3, 4]. Besides all these benefits, PHSs have the ability to provide personalized care and trustworthy feedback, which can be used by patients to improve their health and lead a normal life at their own convenience [5].

Based on the extensive literature conducted, it is observed that literature is sparse on the success factors affecting the QoL of diabetics and their willingness to adopt pervasive healthcare systems (PHSs) for diabetes monitoring. Hence, in this chapter, the evolution of diabetes in Mauritius over the years is presented. Measures that have been taken over the years by health authorities and patients are outlined. Moreover, diabetes management in Mauritius is further gauged through a survey. The findings that elucidate the experiences and reflections of the diabetic patients

G. Huzooree (✉)
Charles Telfair Campus Curtin University, Moka, Mauritius

K. Khedo
University of Mauritius, Moka, Mauritius
e-mail: K.khedo@uom.ac.mu

N. Joonas
Ministry of Health and Quality of Life Victoria Hospital Candos, Quatre Bornes, Mauritius
e-mail: Njoonas@intnet.mu

M. S. Husain et al. (eds.), *Pervasive Healthcare*, EAI/Springer Innovations in Communication and Computing, https://doi.org/10.1007/978-3-030-77746-3_20

are elaborated. Based on the findings, the key technical open issues and challenges are described to better identify the critical success factors for the adoption of PHSs. The implications are then discussed to assess the possibility of PHSs' adoption and acceptance by the Mauritian diabetic patients for better diabetes management and higher QoL.

20.2 Diabetes Management System in Mauritius

There has been a gradual rise in diabetes prevalence over the last 20 years as shown in Fig. 20.1. In 2015, Mauritius ranked second in the world with a prevalence of 22.3%, whereas in 2017, Mauritius ranked fifth with a prevalence of 22.0% [6, 7]. Despite having a very slight decrease in the prevalence of diabetes as far as Mauritius is concerned, the situation is still quite alarming, taking into consideration a small population size of around 1.27 million.

Few studies were identified which investigated the cost of diabetes in Mauritius and sub-Saharan African region. According to the International Diabetes Federation, the total economic cost spent on the treatment of diabetes and its complications in Mauritius in 2015 was USD 65.5 million, or USD 500.2 per person with diabetes per year [7]. The economic burden of the diabetes and its complication is enormous.

To effectively measure and monitor diabetes, regular blood glucose measurements are highly important for effective diagnosis and treatment since the measurements can assist in the identification and prevention of cases of hypoglycemia and

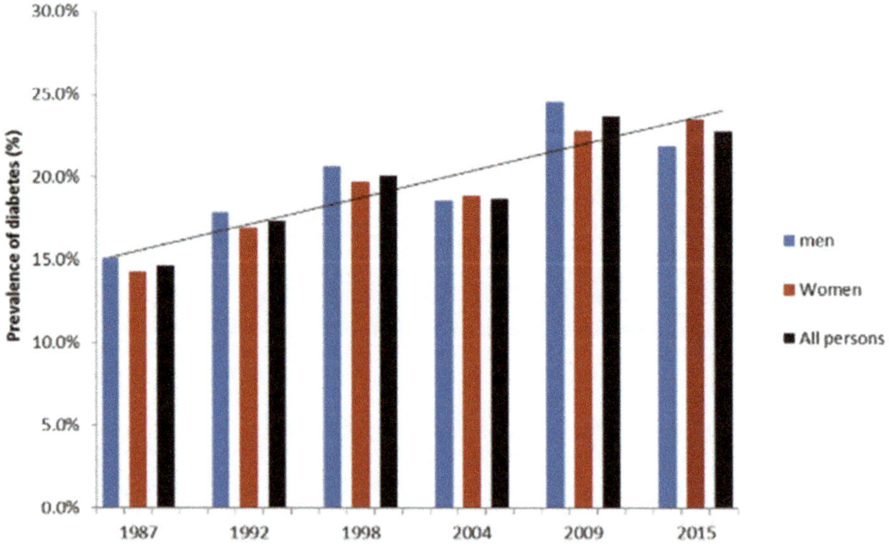

Fig. 20.1 Age-standardized prevalence of diabetes from 1987 to 2015 in Mauritius (Source: Gayan 2015)

hyperglycemia. At present, most of the technologies used in Mauritius for measuring blood glucose levels are technically invasive or minimally invasive.

Due to its high prevalence, the Ministry of Health and Quality of Life (MOHQL) is conscious that diagnosis and management of diabetics remains a major health challenge in Mauritius. The government of Mauritius has expressed the pressing need to take bold, innovative, and preventive measures to address the problems associated with diabetes [8]. Many key stakeholders are working in collaboration with the MOHQL to address this national health concern with the aim of reducing the number of people with uncontrolled diabetes, preventing complications, and improving the quality of life [8].

The National Service Framework for Diabetes (NSFD) is a 10-year program that was set up in 2007 to define strategies for diabetes prevention and standards of diabetes care in Mauritius. The main aim of the NSFD was to (1) reduce new cases of blindness due to diabetes by one third or more, (2) reduce end-stage diabetic renal failure by at least one third, (3) reduce limb amputations for diabetic gangrene by one half, and (4) reduce morbidity and mortality from coronary heart disease through the implementation of 14 key standards [9]. The 14 standards have been regrouped under a total of 10 components, namely, (1) national sensitization and awareness campaign, (2) national diabetes empowerment program, (3) nutritional and physical activity action plan, (4) registration of all people with type 1 and type 2 diabetes, (5) provision of insulin pen-like devices for children with type 1 diabetes, (6) national retinal screening program, (7) podiatry services, (8) provision of self-monitoring blood glucose meters to all pregnant women with diabetes, (9) surveillance for diabetes complications, and (10) strengthening laboratory services. These ten components are categorized into three main interventions, namely, the primary, secondary, and tertiary prevention [10].

20.3 Critical Appraisal of the Diabetes Management System of Mauritius

The National NCD Survey released in 2016 revealed that the prevalence of type 2 diabetes has stabilized for the first time in almost 30 years, a notable progress given diabetes is estimated to account for at least 20% of the national disease burden. However, the report also indicated that the ratio of newly detected diabetes to known cases of diabetes and the proportion of poorly controlled diabetic patients remain high [8].

Despite the fact that a wide range of measures have been taken at the primary, secondary, and tertiary intervention levels in terms of providing (1) screening services around the country, (2) conducting awareness campaigns on healthy lifestyle and the risk factors (such as excessive intake of sugar, poor nutrition, lack of physical activity, and smoking/alcohol abuse) that highly contribute to diabetes, (3) raising regular awareness campaign to foster education about diabetes and its associated complications, (4) conducting mass media campaign, (5) developing and implementing national guidelines, (6) treating diabetes and its associated complications, (7) training multidisciplinary staff to operate the diabetic clinics, and (8) setting up the National Service Framework For Diabetes (NSDF), the NCD surveys showed an increase prevalence of serious complications of diabetes such as kidney failure, blindness, amputations, and coronary heart disease/stroke with heavy cost implications [9].

Prevention, control, and treatment of diabetes and its associated complications remain a difficult and prolonged battle. There is a high need to establish a ratio balance in the allocation of medical resources and primary, secondary, and tertiary intervention services [8]. Diabetes management is still very much doctor-centric in Mauritius, and it is of paramount importance that diabetic patients are empowered and educated so that they can perform effective diabetes self-monitoring and management [9].

20.4 Method

The primary purpose of this cross-sectional study was to (1) assess patient satisfaction about existing diabetes management system in the public healthcare sector, (2) assess the impact of the diabetes disease on the QoL of patients, and (3) assess the critical success factors for the technology adoption level of PHS for diabetes monitoring in Mauritius.

20.4.1 Study Design and Subjects

A cross-sectional study was carried out in the period of August to November 2017 using the widely used Diabetes Treatment Satisfaction Questionnaire (DTSQ) [11], the Audit of Diabetes-Dependent Quality of Life (ADDQoL) questionnaire [12], and Technology Acceptance questionnaire [13], since those three questionnaires have been successfully used in the literature to assess the degree of treatment satisfaction for diabetes patients and the degree any participants is willing to adopt a specific technology. Inclusion and study procedures took place at Victoria Hospital Candos, Mauritius.

The study sample consisted of 50 diabetic patients between 17 and 75 years of age since the diabetic population in Mauritius is quite homogenous and there is no big variance in the profiles of the patients. The sample size covers the different profiles which are representative of the specific categories of the patients (gender, age groups, education level, social status, and diabetes self-management). Participants were from the Indo-Mauritian community, and they all met the inclusion criteria to participate in this study. The inclusion criteria were as follows: patient diagnosed with DMT1. The main exclusion criteria were (1) patients who were diagnosed suffering from DMT2, secondary diabetes, or gestational diabetes. Moreover, a translator was available for those who did not understand the English language.

20.4.2 Instrument

The questionnaire is categorized into five sections, namely, (a) demographic characteristics, (b) general health characteristics, (c) diabetes treatment satisfaction, (d) impact of diabetes on QoL, and (e) patients' intention toward using mobile technology or PHSs to monitor diabetes.

Questions from section c are based on the DTSQ questionnaire, which is a widely used measure and consists of eight items that capture patient satisfaction with the treatment and understanding of diabetes in which each item is scored on a seven-point scales [11]. The six treatment satisfaction items are rated from 0 ("very dissatisfied") to 6 ("very satisfied"), and the summed scores produce a total treatment satisfaction score that ranges from 0 to 36. The other two items measure the perceived frequency of hyperglycemia and hypoglycemia and are considered separately. Both items are rated from 0 ("none of the time") to 6 ("most of the time").

Questions from Section D are based on the Audit of Diabetes-Dependent Quality of Life (ADDQoL), which is a widely used instrument. The main aim is to assess the impact of diabetes on the QoL, considering the significance, importance, and impacts of diabetes on different life domains [12, 14, 15]. It consists of two overview items: one that assesses the current QoL (Q43) (range +3 to −3) and another one that assesses the "impact of diabetes on" the QoL (Q44) (range +3 to −3). For both items, lower scores are associated with poorer QoL. Moreover, the questionnaire consists of 19 items that assess the impact of diabetes on the QoL as follows: leisure activities, working life, local or long-distance journeys, holidays, physical health, family life, friendships and social life, close personal relationships, sex life, physical appearance, self-confidence, motivation to achieve things, people's reactions, feelings about the future, financial situation, living conditions, dependence on others, freedom to eat, and freedom to drink. Respondents rated the importance from 0 (not important at all) to +3 (very important) in attributed importance (importance rating) and rated the impact of diabetes from −3 (very much worse) to +1 (very much better) for the 19 life domains (impact rating). The impact score is multiplied by the importance rating to produce a weighted score for each domain (ranging from −9 to +3). Lower scores are associated with a worse QoL. The weighted score for the domains is divided by all applicable domains to calculate the mean weighed impact (ADDQoL) score (ranging from −9 to +3). Moreover, several items on patients' demographic characteristics are reported.

Questions from section e assess the patients' attitudes and perceptions toward using mobile phones and PHSs for diabetes monitoring using 11 questions. Eight of the eleven questions are answered using a five-point Likert scale (ranging from "strongly disagree" to "strongly agree"). The questions are chosen from past researches that assess patients' perceptions toward the usage of mobile phones and

PHSs for healthcare monitoring [13, 16]. Questions included items assessing their perceptions of diabetes monitoring through mobile phones and PHSs. The other three questions queried the type of mobile phones they possess, their comfort level in using mobile phones and PHSs, and their a priori awareness of mobile health and PHSs for diabetes monitoring.

20.4.3 Ethical Considerations

The follow-up protocol was reviewed and approved by the Ethics Review Committee of the Ministry of Health and QoL of Mauritius prior to the start of the study. Informed and written consent was acquired from all participants prior to enrolment.

20.4.4 Statistical Methods

The data was analyzed using SPSS statistical package (SPSS 21.0, Chicago, USA).

The calculations included frequency and percentage distributions to assess categorical variables (gender, marital status, diabetes self-management, monthly income, smoking status, diabetes duration, diabetes control and education background, age), means, and standard deviations for continuous variables (BMI) to express the sample data. Besides descriptive statistics, the responses were compared using a chi-square test or two-sample t-test for categorical variables and continuous variables, respectively.

Based on the ADDQoL scores, logistic regression analyses are performed to examine statistically significant differences between the patients' demographic characteristics and their QoL. The calculation includes p-value to evaluate which covariates result into a higher or lower QoL. Moreover, quartiles are used to split the patients into two groups based on the ADDQoL score. Lastly, the factors with a p-value lower than 0.05 are statistically significant.

20.5 Results

20.5.1 Sociodemographic Factors and Health Characteristics

Demographic and health-related factors of diabetic patients are illustrated in Table 20.1.

The diabetic participants are in the age group 17–75 years, whereby the majority (62%) aged between 17 and 29 years. Half of the 50 participants were female. Most of the participants are single (30, 60%), have secondary education (37, 74%), and

Table 20.1 Demographic factors and clinical characteristics of the patients

Characteristics	*N* = 50	%	Characteristics	*N* = 50	%
Gender			Smoking status		
Female	25	50	Yes	9	18
Male	25	50	No	41	82
Marital status			Diabetes duration (years)		
Single	30	60	<4 years	8	16
Married	16	32	5–10 years	11	22
Divorced	4	8	>11 years	31	62
Diabetes self-management			Diabetes control		
Yes	45	90	HbA1c ≤ 7.0	25	50
No	5	10	HbA1c >7.0	25	50
Monthly income (Rs)			Education background		
None	19	38	Below primary education	1	2
<Rs 10,000	16	32	Primary education	2	4
Rs 10,000–20,000	8	16	Secondary education	37	74
Rs 20,000 or above	7	14	Tertiary education	10	20
Age			BMI (mean ± SD)	22.03 ± 3.86	
17–29	31	62	<25	40	80
30–44	15	30	25–29	8	16
45–60	3	6	≥30	2	4
61–75	1	2			

are either nonsmoker or ex-smoker (41, 82%). Among the 50 respondents, the majority are unemployed (19, 38%), and very few earn a monthly salary above 20,000 (7, 14%). Most of the patients have DMT1 for 11 years or more (31–62%), and 25 (50%) believe that their diabetes is under control. The BMI has a mean value of 22.03 ± 3.86 kg/m^2, ranging from 16.3 to 32.9. Most of the participants (45–90%) reported that they can manage their diabetes by themselves, and everyone (50–100%) is on insulin therapy. Regarding diabetic complications, 8% have hypertension, 14% have high cholesterol, 18% have poor eye vision, 2% are undergoing kidney dialysis, 1% have suffered from brain stroke, and 8% have heart disease.

20.5.2 Treatment Satisfaction and Patient Characteristics

The mean score of the diabetes treatment satisfaction score (DTSQ) is 26.2 ± 6.26 (ranging from better to worse: 36 to 0) for the study group (Table 20.2). Male patients have a higher DTSQ score than females (26.7 ± 4.72 and 25.6 ± 7.55, respectively).

Patients above 30 years old reported a higher treatment satisfaction than those below 30 years old (26.9 ± 7.28 for >30 years and 25.7 ± 5.62 for ≤30 years). Patients with health complications reported a higher treatment satisfaction than

Table 20.2 Relationship between treatment satisfaction and demographic factors

Patient characteristics	DTSQ score (Mean ± SD)	*p*
Overall (ranging from better to worse: 36 to 0)	26.2 ± 6.26	
Gender		
Female	25.6 ± 7.55	0.562
Male	26.7 ± 4.72	
Diabetes control		
HbA1c ≤ 7	25.8 ± 6.79	0.689
HbA1c > 7	26.5 ± 5.79	
Marital status		
Married	28.9 ± 6.52	0.828
Others	26.3 ± 6.23	
Age		
<30	25.7 ± 5.62	0.492
≥30	26.9 ± 7.28	
Diabetes duration (years)		
≤10 years	28.8 ± 4.81	0.583
>10 years	25.8 ± 7.05	
Health complications		
Yes	27.3 ± 7.59	0.419
No	25.7 ± 5.65	
Income		
Unemployed	24.8 ± 5.50	0.894
<20,000	28.4 ± 5.49	
>20,000	22.0 ± 8.23	

those without health complications (27.3 ± 7.59 for health complications, 25.7 ± 5.65 without health complications).

Patients with HbA1c values higher than 7.0% have higher DTSQ scores, compared to those with HbA1c values below 7.0% (mean ± SD = 26.5 ± 5.79, mean ± SD = 25.8 ± 6.79, respectively). Married subjects reported higher treatment satisfaction scores (28.9 ± 6.52 for married and 26.3 ± 6.23 for others).

According to the findings, DTSQ scores are higher in patients having diabetes for less than 10 years, compared to those having diabetes greater than 10 years (28.8 ± 4.81 for less or equal to 10 years, 25.8 ± 7.05 for greater than 10 years, respectively). Patients earning less than Rs 20,000 reported higher DTSQ scores (28.4 ± 5.49 for <20,000, 24.8 ± 5.50 for unemployed and 22.0 ± 8.23 for >20,000).

20.5.3 Impacts of Diabetes on Different Life Domains

The findings reveal that DTM1 has a negative effect on QoL in 16.7% of diabetics, whereby 91.7% believed that they would have a better life experience if they were not diabetics.

The ADDQoL score was computed ranging from −9.0 to 0 on a specific range of −9 to +3. The median weighted impact ADDQoL score was computed and resulted in −2.9, representing an overall negative effect of DTM1 on the QoL. Twenty-three (46%) participants with DTM1 have a higher QoL (an ADDQoL score higher than −3.0), and 26 (52%) diabetics reported a lower QoL (an ADDQoL score lesser than −3.0). One patient (2%) reported that diabetes does not have any impact on his QoL (an ADDQoL score of 0). The patient is diabetic since birth. The distribution of the weighted impact scores for each life domain is shown in Table 20.3.

The findings highlight that DTM1 has a negative effect on mostly all the domains ranging from −1.0 to −5.9, particularly on the domains "Freedom to eat" (mean −2.5 ± 1.0) and "Freedom to drink" (mean −2.3 ± 1.1).

"Motivation" (mean 2.6 ± 0.8) and "Family life" (mean 2.6 ± 0.7) are rated as the most important domains, while "Dependence on others" (mean 1.5 ± 1.0) and "People's reaction" (1.6 ± 1.2) are rated as the least important QoL domains. After calculating the weighted impact score, the most affected QoL domain is "Freedom

Table 20.3 (ADDQoL) Weighted impact scores

	Impact scores	Importance scores	Weighted impact score
Life domain	Mean ± SD	Mean ± SD	Mean ± SD
Leisure activities (LEI)	−1.6 ± 1.2	2.0 ± 0.9	−3.4 ± 3.3
Working life (WORK)	−1.6 ± 1.3	2.3 ± 1.0	−3.6 ± 3.6
Long-distance journeys (JOR)	−1.4 ± 1.4	1.9 ± 0.9	−3.0 ± 3.3
Holiday (HOL)	−1.5 ± 1.3	1.9 ± 1.0	−3.1 ± 3.5
Physical health (PHY)	−1.6 ± 1.3	2.8 ± 0.5	−4.4 ± 3.9
Family life (FAM)	−1.4 ± 1.4	2.6 ± 0.7	−3.8 ± 3.9
Friendship and social life (FREN)	−1.2 ± 1.3	2.1 ± 0.8	−2.5 ± 3.2
Close personal relationship (PER)	−1.2 ± 1.3	2.3 ± 0.9	−2.9 ± 3.6
Sex life (SEX)	−0.9 ± 1.2	2.0 ± 1.1	−2.0 ± 3.1
Physical appearance (APP)	−1.1 ± 1.2	2.1 ± 0.9	−2.4 ± 3.1
Self-confidence (CONF)	−1.6 ± 1.4	2.5 ± 0.7	−4.2 ± 3.8
Motivation (MOV)	−1.7 ± 1.3	2.6 ± 0.8	−4.6 ± 3.8
People's reaction (RXN)	−1.0 ± 1.1	1.6 ± 1.2	−1.8 ± 2.7
Feelings about the future (FUT)	−1.9 ± 1.3	2.4 ± 0.8	−4.5 ± 3.5
Financial situation (FIN)	−1.2 ± 1.3	2.2 ± 0.9	−2.8 ± 3.4
Living conditions (LIV)	−1.1 ± 1.2	2.3 ± 0.9	−2.5 ± 3.3
Dependence on others (DEP)	−0.8 ± 1.0	1.5 ± 1.0	−1.0 ± 1.9
Freedom to eat (EAT)	−2.5 ± 1.0	2.3 ± 0.8	−5.9 ± 3.1
Freedom to drink (DRINK)	−2.3 ± 1.1	2.2 ± 0.8	−5.1 ± 3.1

Table 20.4 Average weighted impact scores by demographic factors of diabetic patients (t-test)

Patient characteristics	Average weighted impact scores (Mean ± SD)	*p*	Domains with significance
Overall	−3.28 ± 1.82		–
Gender			
Female	−3.66 ± 1.85	0.144	Physical appearance (p=0.014)
Male	−2.90 ± 1.76		
Diabetes control			
HbA1c ≤7	−3.24 ± 1.90	0.882	None
HbA1c >7	−3.32 ± 1.79		
Marital status			
Married	−3.81 ± 2.10	0.162	None
Others	−3.28 ± 1.82		
Age			
<30	−2.70 ± 1.50	0.003	Working life (p = 0.008), friendship and social life (p = 0.045), self-confidence (p = 0.022), Motivation (p = 0.007), people's reaction (p = 0.031), feelings about the future (p = 0.034), and financial situation (p = 0.008)
>=30	−4.23 ± 1.95		
Diabetes duration (years)			
≤10 years	−3.33 ± 1.74	0.895	Financial situation (p = 0.015)
>10 years	−3.26 ± 1.90		
Health complications			
Yes	−3.95 ± 1.59	0.090	Motivation (p = 0.032) and people's reaction (p = 0.001)
No	−3.00 ± 1.86		
Income			
Unemployed	−3.14 ± 1.51	0.926	None
<20,000	−3.54 ± 1.96		
>20,000	−2.78 ± 2.25		

to eat" (mean −5.9 ± 3.1), and the least affected is "Dependence on others" (mean −1.0 ± 1.9).

The comparison of the ADDQoL scores of diabetic patients by gender, diabetes control, marital status, age, diabetes duration level, health complications, and income is shown in Table 20.4. The demographic factor having the most significant impact on the QoL is age among diabetic patients.

Table 20.5 shows the findings of the logistic regression analysis of the ADDQoL scores in the lower quartile. The results highlight that QoL is related only to education background (below primary education, p=0.001, and tertiary education, p = 0.011, respectively).

Table 20.5 Predictors for lower QOL according to the ADDQoL score

	ADDQoL score	P	
	Higher ≥−3.0 n=23 (in %)	Lower <−3.0 *n* = 26 (in %)	
Gender			
Female	36.0	64.0	0.117
Male	56.0	40.0	
Age			
17–29	54.8	41.9	0.11
30–44	33.3	66.7	0.086
45–60	0.0	100.0	0.205
61-75	100.0	0.0	0.093
BMI (mean ± SD)			
< 25	50	47.5	0.842
25–29	37.5	62.5	0.622
≥30	50	50	0.559
Education background			
Below primary education	0	100	0.001
Primary education	0	100	0.342
Secondary education	35.1	62.2	0.174
Tertiary education	100	0	0.011
Monthly income (Rs)			
None	36.8	57.9	0.235
< Rs 10,000	56.3	43.8	0.39
Rs 10,000–20,000	25	75	0.363
Rs 20,000 or above	71.4	28.6	0.174
Marital status			
Single	53.3	43.3	0.344
Married	37.5	62.5	0.164
Divorced	25	75	0.357
Diabetes duration (years)			
<4 years	37.5	62.5	0.762
5–10 years	54.5	45.5	0.559
>11 years	45.2	51.6	0.566
Diabetes control			
HbA1c ≤ 7.0	44	56	
HbA1c >7.0	48	48	0.674
Smoking status			
Yes	55.6	44.4	0.566

However, below primary education has not been taken into consideration since there was only one patient with below primary education in the sample. Besides tertiary education, no other statistically significant relationships are found between QoL and gender, age, BMI, salary, marital status, duration of diabetes, HbA1c, smoking habits, and frequency of medicine intake.

20.5.4 Patient Attitudes Toward Using Mobile Phone Technology to Monitor Diabetes

The majority of the respondents (76%, 38/50) indicated that they already own a smartphone and are comfortable to use a mobile phone (98%, 49/50). Some patients also reported that they have only a basic mobile phone (22%, 11/50), and only one patient mentioned about not having any mobile phone. Only 42% (21/50) had prior awareness of diabetes monitoring using mobile phones and PHSs before they were surveyed (Table 20.6). Additionally, most of the patients thought that mobile technologies and PHSs could help to remind them to follow their doctor's instructions (76%, 38/50).

Furthermore, the majority thought that mobile technologies and PHSs will enable their healthcare professionals to make quicker modifications to their medication if needed (80%, 40/50). Majority of the respondents (84%, 42/50) indicated that if they have access to mobile health devices and PHSs to manage their diabetes at a low cost and are guided on the usage of the systems, they will be willing to accept and adopt the mobile systems and PHSs as directed by the healthcare professionals. Majority of the patients (84%, 42/50) reported that they are comfortable with the remote monitoring of their diabetic conditions using mobile health and PHSs. Additionally, 72% (36/50) felt confident that their privacy will be protected when using mobile health devices and PHSs.

Almost all participants (96%, 48/50) agreed that it is important to follow their doctor's instructions, and 88% (44/50) felt that mobile health technology and PHSs can effectively help them to communicate their medical conditions to their doctors.

Table 20.6 Patient attitudes to using mobile technologies and pervasive healthcare systems

Survey items ($N = 50$)	%	Mean (± SD)
Own a smartphone	76	–
Comfortable using mobile phone	98	1.02 ± 0.141
Prior awareness of mobile health and pervasive healthcare systems	42	1.58 ± 0.499
Would use mobile health and pervasive healthcare systems devices if cost is low	84	4.48 ± 0.863
Willingness to use mobile devices and pervasive healthcare systems if guidance is provided	84	4.34 ± 1.042
Comfortable for having health monitored remotely	84	4.28 ± 0.948
Mobile health and pervasive healthcare systems will help to remind following the doctors' directions	76	4.24 ± 1.098
Mobile technology and pervasive healthcare systems will allow the doctor to make medication changes quicker	80	4.24 ± 1.098
Confident that privacy will be protected when using mobile health devices and pervasive healthcare systems	72	3.98 ± 1.204
Important to follow doctor's directions	96	4.80 ± 0.495
Confident that mobile health technologies and pervasive healthcare systems can effectively communicate medical condition to the doctor	88	4.44 ± 0.929

20.6 Discussion

This survey assesses the influence of several demographic and health-related factors on the QoL of DMT1 patients in Mauritius by using the ADDQoL, which is a broadly used diabetes-specific assessment scale [12].

Several studies conducted in different countries concluded that DMT2 has a negative impact on the QoL [17, 18]. This present research has also indicated a negative impact of DMT1 on the QoL. Several kinds of research have been conducted on the prevalence of diabetes in Mauritius; however, this is the first study conducted that investigate the perception of Mauritian diabetic patients for adopting PHSs to self-manage their disease.

In accordance with prior studies [12, 14, 15, 19], the life domain "Freedom to eat" has the highest negative effect on the QoL of DMT1 patients. This indicates that dietary restriction has a strong influence on the QoL and improvement in dietary habits could lead to an improvement in the QoL of diabetics. As compared to other studies which reported that "People's reaction" has the least impact on the QoL of diabetics, the result of this research showed that "Sex life" has the least effect on the QoL of Mauritian diabetics.

Other studies reported that lower QoL was significantly associated with other health conditions [20]. In this survey, the impact of diabetes duration on the QoL was measured, and no significant relationship was found, which was in accordance with the study of Wang and Yeh [21]. In addition, in agreement with the findings of this research, other studies have shown that younger diabetics reported a better QoL as compared to elder ones. As the age of the diabetics increases, a significant drop in the QoL is noticed [12].

In the present research, the majority of the participants (more than 50%) who have lived with DMT1 for 11 or more years perceive a lower QoL. Furthermore, only 44% who indicated that they could manage their diabetes perceive a high QoL. This finding suggests that more awareness campaigns are needed to increase support and guidance regarding self-management of DMT1 in Mauritius.

An increase in the control of HBA1c was found to have a positive effect on the QoL of patient [22]. However, in this study, no association was found between HbA1c and QoL, which is in concordance with other several research [23, 24]

Finally, the result showed that patients who live alone or are divorced perceive a lower QoL. Moreover, diabetics who earn an income of Rs 20,000 or above have a higher QoL.

Recent studies have shown that PHSs can have a positive influence on the QoL, patient centricity, and ability to monitor health conditions across a wide range of illnesses. The results showed that very few diabetics have knowledge on mobile health monitoring and PHSs before being surveyed. In spite of that, the majority of patients are willing to use mobile and PHSs to manage their diabetes if the mobile devices and PHSs will be at a low cost. The findings showed that mobile technology and PHSs will further assist and help diabetics to follow their medication program. Additionally, the results highlighted that communication with healthcare professionals will be further improved, especially when it concerns changes in their medication. The results of this survey is consistent with prior studies having evaluated the perception using mobile technologies for health monitoring among patients with other health conditions such as hypertension, diabetes, congestive heart failure, and kidney failure [16, 25–27].

Although the majority of the patients were willing to use mobile devices and PHSs to manage their diabetes, a group of patients indicated a less positive attitude. These patients either had a basic mobile phone or were not likely to own a mobile phone. Consequently, this might have an impact on their comfort level in using and adopting new technologies. Thus, this issue could be resolved by ensuring that PHSs are easier to use and trustworthy. PHSs' providers should provide additional support and training programs to assist the patients in learning how to use such systems to monitor their diabetes.

20.7 Future Research Directions

High emphasis is currently being placed on preventative care and diabetes disease management to reduce healthcare expenses and to increase the patients' QoL as this has become a national priority. To address this underlying concern, many PHSDMs have been proposed that can help in the diabetes disease management; however, not all systems were successful on the market, and many had a very low acceptance and adoption rate. These problems were mainly linked to a lack of effectiveness or low QoI of the systems. Despite the fact that many technologies have been researched upon, designed, and developed, the deployment has not proven to be very successful due to several reasons, such as failure to obtain Food and Drug Administration approvals or European Conformity Mark and due to lack of adoption. One of the major causes of such failures remains a lack of QoI [28].

Based on the survey carried out, the following research challenges should be considered for the successful implementation of PHS in Mauritius at the sensor level, communication level, and human-centric level. These issues should be addressed to promote a high degree of QoI in PHSDMs for effective diabetes disease management.

20.7.1 Sensor-Level Challenges

Sensors are key components of PHSDMs as they are mainly used to sense the patients' physiological signs, such as blood pressure, temperature, and BG levels. These sensors are also responsible to process, store, and transmit the sensed information. At the sensor tier level, the QoI is mainly impacted during the data acquisition and sensing from the sensors and the data transmission to the sink (as depicted in Table 20.7).

Table 20.7 Sensor-level challenges

Sensor-level challenges	References	
Data acquisition and sensing	Ensuing accurate and complete measurements from sensor nodes is crucial Loss of data from during data collection will compromise the analysis	[29, 30]
Data transmission	Sensor nodes being disconnected can easily influence real-time decision-making	[31, 32]
Data compression	Preserving the authenticity and accuracy of the data is essential for the acceptance and adoption of the system	[33, 34]
Data acquisition and efficiency	A noisy dataset needs to be smoothed for proper sensing	[35, 36]

Data Acquisition and Sensing

Incorrect data acquisition and sensing has a high impact on the accuracy of PHSDMs and leads to a lower degree of QoI. Inaccurate information is mainly due to faulty sensor readings. Thus, the sensors should have a decent fault processing ability. Data verification algorithms should be further explored to ensure fault checking, measurement error elimination, and data refinement. Moreover, it is important to consider the accuracy and completion of the sensed data to ensure that the data are not plagued.

Data Transmission

Reliable data transfer is another vital process in the healthcare field so that healthcare practitioners can make real-time decisions. Incorrect data transmission affects the degree of completeness and timeliness of QoI. Loss of data or packet from the sensor to the sink leads to incomplete information and consequently results in incorrect data analytics and untimely decisions. Thus, completeness of the information and reliable data transfer is essential for wider adoption of PHSDMs. Additionally, appropriate methods and techniques should be developed to address this underlying concern. Consequently, it is crucial to evaluate the completeness and timeliness of all information transmitted.

Data Compression

Since low-rate wireless communication protocols are used to transfer information from the sensors to the sink, the bandwidth available is quite low and is prone to communication latency. It is very important to consider the qualitative aspect of the communication protocol used for the transmission to ensure wider user acceptance of PHSDMs. The connectivity should be stable and without interference during the exchange of information, so that the systems are efficient, reliable, and ultimately accepted by end users. Delays in the transmission of information can have a substantial impact on the diabetes monitoring of patients, especially in life-threatening and emergency situations. Thus, data compression techniques can be used to significantly reduce the volume of data to be transmitted and the delay in transmission and to consequently promote energy efficiency [37]. Therefore, lightweight data compression algorithms and encryption techniques must be further developed and optimized especially when transmitting huge amount of data in case of emergency. Thus, it is vital to evaluate the degree of QoI after the data has been compressed.

Data Acquisition and Efficiency

Another key technical concern is to enhance the accuracy of information captured since the latter is significantly impacted by the arrangement and position of the sensors and their ability to filter noise from the sensed signals. Real-time data acquisition is essential for reliable continuous monitoring [38]. Furthermore, despite the fact that many techniques are available such as the high-pass and low-pass filters, Fourier transform (FT), Kalman filter, wavelet transform, and piecewise linear representation, denoising the information remains a major bottleneck [39]. Therefore, it is important to find new denoising methods to transform the sensed data while maintaining the accuracy of the information collected. Moreover, it is crucial that accuracy issues are considered to ensure efficiency during data acquisition.

20.7.2 Communication-Level Challenges

As the sensed data are being sent through the communication channel, data are prone to several challenges (as shown in Table 20.8). The different QoI attributes can be affected due to security and privacy issues. Ensuring the confidentiality of these sensed data is a prime concern to promote trustworthiness. Moreover, how fast and reliable the information is being transferred is another important concern that cannot be neglected since healthcare professionals rely on these data for decision-making, especially in emergency cases. Lastly, it is primordial that the information is dependable for effective diagnosis and interventions.

Security and Privacy

Security and privacy constraints have become a global challenge that needs to be addressed due to the pervasive nature of wireless technologies. Body sensors are more prone to security attacks and can be easily compromised by malicious adversaries.

Table 20.8 Communication-level challenges

Communication-level challenges	References	
Security and privacy	Physical theft of medical devices can easily be tampered with Addressing threatening events and security risk in real time is highly needed Data authentication is important to preserve the privacy of medical data	[31, 36, 40, 41]
Reliability of data transmission	Designing effective routing protocol remains one of the major challenges Reliable data transfer is a key challenge in PHS, and the study address can be ensured for using API	[34, 40, 42, 43]
Dependability	False alarms and triggers will eventually lead to unintended consequences Delay in information can lead to frustrated patients	[44, 45]

These security issues include eavesdropping, spoofing, replay attacks, sinkhole attacks, data falsification, denial of service, jamming attack, Sybil attack, and physical attack [31, 46, 47]. While designing and developing PHSDMs to assist diabetic patients, ensuring the security aspect of the system is extremely important since such vulnerabilities will eventually render the entire system unreliable and can even lead to loss of lives. Sensor design needs to be unobtrusive to keep medical conditions discrete. Since health-related information of patients is highly privacy-sensitive, any breach of security will directly influence the privacy of the patients. The sensors must be able to seamlessly integrate and interoperate with other sensor nodes or networks through proper standardization of communication protocols and data storage. Therefore, further research must be carried out to develop cryptographic solutions, intrusion detection systems, and trust management systems to solve these security issues and ensure patients' privacy. Additionally, the aspect of confidentiality will need to be considered to screen any poor data quality pertaining to the lack of security and privacy.

Reliability of Data Transmission

Reliable data transfer is vital in the healthcare field so that healthcare practitioners can make real-time and effective decision-making. Inaccurate and unreliable information can be misleading and can consequently result in incorrect diagnosis, wrong decision-making, unnecessary expenditure, and cause of death. Inaccurate information can be due to incorrect sensed information, lack of calibration of the sensors or errors during data transmission due to noise, path fading, and unstable multi-hop routing paths.

A signal-to-noise ratio (S/N) assesses the level of expected signal to the level of noise power. High S/N is obtained when there is more useful information in the signals rather than noise. Various parameters such as small antenna size of sensor devices and low transmission power affect the S/N, causing more noise and therefore reducing the reliable coverage area. In addition, the placement and orientation of the sensor devices are critical to boosting the S/N. Robust network schemes need to be further developed and studied thoroughly to promote a reliable and resilient network. Furthermore, appropriate set of QoI dimensions will need to be identified to ensure the reliability and timeliness of data transmitted.

Dependability

Dependability is another key challenge since the robustness of PHSDMs impacts the quality of the healthcare services directly and may become a life-threatening matter. Incorrect data, inappropriate handling of exceptional situations, false-alarm triggers, or loss of service needs to be promptly spotted to identify any emergencies and provide timely assistance. It is critical that the data are transmitted with a minimum delay even when there is node failure or malicious modifications especially in emergency situations. Therefore, new mechanisms on emergency data prioritization and fault tolerance techniques should be developed. Moreover, appropriate QoI dimensions should be identified to ensure that accurate data are being transferred within a minimum delay. Furthermore, new researches are required to increase the sensors' battery lifetime to promote user acceptance and better adoption of such systems.

20.7.3 Human-Centric-Level Challenges

After data have been transmitted to the remote server, the data need to be analyzed effectively so that they are represented into meaningful information. Healthcare professionals should be able to rely on the QoI to make important decisions pertaining to the treatment of the patients. Any wrong or incorrect data analytics will compromise the integrity of the diagnosis and formulation of the feedback regarding medication, dietary habits, and exercise changes. Consequently, this will have a negative influence on the acceptance of PHSDMs. Additionally, the patients must be able to interpret the feedback sent by the healthcare professionals easily so that they can take proper actions or make any changes to their medication regime. If the feedback sent to the user is not easily interpreted by both technology-naïve and technology-averse patients, they will quickly lose interest in using PHSDMs. Furthermore, the sensors need to be miniature, unobtrusive, ergonomic, easy to wear, and stylish to gain wider user acceptance. The challenges at the human-centric level are shown in Table 20.9.

Table 20.9 Human-centric-level challenges

Human-centric-level challenges	References	
Data representation	Data should be easily interpretable with appropriate graphical user interface Understanding and learning the analyzed data are crucial appropriate actions	[48, 49]
Personalized feedback	Feedback and responses regarding the patient's status are important for timely decision-making Intuitive visual feedback of the health status is usually helpful and insightful to patients	[29, 50]

Data Representation

Data representation is another challenge since the way the data are represented and interpreted is highly important for effective decision-making. Poor QoI leads to incorrect processing and analysis of information. Consequently, the wrong interpretation of data will compromise the diagnosis. Hence, a higher degree of QoI should be ensured so that healthcare professionals can easily represent, analyze, and interpret the information.

Personalized Feedback

Personalized feedback is critical for the wide adoption of PHSDMs. Relevant feedback concerning the patients' glucose readings is very important to facilitate self-management of the disease. Accurate, helpful, and insightful feedback help the patients to make timely decisions and have trust in using PHSDMs. Thus, innovative ways of personalized feedback can be integrated into PHSDMs that provide customized information, intelligent feedback based on the health data patterns, and personalized medical regime based on the data analytics of the patient's condition. Feedback needs to be clear and well represented so that users can easily understand them and act accordingly. In addition, feedback can be represented using charts and colors to facilitate ease of use.

20.8 Conclusions

Despite all the initiatives taken by the MOHQL to combat diabetes, the prevalence is still high. Thus, in this study, the aim was to assess the impact of the diabetes management system on diabetic patients in Mauritius. Currently, diabetic patients self-monitor their blood glucose (BG) using off-the-shelf glucometers and record their daily BG in a logbook. During their monthly appointment at the hospital, healthcare professionals verify their BG trends and then make necessary adjustments to the patients' medical regime. However, the current diabetes management system is manual. The survey highlighted that very few Mauritian diabetics (42%) had knowledge on mobile health monitoring and pervasive health monitoring before being surveyed. Moreover, this study has highlighted that diabetes led to a lower QoL. However, after being aware of the potentials of PHSDMs, majority of the patients (84%) were willing to use mobile devices and pervasive healthcare systems to manage their diabetes, provided they receive appropriate guidance, their medical data remain confidential, and the services are cost-effective.

Thus, effective diabetes prevention and monitoring will eventually improve the QoL of patients. PHS has the potential to continuously monitor diabetic patients in a real-time manner and can assist patients to better self-monitor their conditions and to be more patient-centric than doctor-centric. Moreover, healthcare professionals can better monitor the vital signs of patients in a real-time manner and perform diagnosis, timely intervention, and effective decision-making. Thus, integrating PHSs in the diabetes management system in Mauritius can prove to be very fruitful in managing the epidemic situation and facilitate communications between healthcare professionals and patients.

References

1. Ng, J. K. Y., Wang, J., Lam, K. Y., Ho, C., Kam, C. C. H. C., & Han, S. (2014). Capturing and analyzing pervasive data for Smarthealth. In *Proceedings of the 28th international conference on advanced information networking and applications (AINA)* (pp. 985–992). IEEE.
2. Huzooree, G., Khedo, K. K., & Joonas, N. (2017). Pervasive mobile healthcare systems for chronic disease monitoring. *Health Informatics Journal, 25*(2), 267–291.
3. Huzooree, G., Khedo, K. K., & Joonas, N. (2019). Data reliability and quality in body area networks for diabetes monitoring. In R. Maheswar, G. Kanagachidambaresan, & R. Jayaparvathy (Eds.), *Body area network challenges and solutions* (pp. 55–86). EAI/Springer Innovations in Communication and Computing.
4. Huzooree, G., Khedo, K. K., & Joonas, N. (2016). Wireless body area network system architecture for real-time diabetes monitoring. In *Emerging trends in electrical, electronic and communications engineering. ELECOM 2016* (pp. 262–271). Springer.
5. Huzooree, G., Khedo, K. K., & Joonas, N. (2018). Low-cost body area network for monitoring of diabetic patient. In *Design and development of affordable healthcare technologies* (pp. 135–164). IGI Global.
6. Gayan, M.. (2015). Mauritius NCD survey 2015 report.
7. IDF. (2018). *IDF SEA members*. Retrieved October 5, 2019, from https://www.idf.org/our-network/regions-members/south-east-asia/members/96-mauritius.html
8. WHO. (2017). *Biennium report 2016|2017*. Retrieved March 20, 2019, from https://www.afro.who.int/sites/default/files/2018-03/WHOMauritius Biennium Report 2016-2017.pdf
9. MOHQL. (2007). *The national service framework for diabetes (NSFD)*. Retrieved March 20, 2019, from https://extranet.who.int/ncdccs/Data/MUS_B6_NSFD.pdf
10. International Diabetes Federation. (2010). *A guide to national diabetes programmes*. Retrieved March 20, 2019, from https://www.idf.org/component/attachments/attachments.html?id=1576&task=download

11. Bradley, C. (1994). The diabetes treatment satisfaction questionnaire: DTSQ. In *Handbook of psychology and diabetes: A guide to psychological measurement in diabetes research and practice* (Vol. 111, p. 132). Routledge.
12. Bradley, C., Todd, C., Gorton, T., Symonds, E., Martin, A., & Plowright, R. (1999). The development of an individualized questionnaire measure of perceived impact of diabetes on quality of life: The ADDQoL. *Quality of Life Research, 8*(1), 79–91.
13. Pinnock, H., Slack, R., Pagliari, C., Price, D., & Sheikh, A. (2006). Professional and patient attitudes to using mobile phone technology to monitor asthma: Questionnaire survey. *Primary Care Respiratory Journal, 15*(4), 237–245.
14. Costa, F. A., Guerreiro, J. P., & Duggan, C. (2006). An audit of diabetes dependent quality of life (ADDQoL) for Portugal: Exploring validity and reliability. *Pharmacy Practice (Granada), 4*(3), 123–128.
15. Holmanová, E., & Žiaková, K. (2009). Audit diabetes-dependent quality of life questionnaire: Usefulness in diabetes self-management education in the Slovak population. *Journal of Clinical Nursing, 18*(9), 1276–1286.
16. McGillicuddy, W. J., et al. (2013). Patient attitudes toward mobile phone-based health monitoring: Questionnaire study among kidney transplant recipients. *Journal of Medical Internet Research, 15*(1), e6.
17. Kuznetsov, L. (2014). Diabetes-specific quality of life but not health status is independently associated with glycaemic control among patients with type 2 diabetes: A cross-sectional analysis of the ADDITION-Europe trial cohort. *Diabetes Research and Clinical Practice, 104*(2), 281–287.
18. Chung, J. O., Cho, D. H., Chung, D. J., & Chung, M. Y. (2013). Assessment of factors associated with the quality of life in Korean type 2 diabetic patients. *Internal Medicine, 52*(2), 179–185.
19. Papazafiropoulou, A. K. (2015). Diabetes - dependent quality of life (ADDQOL) and affecting factors in patients with diabetes mellitus type 2 in Greece. *BMC Research Notes*, 4–9.
20. Turk, E., Rupel, V. P., Tapajner, A., Leyshon, S., & Isola, A. (2013). An audit of diabetes-dependent quality of life (ADDQOL) in older patients with diabetes mellitus type 2 in Slovenia. *Value in Health Regional Issues, 2*(2), 248–253.
21. Wang, H. F., & Yeh, M. C. (2013). The quality of life of adults with type 2 diabetes in a hospital care clinic in Taiwan. *Quality of Life Research, 22*(3), 577–584.
22. Testa, M. A., Simonson, D. C., & Turner, R. R. (1998). Valuing quality of life and improvements in glycemic control in people with type 2 diabetes. *Diabetes Care, 21*(3), 44–52.
23. Weinberger, M. (1995). A nurse-coordinated intervention for primary care patients with non-insulin-dependent diabetes mellitus. *Journal of General Internal Medicine, 10*(2), 9–66.
24. Johnson, J. A., Nowatzki, T. E., & Coons, S. J. (1996). Health-related quality of life of diabetic Pima Indians. *Medical Care, 34*(2), 97–102.
25. Quinn, C. C., Clough, S. S., Minor, J. M., Lender, D., Okafor, M. C., & Gruber-Baldini, A. (2008). WellDoc™ mobile diabetes management randomized controlled trial: Change in clinical and behavioral outcomes and patient and physician satisfaction. *Diabetes Technology & Therapeutics, 10*(3), 160–168.
26. Bostock, Y., Hanley, J., McGown, D., Pinnock, H., Padfield, P., & McKinstry, B. (2009). The acceptability to patients and professionals of remote blood pressure monitoring using mobile phones. *Primary Health Care Research & Development, 10*(4), 299–308.
27. Seto, E., Leonard, K. J., Masino, C., Cafazzo, J. A., Barnsley, J., & Ross, H. J. (2010). Attitudes of heart failure patients and health care providers towards mobile phone-based remote monitoring. *Journal of Medical Internet Research, 12*(4), e55.
28. Sidi, F., Panahy, P. H. S., Affendey, L. S., Jabar, M. A., Ibrahim, H., & Mustapha, A. (2012). Data quality: A survey of data quality dimensions. In *Proceedings of the international conference on information retrieval & knowledge management (CAMP)* (pp. 300–304). IEEE.

29. Pike, M., Mustafa, N. M., Towey, D., & Brusic, V. (2019). Sensor networks and data management in healthcare: Emerging technologies and new challenges. In *International computer software and applications conference* (Vol. 1, pp. 834–839). IEEE.
30. Li, Y., Sperrin, M., Martin, G. P., Ashcroft, D. M., & Staa, T. P. (2020). Examining the impact of data quality and completeness of electronic health records on predictions of patients' risks of cardiovascular disease. *International Journal of Medical Informatics, 133*, 104046.
31. Sun, Y., Lo, F. P., & Lo, B. (2019). Security and privacy for the internet of medical things enabled healthcare systems: A survey. *IEEE Access, 7*, 183339–183355.
32. M. Uzair, M. A. Khan, S. Mann, and M. Imran, "A review: Ubiquitous healthcare monitoring with mobile phone," 2018 9th IEEE annu. ubiquitous comput. electron. mob. commun. conf. UEMCON 2018, IEEE pp. 988–996, 2018.
33. Sindhu, C., & Hegde, N. P. (2017). A novel integrated framework to ensure better data quality in big data analytics over cloud environment. *International Journal of Electrical and Computer Engineering, 7*(5), 2798–2805.
34. Haghi, M. (2020). A flexible and pervasive IoT-based healthcare platform for physiological and environmental parameters monitoring. *IEEE Internet of Things, 7*(6), 5628–5647.
35. Jesus, G., Casimiro, A., & Oliveira, A. (2017). A survey on data quality for dependable monitoring in wireless sensor networks. *Sensors, 17*(9), 2010.
36. Wu, F., Wu, T., & Yuce, M. R. (2019). Design and implementation of a wearable sensor network system for IoT-connected safety and health applications. In *IEEE 5th world forum on internet of things* (pp. 87–90). IEEE.
37. Chen, M., & Fowler, M. L. (2003). The importance of data compression for energy efficiency in sensor networks. In *Proceedings of the conference on information sciences and systems* (p. 13). IEEE.
38. Alemdar, H., & Ersoy, C. (2010). Wireless sensor networks for healthcare: A survey. *Computer Networks, 54*(15), 2688–2710.
39. Lai, X., Liu, Q., Wei, X., Wang, W., Zhou, G., & Han, G. (2013). A survey of body sensor networks. *Sensors, 13*(5), 5406–5447.
40. Dhagarra, D., Goswami, M., & Kumar, G. (2020). Impact of trust and privacy concerns on technology acceptance in healthcare: An Indian perspective. *International Journal of Medical Informatics, 141*, 104164.
41. Pramanik, I., Lau, R. Y. K., Kalam, A., Hossain, S., Hossain, K., & Karmaker, B. K. (2020). Healthcare informatics and analytics in big data. *Expert Systems with Applications, 152*, 113388.
42. Triantafyllidis, A., Koutkias, V. G., Chouvarda, I., & Maglaveras, N. (2014). Development and usability of a personalized sensor - based system for pervasive healthcare. In *Proceedings of the 36th annual international conference of the IEEE engineering in medicine and biology society* (pp. 6623–6626). IEEE.
43. Jeong, I. C., Bychkov, D., & Searson, P. C. (2019). Wearable devices for precision medicine and health state monitoring. *IEEE Transactions on Biomedical Engineering, 66*(5), 1242–1258.
44. Rodbard, D. (2016). Continuous glucose monitoring: A review of successes, challenges, and opportunities. *Diabetes Technology & Therapeutics, 18*(2), 2–13.
45. Alaiad, A., & Zhou, L. (2017). Patients' adoption of WSN-based smart home healthcare systems: An integrated model of facilitators and barriers. *IEEE Transactions on Professional Communication, 60*(1), 4–23.
46. Kumar, M. (2014). Security issues and privacy concerns in the implementation of wireless body area network. In *Proceedings of the international conference on information technology (ICIT)* (pp. 58–62). IEEE.
47. Touati, F., & Tabish, R. (2013). U-healthcare system: State-of-the-art review and challenges. *Journal of Medical Systems, 37*(3), 9949.
48. Karkouch, A., Mousannif, H., Al Moatassime, H., & Thomas, N. (2018). A model-driven framework for data quality management in the Internet of Things. *Journal of Ambient Intelligence and Humanized Computing, 9*(4), 977–998.

49. Mashoufi, M., Ayatollahi, H., & Khorasani-zavareh, D. (2018). A review of data quality assessment in emergency medical services. *The Open Medical Informatics Journal, 12*, 19–32.
50. Bai, L., Meredith, R., & Burstein, F. (2018). A data quality framework, method and tools for managing data quality in a health care setting: An action case study. *Journal of Decision Systems, 27*(1), 144–154.

Chapter 21
Aiding IoT and Cloud to Control COVID-19: A Systematic Approach

N. Ambika

21.1 Introduction

Internet of things [1] is shortly known as IoT [2]. It is an assembly of multiple types of equipment of different caliber and functionality working toward a single goal. The collection aims to communicate with each other, utilizing the common platform provided to them. The medical system [3] engages in continuous monitoring of the patient. Notwithstanding regular clinical assessment, the patient's body states, including pulse, diabetes, electroencephalogram, and other crucial biomedical signs, are checked by applying different clinical GPS beacons for finding or improving well-being quality. The sharing of such a tremendous measure of information among associations can encourage clinical findings, biomedical research, and approach-making. Blockchain [4] aids in bringing more reliability to the system. These are hash codes derived from the data. Any change in the transmitted data is notified at an early stage using this methodology.

The work [5] investigates and features the general uses of the IoT theory by contributing a viewpoint guide to handle the epidemic. The framework recommends embracing four phases of the methodology—well-being information monitoring in remote areas, virtual administration, examination of information obtained, and control and follow-up reporting.

MedChain [6] develops on a decentralized system. It associates all medical services suppliers, including emergency clinics, clinical focuses, centers, and social insurance corporates. The MedChain arrangement contains two kinds of friend hubs. Super companions comprise the servers from enormous social insurance suppliers, for example, national emergency clinics, which are progressively fit in figuring and capacity, giving the principal foundation of information sharing. The edge

N. Ambika (✉)
Department of Computer Applications, SSMRV College, Bangalore, India

M. S. Husain et al. (eds.), *Pervasive Healthcare*, EAI/Springer Innovations in Communication and Computing, https://doi.org/10.1007/978-3-030-77746-3_21

hubs are the servers from little suppliers. For example, network centers store real patient information. The assets of a super-peer partition are divided into three modules. The blockchain server keeps up the blockchain [7] for checking information trustworthiness and reviewing exercises. The index server keeps up the stock of client social insurance information, maps them to the legitimate area of capacity, and oversees meetings during information sharing. The servers of both kinds on every single super-peer structure consist of two subsystems. HDB stores the genuine medical services information of patients.

The framework [8] comprises five sections: overlay configuration, cloud stockpiling, healthcare suppliers, smart agreements, and patients furnished with human services wearable IoT gadgets. The distributed storage bunches client's information into indistinguishable squares. These mists are associated with overlay systems when the data is put away in a block. The system worker transmits the hashed information squares to the protective covering arrangement. The hashed data in the individual block is determined using the Merkle tree. A protective cover is a shared system that depends on circulated engineering. The hubs associated with the system could be a PC, cell phone, tablet, or some other IoT gadgets. It comprises an explicit device. They have to demonstrate significant authentication in order to affirm. Such declaration can be transferred or confirmed before making a record on the system. When approved, he/she will have the option to sign information/exchange. Therapeutic services suppliers are named by policy agencies or by a sick person to execute clinical trials or give clinical medicines. Social insurance specialist co-ops manage the treatment of patients once they get a caution from the system. Smart agreements permit the production of understandings in any IoT gadget execution when the given conditions are met. They have used both encryption plans—symmetric and asymmetric.

The proposal consists of two phases. In the first phase, the deceased data is collected by the respective personnel and fed into the system. The hash value derivation happens at two levels. In the first step, the hospital's hash value obtained increases reliability to the system. The aggregated data from the patient undergoes affixation with the hash value. The procedure adds more trust to the system. In the second phase, the data undergoes sharing among various communities. Some of the groups considered are hospital authorities, media, and researchers. The highly confidential information is restricted based on the need of the individual and their authentication rights. The personnel diagnosing similar cases are into this set.

Section 21.2 narrates the contribution provided by previous authors. Section 21.3 explains the proposed work. Analysis of the work is in Sect. 21.4. The work concludes in Sect. 21.5.

21.2 Literature Survey

This section describes the various contributions in detail. MedChain [6] develops on a decentralized system. It associates all medical services suppliers, including emergency clinics, clinical focuses, centers, and social insurance corporates. The MedChain arrangement contains two kinds of friend hubs: super companions and edge hubs. Super companions comprise of the servers from enormous social insurance suppliers, for example, national emergency clinics, which are progressively fit in figuring and capacity, giving the principal foundation of information sharing. The edge hubs are the servers from little suppliers, for example, network centers, which just store the real patient information. The assets of a super-peer are partitioned into three modules: blockchain administration, catalog administration, and human services database (HDB). The blockchain server keeps up the summation of blockchain [7] for checking information trustworthiness and reviewing exercises. The index server keeps up the stock of client social insurance information, maps them to the legitimate area of capacity, and oversees meetings for data sharing. The servers of both kinds on every single super-peer structure consist of two subsystems. It stores the genuine medicinal services information of patients.

Healthcare Data Gateways [9] typically models the transfer of information once. Information is changeless once transferred. In this way, rather than arranging tolerant information into tables, the creators have proposed to utilize one basic diagram to show a wide range of data and free the clients from the mapping issue. Every patient has one such mapping table that accepts the data as a table name. The deceased is recognized by a blueprint. The strategy is known as the Indicator-Centric Schema model. A staggering list of multidimensional methodology is proposed. In one kind of indexing, information is first recorded dependent on the indicator utilizing the hash file. Every pointer is additionally filed on time using a B+ tree list. The index is a list as well as a registry to arrange the information. Data recovery analyzes the hash file, B+ tree file, and data on the leaf hub.

Social insurance exchanges related to a partner are arranged into a chain of human services exchange squares [10]. The chain can be viewed as an account of an individual's medicinal services way through life. When an exchange is led, a comparison of social insurance boundaries is sent to at least one approval gadget. The gadgets build up the legitimacy of the exchange and produce another square employing proof-of-work standard. When a new square is determine, it tends to annex to the partner social insurance blockchain.

The framework [11] equipment engineering comprehensively comprises four significant constituents. It is indicated as a wristwatch, passage, cell phone application, and cloud. The sensor gadget consolidates a SpO_2 and an HR detector. It speaks with the channel utilizing an 868-MHz MiWi convention. The entrance transmits the detected information to a cell phone over Bluetooth. The wristwatch-incorporated accelerometer awakens the radio and preparing units when the client moves. The information produced by the SpO_2 and pulse sensor is transmitted to the processor. It follows the transmission of handled knowledge to an 868-MHz radio handset. The radio unit utilizes an ATSAMR30E18A microcontroller. It incorporates ultra-depleted force sub-GHz band AT86RF212B handset. When moved by a client, the wristwatch-coordinated measuring instrument awakens the communication system and handling units.

The proposed model [12] uses propelled methods and administrations. Occasion activation based on content communication philosophy is accepted to the procedure of the sick continuous content at fog region. The mining idea investigates the occasion's affliction by figuring the transient well-being record (THI) of the patient. The health content of 67 patients is IoT-based on smart domiciliary conditions produced for 30 days. The planned stratified methodology for fog-based shrewd far off patient observation is five layers. Information acquisition layer plays out the errand of information recovery from IoT gadgets about different occasions inside home conditions identified with the patient straightforwardly or in a roundabout way. Information is recovered pervasively from divergent remote equipment gadgets. It implants in various areas at habitation and from the physical structure detecting system of the sufferer. These equipment gadgets deal with isolate detecting marvels and can detect and transmit information progressively. The patient speaks with this framework by initially enrolling his/her data from the outset case by responding to addresses identified with a health history and individual subtleties. After enlistment, a recognizable proof count is given to the sufferer by the system worker. Data mining layer targets separating helpful information from haze information administrations progressively. The haze layer decides the patient's well-being state as a sheltered state.

Service-oriented architecture (SOA) [13] concentrates on actualizing solicitation reaction cooperation to associate parts in appropriated frameworks. EDA depends on an offbeat message-driven correspondence model to spread data all through the framework layers. It portrays occasion preparing applications. The extent of nearby self-governance is required and does not tie practically different segments into the equivalent incorporated administration model. The theoretical model of an occasion handling framework presented gives important ideas to enhance the reference design. There are the event processing network and the event channel. An EPN depicts how occasions got from makers are coordinated to the shoppers through specialists/administrators that process these occasions by performing change, approval, or enhancement. An EC is a component for conveying streams from occasion-makers and occasion administrators to occasion purchasers and other occasion supervisors.

It is the vitality proficient IoT-well-being observing framework [14] that requires a scientific compromise between the nature of the reproduced communication and the vitality exhausted in the process and connection schemes. The sensing subsystem involves the AD8232 ECG screen that positions the arrangement of trio terminals. It is a devoted foremost goal to coordinate with electrical device pulse screen. It intends to remove and enhance a channel with little biological signals in the sight of noisy conditions, for example, those made by movement antiquities or far off terminal arrangement. The screen contains an ultra-low-force analog-to-digital converter. The yield communication is obtained on an installed microcontroller.

Information signals are taken from the rightmost limb. The leftmost limb and right leg shape is an Einthoven triangle. To build up the processing subsystem, the authors use Arduino Uno R3, which expels commotion from gained biosignals, modifies baselines, enciphers communications utilizing abnormal coefficients, and streamlines framework boundaries to devour the least vitality. Arduino Uno includes a low-force component, an effectual microcontroller in ADC, and a USART correspondence highlight. The WiFi component in Arduino communicates continuous information to a worker found commonly out in the open/private cloud. That information undergoes recovery by the doctors' or clinics' faculty. This Arduino-based WiFi protective cover, ESP8266, is utilized in this framework to plan the connection scheme.

There are two wearable sensor hubs [15]: the safe node for natural checking and the health node for physiological boundary estimations. The health node includes a Bluetooth Low Energy (BLE) module empowering WBAN correspondence, a PPG sensor for pulse checking, and an internal heat-level sensor. There are four natural sensors on the safe node to quantify the encompassing temperature, relative dampness, CO_2, and UV sensor. The safe node involves two remote modules—the BLE for correspondence inside the WBAN and LoRa for transmission in the LPWAN. The BLE in the safe node is liable for getting sensor information from the health node inside the WBAN communicates to a far off door through the LoRa organizer. BLE can send data at low-force utilization and a high information rate. LoRa transmits information over a significant distance while relinquishing the information rate and expanding power utilization. The IoT cloud worker gets the data from the IoT door and stores it into the cloud database: MySQL. The information was put away in the database for additional investigation.

The framework [16] requires dynamic correspondence channels to send health information for observation and cautions. The RPi3 has onboard WiFi, Bluetooth, and USB booting abilities. The modem utilizes a SIM card and works over a bought-in portable administrator to send information utilizing a messaging service. The interface and RPi3 use circuit changing to set up a correspondence way between them. A significant overhaul in the RPi3 component is an inserted network with an onboard WiFi. MQ telemetry transport convention communicates information through WiFi. The sunroom circulatory strain/beat rate sensor and RPi3's in-manufactured BLE compartment require a UART computer circuit. RPi3 accompanies a remote UART transfer. These three modes impart multiplexed information for observing sick imperative signs—internal heat level, pulse, and circulatory strain to a clinician.

It is a structure made of a clothing IoT cloud-based wellness checking framework (WISE) [17]. It embraces various interrelated clothing detectors to watch the health state of the topic. The signs include circulatory strain, pulsation, and internal heat level. Because of the constrained memory and figuring limit of the sensor hubs, so as to maintain a strategic distance from the utilization of an advanced mobile language unit as a preparing unit, the sensor information gathered from those wearable sensors will be communicated to the storage worker straightforwardly. The WBAN comprises three classifications of detecting gadgets. The heartbeat sensor information shows the normality of the pulses, which can likewise mirror the myocardial exercises. Such sensors check patients with coronary illness. The fundamental measure device in the circuit will peruse the fundamental measure from the environmental factors and demonstrated the fundamental quantity in the form of Celsius. The pulse sensor is a nonintrusive detector intended to quantify human circulatory strain. It estimates pulsation, diastolic, and average blood vessel force using the oscillometric strategy.

LoRaWAN [18] is a protected and productive transmission innovation covering huge territories active from 1 km in an urbanized geographical area to 60 km in an open space land. The framework depends on a passage that gets information from sensor hubs furnished with LoRa handsets and advances it to a worker in encoded IP parcels employing Ethernet. It comprises four segments. The LoRa end hub is an observing module that uses e-well-being sensors associated with a LoRa handset. The LoRa end hub gathers health boundaries, for example, glucose level, pulse, and temperature. It sends them as per LoRaWAN particulars to the LoRaWAN Gateway. The LoRaWAN door changes over receiver rate bundles to IP parcels. RF parcels obtained by the concentrator is sent to the host. The LoRaWAN worker assembles information bundles originating from closing hubs through the entranceway. The worker analyzes their trustworthiness, decodes their substance, and stocks them in NoSQL information for approaching investigation. The dashboard is an electronic interface that appears on two PCs, and cell phones permit fitness experts to follow patients.

The checking framework [19] incorporates patients, health observing unit, cloud for information stockpiling, and gatekeepers with the assistance of some equipment units, different sensors, and gadgets with a web association. The framework has three modules. The detecting module comprises some submodules called the mind hub. It is relevant information to communicate structure sensors to the cerebrum hub through the entryway. All gathered information is put away into impermanent memory of detecting a module called mind hub. Branch creation, demand coordinating, and information base are the submodules in the main module. The database is for the lasting stockpiling of information. The information in-branch hub circulates into the unique branch. It is put away in the database using the web. The solicitation taken from the client coordinates with the capacity to have some job-based validation process. Application interpretation and circumstance procurement are the submodules in the association module. The circumstance boundary includes a date, time, area, and application necessities. The confirmed client interface with the framework coordinates, and the application allows access to associate with the framework.

The framework [20] makes associate in nursing humanoid stage transferable program for the oriented area that utilizes the technology and diffused computation. It is a non-nosy strategy using the boundaries remembered for the framework to identify type II diabetes, driving the pattern of non-meddling human services checking. It comprises three social insurance sensors used to measure temperature, beat, and blood. The client wears all the sensors to gather information for transmission. The cloud prepares the transferred data. On the off chance that the health status shows unfortunate, the framework will mention to the client what is the infection he may confront and what avoidances he should take.

The general engineering of IReHMo [21] comprises five layers. The detecting layer includes home computerization gadgets, for example, sensors and actuators. The attention is on the information assortment, separating, pre-handling, and encoding in the internal passage. Sensor information is gathered and put away locally and is sent to the far off workers. Utilizing openHAB—a middleware for incorporating a few home mechanization arrangements—the home passage can cooperate with a few kinds of IoT conventions, for example, Z-wave, KNX, and Insteon. Information from the home door is sent to the onlooker. The cloud is the less desirable finish of the information stream from the sensors. The uppermost region of the pile is the utilization part, where applications connect with clients using the net intersection. Since sensor information is gathered, put away, and handled consistently, clients can get an all-encompassing image of the circumstance and convey activities in like manner.

The framework [22] uses the IoT to identify catching voice, internal heat level, electrocardiogram, and encompassing dampness. They prohibit gadgets like laryngoscope and stroboscope. The information is sent by Bluetooth innovation to the sick cell utilizing a created application. For validation purposes, it is installed into the signs. The mark is a customized recognizable proof of the deceased person, which is made by the deceased himself. Watermark installing is a significant advance in the planned framework since it ensures the responsibility for individual information. The watermarking plan uses a distinct riffle change and a particular worth deterioration-based calculation. The patient ID uses the watermark and the technology in the defined coefficients' subband at tier 2 of the sound, which communicates disintegration utilizing separate communication. The mark communicates to the cloud through the Internet. It has the accompanying primary components—authentication supervisor, information chief, highlight extraction worker, characterization worker, and capacity. The verification director examines the patient for joining up with the framework. Whenever enlisted, it separates his/her personality. It moreover deals with the solicitation entree by the specialists by checking their character. The information supervisor commands the progression of information to and from the workers. The highlight extraction worker highlights separately from the symbol. The highlights use a classifier to arrange the sign. The information chief receives it, and models of the classifier are put away in the capacity.

The work [23] is a flexible and adaptable IoT framework. It gathers the information expected to encourage the free living of seniors and residents to improve their satisfaction. The proposed framework structure reasons aim to have a reduced-power framework that can be worn during the daytime and be turbocharged as fundamental. It intends to be light and agreeable to wear. It has six segments. A heartbeat oximeter sensor quantifies the measurement of oxygen bust-up in the customer's liquid body substance. The identity of hemoprotein and deoxyhemoprotein is under consideration. An electrocardiogram detector is an organization of cardiovascular information, for instance, the rate and cadence of the heart. The second module of the planned framework is a Bluetooth degraded-energy iLighthouse, which is generally utilized for interior situating. When the client relocates to the vicinity of an iLighthouse, its ID is perused by the microcontroller. The iLighthouse identification is transmitted to the storage worker to acquire the client's area. The BLE innovation permits the iBeacon to be controlled by remote cell batteries for expanded time stretches.

The proposal [5] is endeavoring to investigate and feature the general uses of the IoT theory by giving a viewpoint guide to handling the COVID-19 epidemic. The framework recommends embracing four phases of the methodology—well-being information monitoring in remote areas, virtual administration, examination of information obtained, and control and follow-up reporting.

It is the actuation of caution to give the recommended medication in time shown in the LCD [24]. This alert warning will lessen the man's mistake and assist the clinical colleague or dependable independent to agree with the long suffering. The excess useful part of the structure is the mode toward transmitting an electronic mail warning device and messaging service ready using a Python collection to the expert, clinical auxiliary, and family members of the long suffering if any of the intentional physiological boundaries pass over the boundary. The ideal environmental factor essential to a sick person's welfare state is accomplished by sending a regular message to the command portion of the model. It is similar to a cryptography material that will impart to the machines of the affected role's space to make perfect room status. It is categorized into four fundamental modules. The health monitoring and information assortment module comprises critical well-being boundaries like pulsation, circulative stress, breath, fundamental measure, glucose level, improvement of the patients, and saline level. In the wake of accepting the signs from these sensing elements, it will be sent to the Raspberry Pi. Raspberry Pi runs on a Linux-based working framework named Raspbian, and it can work as a little PC. In the proposed framework, a stage down transformer works on the sensors, as the force prerequisite is diverse for various sensors. The graceful voltage of 230 V changes over into 0–9 V and 15–0–15 V. It will send to an exchanged mode power gracefully (SMPS). Diodes will be required to change over AC voltage to DC voltage. The changes over DC voltage will undergo undulation. Along these lines, a 1000 μf capacitor will likewise be utilized for power gracefully associated with the sensors. In this framework, two thermistors will associate with the resistor organization for breath estimation. One thermistor will quantify the breath, while the other one will be used for area fundamental measure estimation. The body development of a patient is observed by utilizing MMA7260QT.

Structure health monitoring (SHM) [25] is furnished with different sensors for observing any preliminary changes. In the proposed framework, at first, all the observed information from introduced sensors is gathered at a neighborhood passage for pre-handling, sifting, and information game plan. The design is taken care of to a blockchain-based keen agreement to break down the condition of the structure. In Ethereum, Oracle is the most well-known believed outsider help that runs over the entryway to enter blockchain-based brilliant agreements just as associate keen accord with this present reality. The blockchain timestamps the assembled data, and the smart assent assesses against pre-characterized limits for independent dynamic. After gathering the notice or ready conditions, intelligent contracts naturally speak with appended gadgets for premature reprimand and concerned offices.

21.3 Proposed Work

COVID-19 is a virus that originated from Wuhan, China. It has taken the entire world under its control, increasing the death rate. The ailment has spread to all the categories irrespective of their gender, blood group, or age. Any infection can be brought into control when the appropriate medicine can be advised based on the symptoms analyzed by the personnel. The personnel are not yet certain about the signs. Hence, primary indications have to be jolted down to bring the spread into control. There has to be a confirmation of the symptoms and the methodology adopted to cure the infected. Hence, a trusted system has to be developed. The proposal is the procedure to be followed in order to build trust among the stakeholders. Reliability is a property of the system that ensures trust among the stakeholders. The Internet is an enormous web that connects devices of different capacities. The architecture provides a foundation for various devices to communicate in the programmed language (Table 21.1). The protocol has two major phases:

Table 21.1 Notations used in the proposal

Notations used in the study	Description
H_i	Hash code of the hospital *i*
L_i	Location of the hospital *i*
C_{id}	Certificate identification provided by respective government authorities
P_i	Thumb print of the personnel in-charge of the processing
D_i	Device identity used in processing
$Addr_i$	IP address of the device used in processing
S_{id}	Specialist (doctor) identity
I_{id}	Identity of the patient
$Data_i$	Analyzed case study
R_i	Resultant data
M_i	Authenticated data
G	Global cloud server
Req_i	Request data *i*
Req_data_i	Requested data *i*

21.3.1 Data Collection Phase

In this phase, the deceased data is collected by the respective personnel and fed into the system. The hash value derivation happens at two levels. In the first step, the hospital's hash value obtained increases reliability to the system. In further steps, the aggregated data from the patient undergoes affixation with the hash value. The procedure adds more trust to the system.

Step 1: Every established and authenticated organization has its own identity provided by the respective government authorities. Hence, the hospital or specialized clinics have to undergo registration using their credentials:

$$H_i \rightarrow \text{hash}\left(L_i, C_{id}, T_i, P_i, \text{Addr}_i, D_i\right) \tag{21.1}$$

In Eq. (21.1), the hospital is using L_i (location of the hospital obtained by the GPS system), C_{id} (certificate identity given by the government authority), T_i (time of registration), P_i (personnel identification), D_i (device identity), and Addr_i (the IP address of the device).

Step 2: The patient detected for the virus has to be analyzed. In this study, a specialized team of doctors (with different capabilities) has to be formed. This person has to prepare a case study analyzing the symptoms of the infected. The case study encompasses reading taken, the patient's daily routine, the medication he is given, any other illnesses he is suffering from, and symptoms observed. The practitioner has to upload the same into the system. Cloud systems can provide better storage and maintenance to the MedChain system. To obtain the resultant data, the identity of the doctor and the identity and case study of the diseased are considered. In Eq. (21.2), the doctor identity S_{id}, the case study w.r.t patient Data_i, the patient identity I_{id}, and time T_i are represented. The patient data also contains the images obtained during the diagnosis and the treatment provided:

$$R_i \rightarrow \text{hash}\left(S_{id}, \text{Data}_i, I_{id}, T_i\right) \tag{21.2}$$

Step 3: The hash code w.r.t to the hospital is affixed to the resultant data to make the data more reliable. In Eq. (21.3), the authenticated data M_i is generated by affixing the hash code of the respective hospital H_i to the resultant data R_i and encrypted data Data_i:

$$M_i \rightarrow H_i \| R_i \| \text{En}\left(\text{Data}_i\right) \tag{21.3}$$

Step 4: The data is uploaded to the global cloud system G after registration and authentication. The same is represented in Eq. (21.4). Figure 21.1 is the flowchart for phase I:

$$M_i \rightarrow G \tag{21.4}$$

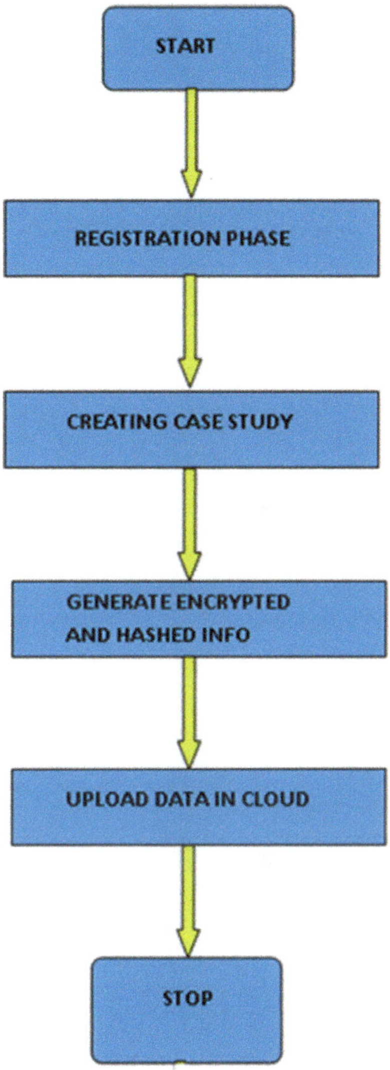

Fig. 21.1 Flowchart of data collection phase

21.3.2 Sharing the Data Among Various Personnel

In this phase, the data undergoes sharing among various communities. Some of the groups considered are hospital authorities, media, and researchers. The highly confidential information is restricted based on the need of the individual and their authentication rights. The personnel diagnosing similar cases are into this set.

Step 1: The group is a set of personnel working on the case where they require some assistance from the previous studies. The authorities use the hospital hash value with their identities. It accesses information from the earlier case study. The

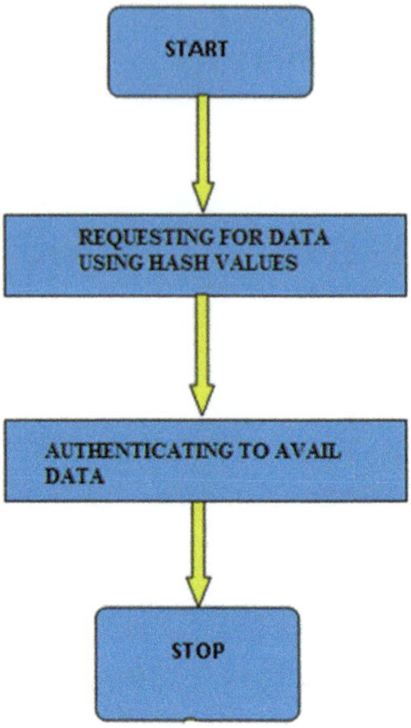

Fig. 21.2 Representation of sharing data to the requested users

personnel avail with the entire dataset with medication provided (doses, improvement shown by the patient, side effects the patient is shown, images of the diagnosis at various stages including X-ray, scanning report, etc.).

$$H_j T_j \text{Req}_j \rightarrow G \tag{21.5}$$

In Eq. (21.5), H_j is the hospital hash value where the personnel T_j is requesting the data Req_j to the cloud system G. The rest of the communities considered fall into another group. Similar procedure is adopted to extract the necessary data, but the data shared is minimal among other groups.

Step 2: The requested data is authenticated, and based on the availability terms, the individual is given data. In Eq. (21.6), the cloud server G is transmitting the requested data Req_data_i to the requested T_j. Figure 21.2 is the flowchart used to represent the sharing of the data phase:

$$G : \text{Req\_data}_i \rightarrow T_j \tag{21.6}$$

21.4 Analysis of the Work

The illness is well treated when the symptoms occur after analysis. The physicians do not have the complete COVID-19 indications as some infected do not show any symptoms. The infection shows its signs at a particular stage. These pale symptom records create awareness among others. The proposal is an attempt to record all the reliable indications.

MedChain [6] developed a decentralized system which associates all medicinal services suppliers, including emergency clinics, clinical focuses, centers, and social insurance corporates. The MedChain arrangement contains two kinds of friend hubs. Super companions comprise the servers from enormous social insurance suppliers, for example, national emergency clinics, which are progressively fit in figuring and capacity, giving the principal foundation of information sharing. The edge hubs are the servers from little suppliers. For example, network centers store real patient information. The assets of a super-peer fall into three modules: blockchain administration, catalog administration, and human services database. The blockchain server keeps up the sum [7] for checking information trustworthiness and reviewing exercises. The index server keeps up the stock of client social insurance information, maps them to the legitimate area of capacity, and oversees meetings for information sharing. The servers of both kinds on every single super-peer structure consist of two subsystems. HDB stores the genuine medicinal services information of patients.

The framework [8] comprises five sections: overlay arrange, Cloud stockpiling, Healthcare suppliers, Smart agreements, and patient furnished with human services wearable IoT gadgets. The distributed storage bunches client's information in indistinguishable squares related to a one of a kind section number. These mists are associated with overlay systems when the data is put away in a block. The storage worker transmits the hash of the learning squares to the overlay arrange. The hashed of the knowledge in the individual piece is determined to utilize Merkle Tree. An overlay is a shared system that depends on circulated engineering. The hubs associated with the system could be a PC, cell phone, tablet, or some other IoT gadget. It comprises an explicit device. They have to demonstrate to affirm with significant authentication. Such a declaration can be transferred or confirmed before making a record on the system. When approved, he/she will have the option to sign information/exchange. Therapeutic services suppliers are named by security agencies or by long-suffering to carry through a clinical trial. Social insurance specialist co-ops manage the treatment of patients once they get a caution from the system. Smart agreements permit the production of understandings in any IoT gadgets execution when given conditions satisfies. They have utilized used both encryption plans—symmetric and asymmetric.

The proposal consists of two phases. In the first phase, the deceased data is collected by the respective personnel and fed into the system. The hash value derivation happens at two levels. In the first step, the hospital's hash value obtained increases reliability to the system. In further steps, the aggregated data from the patient undergoes affixation with the hash value. The procedure adds more trust to the system. In the second phase, the data undergoes sharing among various communities. Some of the groups considered are hospital authorities, media, and researchers. The highly confidential information is restricted based on the need of the individual and their authentication rights. The personnel diagnosing similar cases are into this set. The work simulates using NS2. Table 21.2 consists of parameters used in the simulation.

Table 21.2 Parameters used in the simulation

Parameters	Description
Number of devices used	20 (5 hospitals × 4 devices each)
Number of hospitals considered	5
Length of time duration	16 bits
Length of the identity of personnel or patient (biometric reading)	32 bits
Maximum length of data (at a time)	1200 bits
Length of the location information	16 bits
Certificate identity given by the government authority	20 bits
Simulation time	60 ms
Length of IP address	36 bits

21.4.1 Reliability

The proposal provides better reliability by 1.014% when compared to [8] and by 3.1% when compared to [6]. As the proposal uses the hash value of the hospital and all the transmitted data, the procedure adds better trust to the system. The same is represented in Fig. 21.3.

21.4.2 Availability

The proposed work is available globally, while the previous contribution is restricted to a number of individuals. Global authentication is helping the professionals by sharing with various groups. Data is shared among insurance companies and personnel of the hospital [8]. In [6], it is a decentralized system. The same is represented in Fig. 21.4.

21.4.3 Scalability of Information

The proposal [5] is endeavoring to investigate and feature the general uses of the IoT theory [26] by contributing a viewpoint guide to handle the COVID-19 epidemic. The framework recommends embracing four phases of the methodology—wellbeing information observing in remote areas, virtual administration, and examination of information obtained and controlling and following up report got. The proposed work will aggregate the data in the cloud server and will be available to all personnel after authentication. As compared to [5], the proposal provides 75% more information. The same is represented in Fig. 21.5.

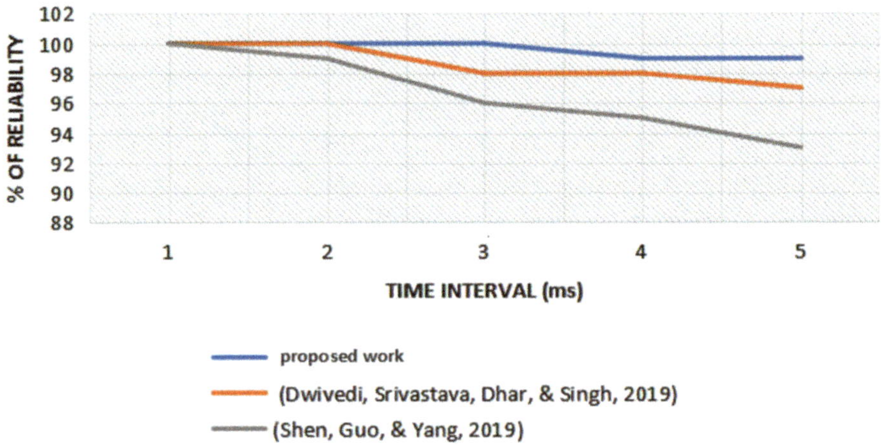

Fig. 21.3 Comparison of the proposed work with other contributions

Fig. 21.4 Availability of the proposed work and other contributions

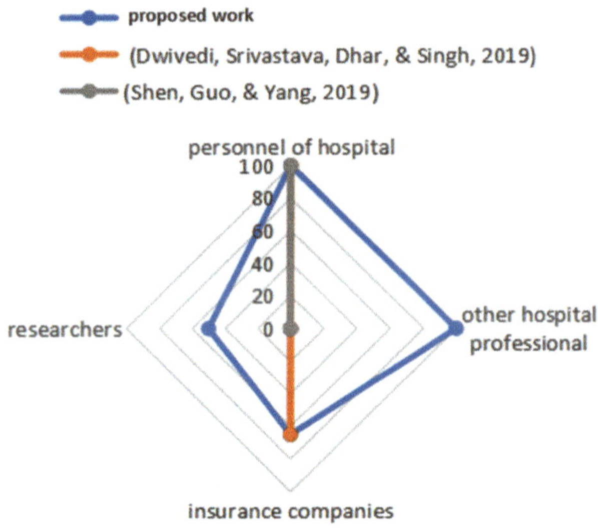

21.5 Conclusion

IoT is used to aid many applications, minimizing human efforts. These devices assemble process data and communicate them to the predefined destination to accomplish the task. The proposal consists of two phases. In the first phase, the deceased data is collected by the respective personnel and fed into the system. The hash value derivation happens at two levels. In the first step, the hospital's hash value obtained increases reliability to the system. In further steps, the aggregated data from the patient undergoes affixation with the hash value. The procedure adds more trust to the system. In the second phase, the data undergoes sharing among

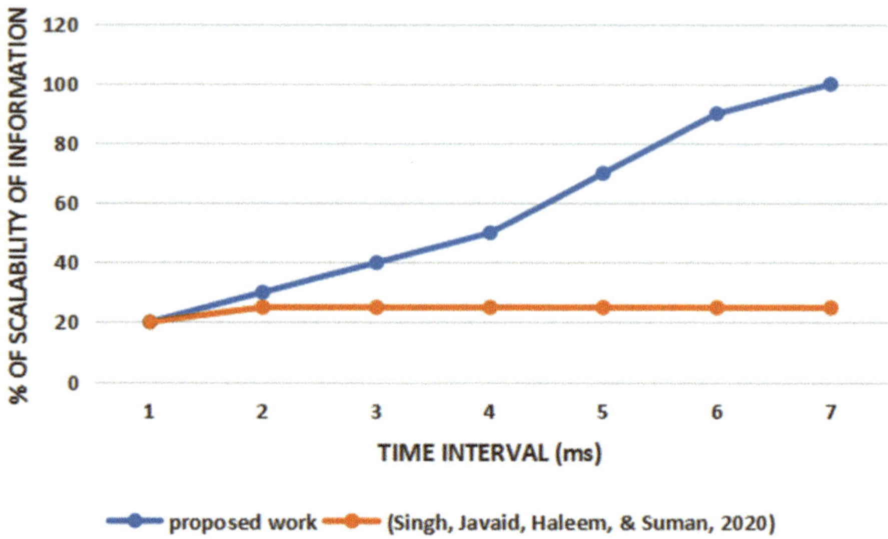

Fig. 21.5 Comparison of the proposal with other contributions [5]

various communities. Some of the groups considered are hospital authorities, media, and researchers. The highly confidential information is restricted based on the need of the individual and their authentication rights. The personnel diagnosing similar cases are into this set.

The proposal provides 1.014% and 3.1% reliability against previous contributions. It provides better availability of data and scalability of the information under a single roof.

References

1. Balandina, E., Balandin, S., Koucheryavy, Y., & Mouromtsev, D. (2015). IoT use cases in healthcare and tourism. In *IEEE 17th conference on business informatics* (Vol. 2, pp. 37–44). IEEE.
2. Ambika, N. (2020). Encryption of data in cloud-based industrial IoT devices. In *IoT: Security and privacy paradigm* (pp. 111–129). CRC Press.
3. Ambika, N. (2020). Methodical IoT-based information system in healthcare. In C. Chakraborthy (Ed.), *Smart medical data sensing and IoT systems design in healthcare* (pp. 155–177). IGI Global.
4. Cachin, C. (2016). Architecture of the hyperledger blockchain fabric. In *Workshop on distributed cryptocurrencies and consensus ledgers* (Vol. 310, p. 4). IEEE.
5. Singh, R. P., Javaid, M., Haleem, A., & Suman, R. (2020). Internet of things (IoT) applications to fight against COVID-19 pandemic. *Diabetes & Metabolic Syndrome: Clinical Research & Reviews, 14*(4), 521–524.
6. Shen, B., Guo, J., & Yang, Y. (2019). MedChain: Efficient healthcare data sharing via blockchain. *Applied Sciences, 9*(6), 1207.
7. Atlam, H. F., & Wills, G. B. (2019). Technical aspects of blockchain and IoT. In *Role of blockchain technology in IoT applications* (p. 115). Elsevier.

8. Dwivedi, D., Srivastava, G., Dhar, S., & Singh, R. (2019). A decentralized privacy-preserving healthcare blockchain for IoT. *Sensors, 19*(2), 326.
9. Yue, X., Wang, H., Jin, D., Li, M., & Jiang, W. (2016). Healthcare data gateways: Found healthcare intelligence on blockchain with novel privacy risk control. *Journal of Medical Systems, 40*(10), 1–8.
10. Witchey, N. J. (2019). Healthcare transaction validation via blockchain, systems and methods, 10,340,038.
11. Kumar, S. (2020). A wristwatch-based wireless sensor platform for IoT health monitoring applications. *Sensors, 20*(6), 1675.
12. Verma, P., & Sood, S. K. (2018). Fog assisted-IoT enabled patient health monitoring in smart homes. *IEEE Internet of Things Journal, 5*(3), 1789–1796.
13. Zamfir, M. (2016). Towards a platform for prototyping IoT health monitoring services. In *International conference on exploring services science* (pp. 522–533). Springer.
14. Ghosh, Raha, A., & Mukherjee, A. (2020). Energy-efficient IoT-health monitoring system using approximate computing. *Internet of Things, 9*, 100166.
15. Wu, F., Wu, T., & Yuce, M. R. (2019). An internet-of-things (IoT) network system for connected safety and health monitoring applications. *Sensors, 19*(1), 1–21.
16. Swaroop, K. N., Chandu, K., Gorrepotu, R., & Deb, S. (2019). A health monitoring system for vital signs using IoT. *Internet of Things, 5*, 116–129.
17. Wan, J., et al. (2018). Wearable IoT enabled real-time health monitoring system. *EURASIP Journal on Wireless Communications and Networking, 2018*(1), 298.
18. Mdhaffar, T., Chaari, K., Larbi, M. J., & Freisleben, B. (2017). IoT-based health monitoring via LoRaWAN. In *IEEE EUROCON 2017-17th international conference on smart technologies* (pp. 519–524). IEEE.
19. Ghosh, M., Halder, D., & Hossain, S. A. (2016). Remote health monitoring system through IoT. In *5th international conference on informatics, electronics and vision (ICIEV)* (pp. 921–926). IEEE.
20. Saha, H. N. (2017). Health monitoring using internet of things (IoT). In *8th annual industrial automation and electromechanical engineering conference (IEMECON)* (pp. 69–73). IEEE.
21. Khoi, N. M., Saguna, S., Mitra, K., & Åhlund, C. (2015). IReHMo: An efficient IoT-based remote health monitoring system for smart regions. In *17th international conference on E-health networking, application & services (HealthCom)* (pp. 563–568). IEEE.
22. Muhammad, G., Rahman, S. M. M., Alelaiwi, A., & Alamri, A. (2017). Smart health solution integrating IoT and cloud: A case study of voice pathology monitoring. *IEEE Communications Magazine, 55*(1), 69–73.
23. Abdelgawad, Yelamarthi, K., & Khattab, A. (2016). IoT-based health monitoring system for active and assisted living. In *International conference on smart objects and technologies for social good* (pp. 11–20). IEEE.
24. Saha, J., et al. (2018). Advanced IOT based combined remote health monitoring, home automation and alarm system. In *8th annual computing and communication workshop and conference (CCWC)* (pp. 602–606). IEEE.
25. Jo, W., Khan, R. M. A., & Lee, Y. S. (2018). Hybrid blockchain and internet-of-things network for underground structure health monitoring. *Sensors, 18*(12), 4268.
26. Nagaraj, A. (2021). *Introduction to sensors in IoT and cloud computing applications*. Bentham Science Publishers.

Index

M. S. Husain et al. (eds.), *Pervasive Healthcare*, EAI/Springer Innovations in Communication and Computing, https://doi.org/10.1007/978-3-030-77746-3

Q

R